Empowering Vulnerable Populations

Also Available from Lyceum Books, Inc.

Advisory Editors: Thomas M. Meenaghan, *New York University*
                   Ira C. Colby, *University of Houston*

NONPROFITS AND TECHNOLOGY: EMERGING RESEARCH FOR USABLE KNOWLEDGE
   by Michael Cortés and Kevin M. Rafter, foreword by Tessie Guillermo

A PRACTICAL GUIDE TO SOCIAL SERVICE EVALUATION
   by Carl F. Brun

SOCIAL WORK WITH VOLUNTEERS
   by Michael E. Sherr, foreword by John G. McNutt

ADVOCACY PRACTICE FOR SOCIAL JUSTICE
   by Richard Hoefer

TEAMWORK IN MULTIPROFESSIONAL CARE
   by Malcolm Payne, foreword by Thomas M. Meenaghan

STRAIGHT TALK ABOUT PROFESSIONAL ETHICS
   by Kim Strom-Gottfried

ADVOCACY, ACTIVISM, AND THE INTERNET: COMMUNITY ORGANIZATION AND SOCIAL POLICY
   by Steven F. Hick and John G. McNutt

WHAT IS PROFESSIONAL SOCIAL WORK?
   by Malcolm Payne

Empowering Vulnerable Populations

COGNITIVE-BEHAVIORAL INTERVENTIONS

MARY KEEGAN EAMON
University of Illinois at Urbana-Champaign

LYCEUM
BOOKS, INC.

5758 South Blackstone Avenue
Chicago, Illinois 60637

© Lyceum Books, Inc., 2008

Published by

LYCEUM BOOKS, INC.
5758 S. Blackstone Ave.
Chicago, Illinois 60637
773 + 643-1903 (Fax)
773 + 643-1902 (Phone)
lyceum@lyceumbooks.com
http://www.lyceumbooks.com

All rights reserved under International and Pan-American Copyright Conventions. No part of the publication may be reproduced, stored in a retrieval system, copied, or transmitted in any form or by any means without written permission from the publisher.

12 11 10 09 08   1 2 3 4 5

ISBN 978-1-933478-21-0

Library of Congress Cataloging-in-Publication Data

Keegan, Eamon, Mary.
  Empowering vulnerable populations : cognitive-behavioral interventions / Mary Keegan Eamon.
    p. cm.
  Includes bibliographical references and index.
  ISBN 978-1-933478-21-0
  1. Cognitive therapy. 2. Psychiatric social work. I. Title
RC685.C6K345   2008
616.89'142—dc22

                                           2007038129

To Thomas Raymond Keegan, Mae Deutsch Keegan, and Jennie Gilge Eamon, my role models for courage, self-sacrifice, hard work, and dedication to and love of family

Contents

Tables   xiii
About the Author   xiv
Preface   xv
    Objectives of This Book   xv
    Audience for This Book   xvi
    Organization and Content   xvi
    How to Use This Book   xviii
    Acknowledgments   xix

PART ONE
Vulnerable Populations, Cognitive-Behavioral Methods, and Empowerment

Chapter 1   Vulnerable Populations   3
    Definition of Vulnerable Populations   3
      Disabilities   4
      Racial/Ethnic Minorities   5
      Sexual Minorities   5
      Females   6
      Older Individuals   7
      Individuals with Low Income   7
    Risk Factors   8
    Additional Readings and Resources   10

Chapter 2   Cognitive-Behavioral Theory and Methods   11
    Definition of Terms and Cognitive-Behavioral Therapies   11
      Definition of Terms   11
      Defining Characteristics   12
    Cognitive-Behavioral Theories   13
      Behavioral Theories   13
      Social Learning and Cognitive Theory   15
    Cognitive-Behavioral Assessment   17

Common Interventions 19
   Behavioral Interventions 19
   Cognitive-Behavioral Interventions 25
Additional Readings and Resources 27

Chapter 3 Empowerment and Cognitive-Behavioral Methods 28
Empowerment and Selection of Intervention Goals 28
Criticisms of Cognitive-Behavioral Methods and Their
     Consistency with Empowerment and Social Work
     Practice 30
   Do Cognitive-Behavioral Methods Constrain Individual
      Freedom through Expert Control? 30
   Are Cognitive-Behavioral Methods Inconsistent with a Social
      Justice Perspective? 34
   Do Cognitive-Behavioral Methods Lack Social
      Relevance? 37
   Summary 000
Overview of Parts II through V 41
Additional Readings and Resources 41

PART TWO
Accessing and Increasing Social Resources

Chapter 4 Enhancing Social Interactions 45
Acquiring Basic Communication and Other Social Skills 45
Interventions for Vulnerable Children and Youths 46
   Children and Youths with Physical Disabilities and Sensory
      Impairments 47
   Children and Youths with Learning, Cognitive, and
      Developmental Disabilities 51
   Children and Youths with Behavioral/Emotional
      Disorders 59
   Children and Youths with Multiple Disabilities 61
   LGB Youths 66
Interventions for Vulnerable Adults 67
   Adults with Physical Disabilities 68
   Adults with Mental Retardation 69
   Adults with Severe Mental Illness 72
   Adults with Multiple Disabilities 77
   The Elderly 78
   Gay Men 80
Analysis and Critique for Practice and Research 82
   Effectiveness and Additional Applications 83

Freedom, Control, and Social Justice   85
Social Validity   86
Additional Readings and Resources   93

Chapter 5   Increasing Leisure, Recreational, and Related Activity   95
Interventions for Vulnerable Children and Youths   95
Children and Youths with Physical Disabilities   96
Children and Youths with Learning/Developmental Problems   97
Children and Youths with Multiple Disabilities   99
Interventions for Vulnerable Adults   102
Adults with Physical Disabilities   103
Adults with Mental Retardation   103
Adults with Severe Mental Illness   106
Adults with Multiple Disabilities   107
The Elderly   108
Analysis and Critique for Practice and Research   109
Effectiveness and Additional Applications   110
Freedom, Control, and Social Justice   111
Social Validity   113
Additional Readings and Resources   118

Chapter 6   Recruiting Assistance to Enhance Personal Well-Being   119
Enhancing Social and Emotional Support   119
Poor, Minority Pregnant Adolescents or Parenting Adolescent Mothers   120
Women with Low Income   121
Lesbians   124
Meeting Medical and Emergency Needs   125
Adults with Chronic Disease   125
Adults with Mental Retardation   126
Adults with Severe Mental Illness   127
The Elderly   128
Performing Routine or Daily Activities   129
Adults with Physical Disabilities and Visual Impairments   129
Individuals with Learning, Cognitive, and Developmental Disabilities   131
Individuals with Multiple Disabilities   132
The Elderly   133
Attaining Individually Defined Goals   133
Adults with Physical Disabilities and Sensory Impairments   134

African American Youths   136
Youths with Behavioral/Emotional Disorders and Learning
    Disabilities   137
Analysis and Critique for Practice and Research   138
    Effectiveness and Additional Applications   138
    Freedom, Control, and Social Justice   140
    Social Validity   141
Additional Readings and Resources   145

PART THREE
Acquiring and Increasing Economic Resources

Chapter 7   Obtaining Employment   149
Economic Resources of Vulnerable Populations   149
Securing Employment by Learning Job-Seeking Skills   152
    Interviewing Skills   153
    Recruiting Skills   156
    The Job Club Method   157
Analysis and Critique for Practice and Research   163
    Effectiveness and Additional Applications   163
    Freedom, Control, and Social Justice   165
    Social Validity   166
Additional Readings and Resources   170

Chapter 8   Maintaining and Advancing in Employment   171
Supported Employment   171
Increasing Work Productivity and Quality   173
    Workers with Physical Disabilities   174
    Workers with Mental Retardation   175
    Workers with Severe Mental Illness   183
Enhancing Employment-Related Social Skills   184
    Workers with Developmental and Physical Disabilities   185
    Workers with Severe Mental Illness   188
Analysis and Critique for Practice and Research   190
    Effectiveness and Additional Applications   190
    Freedom, Control, and Social Justice   191
    Social Validity   192
Additional Readings and Resources   196

Chapter 9   Accessing Public and Private Sources of
                 Economic Resources   197
Public and Private Sources of Economic Assistance   197

Assisting Vulnerable Populations in Accessing Public and Private
    Assistance   199
Adults with Severe Mental Illness   199
Minority Youths and Youths with Disabilities   200
Females with Low Income   200
Analysis and Critique for Practice and Research   202
Summary   204
Additional Readings and Resources   205

PART FOUR
Increasing Self-Determination

Chapter 10 Enhancing Personal Control and Input into Decision Making 209
Self-Determination of Vulnerable Populations   210
Enhancing Control over Personal Decision Making   212
    Decision Making in Multiple Areas and Participating in
        Educational Conferences   212
    Establishing and Attaining Personal Goals   216
    Analysis and Critique for Practice and Research   221
    Effectiveness and Additional Applications   222
    Freedom, Control, and Social Justice   223
    Social Validity   224
Additional Readings and Resources   228

Chapter 11 Increasing Choice Making in Daily and Long-Term Decisions 229
Recreational and Leisure Activity   229
    Individuals with Mental Retardation   230
    Individuals with Multiple Disabilities   232
Routine and Daily Activities   234
    Individuals with Mental Retardation   234
    Individuals with Multiple Disabilities   236
Community Residence   240
Analysis and Critique for Practice and Research   242
    Effectiveness and Additional Application   242
    Freedom, Control, and Social Justice   243
    Social Validity   244
Additional Readings and Resources   248

Chapter 12 Securing Legal and Personal Rights 250
Securing Legal Rights   251
    General Legal Rights   252
    Workplace Accommodations   253
    Educational Accommodations   255

Right to Refuse Unwanted and Unprotected Sexual
    Behavior   259
  Females   261
  African American Youths   266
  Sexual Minorities   267
  Individual with Severe Mental Illness   270
Analysis and Critique for Practice and Research   272
  Effectiveness and Additional Applications   272
  Freedom, Control, and Social Justice   275
  Social Validity   276
Additional Readings and Resources   283

PART FIVE
Increasing Involvement in Macro Decision Making and Summary

Chapter 13 Changing Social Policies and Community and Organizational Practices   287
Macro Decision Making among Vulnerable Populations   288
  Constrained Involvement   288
  Beneficial Outcomes from Macro Involvement   290
Increasing Involvement in Macro Decision Making   291
  Skills Training and Increasing Group Attendance   292
  Government- and Foundation-Sponsored Programs   300
Analysis and Critique for Practice and Research   310
  Effectiveness and Additional Applications   311
  Freedom, Control, and Social Justice   312
  Social Validity   313
Additional Readings and Resources   317

Chapter 14 Summary, Practice Implications, and Future Research   319
Effectiveness and Additional Applications   319
Empowerment and Cognitive-Behavioral Interventions   322
  Individual Freedom and Control   322
  The Social Justice Perspective   326
  Social Validity   328
Concluding Comments   348
Additional Readings and Resources   349

References   351

Index   379

Tables

4.1	Example of Receiving, Processing, and Sending Skills	94
5.1	Questions and Statements Trained for Decoding, Decision, Performance, and Evaluation Skills for Ordering Drinks	105
6.1	List of Help-Recruiting Skills	135
11.1	Sequence for Providing Choice Opportunities	237
11.2	Offering Choice and Prompting Performance	238

About the Author

Mary Keegan Eamon, MSW, MBA, PhD, is associate professor in the School of Social Work at the University of Illinois at Urbana-Champaign. She worked as a practitioner for twelve years in the child welfare field and providing mental health services to adults diagnosed with chronic mental illness and to children and families. Professor Eamon teaches courses in the areas of direct practice and theories of social work practice. She has written numerous articles on the ways in which poverty affects the well-being of children and families and the effectiveness of the services they receive. Recently her research interests involve the design and evaluation of training programs that assist individuals and families in accessing public benefits programs and in increasing involvement in political activity.

Preface

OBJECTIVES OF THIS BOOK

This is a source book of cognitive-behavioral (CB) interventions that facilitate empowerment of vulnerable populations. The book has three objectives: (1) to present and evaluate a broad range of CB interventions that assist vulnerable populations in attaining empowerment-related goals, (2) to demonstrate the consistency of CB applications with an empowerment perspective, and (3) to direct future research on CB interventions that can assist vulnerable groups in attaining empowerment outcomes.

While an extensive literature of CB applications for vulnerable populations is available in professional and applied journals, no current source documents the breadth and depth of those applications as a means to achieve empowerment outcomes. Presence of such content is critical. The Council on Social Work Education's "Educational Policy and Accreditation Standards" requires that social work education programs integrate content on vulnerable populations, including strategies to increase more equitable access to societal resources. The Code of Ethics of the National Association of Social Workers gives to the social work profession the primary mission to enhance individual well-being and to assist individuals in meeting their basic needs, with an emphasis on meeting the needs and empowerment of vulnerable groups. The importance of including course content on interventions that empower vulnerable populations, and the scarcity of such content in current CB texts, led me to locate and integrate additional relevant readings into my own CB course. This book is the product of those efforts.

In addition to providing examples of applications of CB techniques, I also address criticisms of CB approaches that attempt to identify contradictions between CB interventions and an empowerment perspective. Some scholars and practitioners, particularly from social justice, feminist, and strengths-based perspectives, have argued that CB methods constrain client freedom, focus on individual deficits rather than the unfavorable or unjust environments that cause the problems, and frequently ignore the socioeconomic and cultural contexts in which behaviors occur. In this book I provide examples and a rationale that I hope are responsive to those concerns.

AUDIENCE FOR THIS BOOK

Students, instructors, and practitioners in the field of social work, as well as in other professions, including education, counseling, clinical and school psychology, and vocational and physical rehabilitation, should find this book useful. The interventions presented here were specifically selected for their applicability to direct practice with individuals or groups in settings in which social workers, educators, and other professionals work. The interventions do not require practitioners or other professionals to mobilize community members or to directly influence macro policies or practices. However, because some of the interventions assist vulnerable populations in learning knowledge and skills for influencing macro decision making and community and organizational practices, the use of these interventions might help bridge the gap between micro and macro practice that historically has produced tension within the social work profession (Austin, Coombs, & Barr, 2005).

Professionals involved in administration, social policy, and community practice who are responsive to the special needs of vulnerable populations, as well as researchers, also will find applicable content. Administrators are in a position to select and encourage the adoption and use of relevant programs and interventions in their agencies, organizations, and schools. Social workers and other professionals involved in social policy formation and implementation are in a position to advocate for training programs, such as those discussed in this book, that teach vulnerable populations the knowledge and skills to influence the macro decisions and policies that define the services they receive and that affect other aspects of their lives. Although community organizers directly mobilize people to influence macro policies and decision-making processes, they also teach political and advocacy skills to community members. Interventions to achieve those goals are included in this book. Finally, current and future researchers, including doctoral and MSW students and practitioners, who are interested in developing and evaluating CB interventions that empower vulnerable populations will find this book useful. The book provides numerous examples of such interventions, discusses the limitations of current research, and makes suggestions for designing and evaluating CB interventions that empower vulnerable groups.

ORGANIZATION AND CONTENT

This book is divided into five parts. Part I contains three chapters providing an introduction to the book. Chapter 1 defines vulnerable populations, and chapter 2 briefly discusses CB terms, theory, assessment, and commonly used interventions. Chapter 3 examines the consistency of CB methods with empowerment and social work practice, including issues of personal freedom and control, social justice, and social relevance. Parts II through V describe and critically examine a wide range of CB interventions for vulnerable populations. Each part contains chapters that focus on interventions designed to achieve a specific outcome consistent with an empowerment perspective. In part II the outcomes are accessing and increasing social resources. In part III, the outcomes are acquiring, maintaining, and increasing economic resources. In part IV, the goals are enhancing self-determination. In the first chapter in part V, the focus outcomes are influencing macro decision making, including social policy and community and organizational practices. The final chapter in part V provides an overview of the effectiveness of the CB interventions described in the ten intervention chapters, returns to a discussion of the consistency between CB methods and empowerment, and makes suggestions for practice and future research.

The interventions described in parts II through V are organized by intervention goal and vulnerable population. Vulnerable populations include individuals with disabilities, including severe mental illness, mental retardation, and sensory, learning, and physical disabilities; the poor; racial/ethnic and sexual minorities; the elderly; and females. The CB interventions presented in the ten intervention chapters are not exhaustive but were chosen for two main reasons. First, the interventions provide examples of a range of CB interventions designed to assist vulnerable populations in attaining the identified goals. Second, many of the interventions demonstrate applications that are specifically developed to accommodate the special needs of the identified population. As reflected in the intervention chapters, considerable variation exists in the number of CB interventions that researchers have designed and evaluated to assist particular vulnerable populations in achieving the identified outcomes.

To facilitate both instructional and practical applications of the material presented in this book, I attempted whenever possible to describe the interventions in sufficient detail to allow practitioners with knowledge of commonly used CB interventions to implement them. Consistent with the increased requirement of social workers to use evidence to inform practice decisions, the research design and the results of the evaluations for the CB interventions are provided. At the end of each chapter, I discuss and analyze the interventions and their evaluations, identify possible additional applications, and suggest areas of future research. Issues that are of particular concern to practitioners, instructors, and researchers in social work and related fields also are discussed. These include issues related to freedom and control of the intervention process, social justice, and the social relevance of the intervention goals, results, and procedures, as well as transfer and maintenance of treatment gains. For interventions or programs involving detailed multicomponents or treatment manuals, sources for additional information on the interventions are provided at the end of each chapter.

HOW TO USE THIS BOOK

This book is not a textbook on CB methods. Although chapter 2 provides a brief overview of commonly used CB terms, theories, assessment procedures, and interventions, readers of this book are assumed to have some knowledge of these issues. This book can be used as a companion book in CB courses and in practice courses that contain content on CB theories and interventions. The organization of the book allows instructors, students, practitioners, and researchers to readily identify interventions that are applicable for attaining particular outcomes for specific vulnerable clients and to assess the effectiveness of the interventions.

The CB interventions described in this book (e.g., prompting, reinforcement, social skills training, cognitive restructuring, and problem solving) are considered by texts, books, and articles on CB applications as accepted practices for treating many common problems. Chapter 2 also briefly discusses the large number of CB therapies identified as evidence-based practices for treating children, youths, and adults with a variety of problems. Despite the evidence for the effectiveness of many CB interventions, the interventions described in this book are combined in unique ways and make special adaptations for the special needs of vulnerable clients. The quality of the research evaluating the interventions varies considerably. Only a few of the evaluations compared the effectiveness of different types or combinations of CB interventions to achieve a specific intervention goal, and even fewer compared the effectiveness of CB interventions with other types of interventions. For all of these reasons, I make no claim that specific CB interventions or multicomponent programs included in this book are equally or more effective in achieving specific outcomes for particular vulnerable groups, compared with other CB interventions or alternative types of interventions.

I make five assumptions about the use of this book for the purpose of selecting particular goals and interventions for a given client. First, the process of identifying problems and behaviors to modify, establishing goals, and selecting interventions must be conducted using sound clinical judgment and information gathered from a thorough individualized assessment, including a functional analysis. Second, the identification of problems, goals, and outcome measures will be negotiated with clients and others involved in the intervention process. Third, consistent with evidence-based practice, practitioners will draw on multiple sources of information to evaluate the evidence for the effectiveness of different interventions to attain the identified goal. Fourth, depending on the results of this process, the interventions described in this book can be presented to clients as options for attaining the agreed upon goals, including evidence for their effectiveness and the realistic expectations of the potential benefits and risks. Fifth, the interventions will be implemented within the value base and ethics of social work and related professions

ACKNOWLEDGMENTS

This book is the product of the work of multiple researchers in many different fields, including social work, education, vocational and physical rehabilitation, psychiatry, and clinical, community, and school psychology. Without the effort and dedication of these researchers in applying CB methods to assist vulnerable populations in achieving the identified empowerment goals, this book could not have been written.

I also acknowledge the reviewers of a previous draft of this book for their insightful and helpful comments, and my husband, Doug Eamon, for his editing suggestions. Finally, I acknowledge Saijun Zhang, Cray Mulder, Sachiko Bamba, and Samantha Hack-Ritzo, doctoral students at the University of Illinois at Urbana-Champaign School of Social Work, who assisted with various aspects of this book.

PART

ONE

Vulnerable Populations, Cognitive-Behavioral Methods, and Empowerment

1 Vulnerable Populations

Cognitive-behavioral (CB) interventions that assist vulnerable populations in achieving four main types of empowerment goals are discussed and evaluated in this book. The goals are (1) accessing and enhancing social resources, (2) acquiring and increasing economic resources, (3) increasing self-determined behavior, and (4) influencing the social policies and organizational and community practices that affect the lives of vulnerable groups. This chapter defines vulnerable populations and examines the reasons for their vulnerability, as well as the applicability of CB interventions to assist them in attaining empowerment goals. The second chapter discusses CB theories, assessment procedures, and strategies that are frequently combined into the multicomponent interventions and programs described in the next four parts of this book. The final chapter in part I considers common criticisms of CB methods and discusses consistencies of the methods with empowerment and social work practice.

DEFINITION OF VULNERABLE POPULATIONS

This book evaluates CB interventions for populations frequently referred to by social work educators and scholars as *at risk, vulnerable,* or *oppressed* (Council on Social Work Education [CSWE], 2001; Gitterman, 1991; Greif & Ephross, 2005; National Association of Social Workers [NASW], 1999). The terms commonly are used interchangeably and have been used to describe different groups of people. Generally the terms apply to individuals who share certain characteristics that differentiate them from younger, able-bodied, heterosexual, white men with higher socioeconomic status, a group possessing a disproportionate amount of societal resources and influence. Common characteristics of populations that place them at risk of discrimination, oppression, possessing few social and economic resources, and exclusion from decision-making processes include a variety of disabilities, poverty, female gender, culture, religion, minority racial/ethnic background, minority sexual orientation, and older age.

This book uses the term *vulnerable populations* to describe individuals with disabilities, racial/ethnic minorities (including recent immigrants), sexual minorities, females, older individuals, and persons with low income.

Disabilities

The Americans with Disabilities Act (ADA) of 1990 (PL101–336) defines a disability as a physical, cognitive, psychological, or behavioral condition that substantially interferes with the performance of one or more daily activities. Examples of daily activities include communicating, self-care, seeing and hearing, and physical mobility. Multiple criteria have been used to identify and differentiate diverse populations of individuals with disabilities (Msall et al., 2003; Westbrook, Silver, & Stein, 1998). This book defines four main categories of disabilities related to specific interventions discussed in subsequent chapters. First, physical disabilities include children and adults with mobility limitations (e.g., resulting from paralysis, multiple sclerosis, or cerebral palsy) and sensory (i.e., visual and hearing) impairments, and chronic diseases, such as acquired immune deficiency syndrome (AIDS) and diabetes. Second, learning, cognitive, and developmental disabilities apply to young children with developmental delays; children and adults with mental retardation, a learning disability, or autism; and adults with dementia. Third, mental health disabilities pertain to children diagnosed with a behavioral/emotional disorder and adults diagnosed with severe mental illness (e.g., schizophrenia, bipolar disorder, and major depression). Finally, multiple disabilities refer to individuals experiencing at least two types of disabilities, such as a combination of mental retardation and a physical disability.

Regardless of the criteria used to categorize them, individuals with disabilities are the largest and most vulnerable group in this country (Kopels, 1995). Although disability rates vary by definition (Westbrook et al., 1998), an estimated 54 million persons in this country (approximately 20% of the population) have a disability. The disability rate also is increasing, particularly among adults age 65 years and older (U.S. Department of Health and Human Services, 2000). As discussed in subsequent chapters of this book, in addition to experiencing physical and emotional pain, individuals with disabilities have an increased risk of experiencing negative outcomes in multiple areas of their lives. The areas include education; social interactions and relationships; recreation/leisure; employment; access to appropriate services, medical care, and other community activities; communicating and making choices; and participating in the macro decisions that affect the services they receive and other important aspects of their lives.

These multiple risks are a reason for the large number of CB interventions developed for this population. The CB interventions are designed to assist children, youths, and adults with a variety of disabilities in increasing their social interactions and relationships, leisure/recreational activity, and social integration into school, work, and community settings. The interventions can assist individuals with disabilities in meeting their medical and emergency needs, obtaining necessary information, and recruiting assistance to perform daily and routine activity and to attain their personal goals. CB strategies also can increase the economic well-being of adults with disabilities and enhance the self-determined behavior of adults and youths with disabilities in school, work, family, and residential settings. Self-determined outcomes consist of setting and achieving personal goals, actively participating in educational conferences, advocating educational and work accommodations and other legal rights, and increasing choice making in routine and daily activities and in longer-term decisions. Finally, CB interventions can teach political and advocacy skills for groups with disabilities to change the macro policies and practices that define the services they receive and influence their ability to fully integrate into society.

Racial/Ethnic Minorities

Three-fourths of this country's population identify themselves as "white," with Latinos (12.5%) and African Americans (12.3%) constituting the two largest racial/ethnic minority groups (U.S. Census Bureau, 2001). The population in the United States is becoming more diverse, with the number of foreign-born people more than doubling between 1980 and 2000 (Tumlin & Zimmermann, 2003). Social workers historically have assisted recent immigrants in making a successful transition into this society and also have long recognized the unique challenges faced by African Americans because of widespread discrimination (Diner, 1970).

Discrimination, residential and educational segregation, residing in low-resource communities, and attending low-quality schools can place racial/ethnic minorities at risk of failing to attain their educational, employment, and other personal goals. Latinos, African Americans, native populations, and individuals who are foreign born also are disproportionately represented in other vulnerable groups, including those who are poor or have a disability (U.S. Census Bureau, 2005, 2006). In addition to describing CB interventions designed to assist individuals with disabilities in attaining multiple empowerment goals, this book discusses CB strategies that can assist racial/ethnic minority groups in securing employment, obtaining economic assistance from public and private sources, and recruiting mentors to achieve their personal goals. CB interventions designed to teach African American youths, adults, and homosexual and bisexual men, groups at heightened risk for HIV infection, in asserting their right to refuse unwanted or unsafe sexual activity also are described.

Sexual Minorities

In this book, sexual minorities are considered to be individuals who identify themselves as lesbian, gay, or bisexual (LGB). The transgender population also can be considered vulnerable, but no CB interventions could be located that assist these individuals in achieving the goals identified in this book. Although the *Diagnostic and Statistical Manual of Mental Disorders (DSM-II)* eliminated homosexuality as a disorder more than three decades ago, LGB individuals continue to be an "invisible" and stigmatized population (Martell, Safren, & Prince, 2004). Lesbian, gay, and bisexual youths and adults can experience social isolation, discrimination, and few opportunities to observe and learn social skills that can assist them in establishing social support and meaningful relationships.

The CB interventions discussed in these chapters assist LGB youths and adults in coming to terms with their sexual identity, negotiating the coming-out process, establishing personal relationships, and increasing social support. CB interventions also are described that teach LGB populations skills for asserting their right to refuse unwanted and unprotected sexual behavior, which can result in sexually transmitted diseases (STDs), including HIV infection.

Females

As documented in subsequent chapters, females face greater risks compared with males. Regardless of age, women are more likely to live in poverty, with the most striking differences existing between unmarried women and women with children and their male counterparts. As discussed in chapter 7, securing employment and the economic well-being of single mothers are particularly important since the passage of the Personal Responsibility and Work Opportunity Reconciliation Act (PRWORA), which forces most mothers receiving welfare benefits into paid employment. Pregnant and female parenting adolescents and women with few economic resources are vulnerable to high stress levels, low levels of social support, and psychological problems such as depression. Elderly women are more likely than elderly men to experience a disability and to reside in an institutionalized setting (U.S. Census Bureau, 2005). Women, particularly those with few economic resources, also are at a disadvantage to negotiate with their male partners whether to engage in sexual or in safe sexual behavior. As described in more detail in chapter 13, women historically have had low levels of involvement in medical research and in influencing policy on health issues, particularly involving problems that disproportionately affect them, such as breast cancer.

The CB interventions described in this book are designed to enhance the social, emotional, and instrumental support of pregnant and parenting adolescent mothers and women with low income. These strategies can increase women's employment and economic assistance from their social networks and other community sources. Such interventions also can teach female adolescents and adults skills for asserting their rights to refuse unwanted and unprotected sexual behavior, behaviors which can result in unwanted pregnancies and STDs. Finally, the chapters describe CB interventions that can increase women's involvement and influence in decision making related to medical research and policy.

Older Individuals

The number of older persons in the United States dramatically increased during the twentieth century. There are now more than 35 million individuals age 65 years and older (12% of the total population). This age group is projected to double between 2000 and 2030, an increase that is primarily the result of the first baby boomers reaching the age of 65 in 2011. The older population is expected to become more racially/ethnically diverse, reflecting the recent demographic increases in Latinos and Asians in this country. Older individuals are more likely to live alone and to experience sensory, physical, mental, self-care, and mobility impairments, compared with other individuals. Although disability rates among older individuals are declining, an estimated 80% of older individuals have at least one chronic health condition, and 50% have at least two. Though nursing home care has recently decreased among whites (it has increased among African Americans), and the overwhelming majority of the elderly receive home- and community-based care, nursing homes remain the most common type of institutionalized care for this population. More than 90% of institutionalized elders in this country live in nursing homes (U.S. Census Bureau, 2004, 2005).

The increase in the older population, their longer life span compared with previous generations, and the associated risks of their becoming disabled, socially isolated, and institutionalized present many challenges to older individuals and to policy makers, families, health-care providers, social agencies, and practitioners working in the area of aging. The CB interventions discussed in this book empower older individuals by addressing many of these risks. The interventions can assist older individuals in enhancing their social interactions, increasing their leisure/recreational activity, meeting their medical and emergency needs, requesting assistance, securing employment for those who desire to continue working or rely on employment for economic reasons, and learning political and advocacy skills for influencing macro decision making on issues related to aging.

Individuals with Low Income

Approximately 13% of the people in this country live in poverty (U.S. Census Bureau, 2006). Other populations described here as vulnerable, including racial/ethnic minorities, women, individuals with disabilities, and older individuals who are foreign born, noncitizens, and from minority racial/ethnic backgrounds, also are disproportionately poor. The CB interventions described in this book are designed to increase the economic well-being of vulnerable populations who are unemployed and have few economic resources in three ways. First, the interventions can assist vulnerable groups in learning job-seeking skills to secure employment. One intervention is specifically designed to teach former Asian refugees appropriate social skills to obtain employment. Second, the interventions teach vulnerable populations skills for increasing their productivity, work quality, and relevant social skills, which can result in maintaining and advancing in employment. Third, the interventions assist vulnerable groups in learning the knowledge and skills needed for obtaining economic resources from public benefits programs and private sources, including their social networks and nonprofit private agencies.

Finally, the CB interventions described are designed to enhance the social support of women with low income, assist policy board members of low-income self-help groups in increasing their problem-solving skills to resolve community problems, improve the public speaking performance of neighborhood service center staff in low-income communities, and enhance the leadership skills of chairpersons of executive boards serving low-income neighborhood centers.

RISK FACTORS

Classifying individuals with particular characteristics into groups, such as racial/ethnic minorities, or broad categories, such as *vulnerable*, should not be taken as pejorative or stereotypical. Individuals placed into these groups and referred to as vulnerable have many differences and multiple strengths, and the majority are successful, happy, and productive members of society. However, as the introductions to the CB intervention chapters in this book demonstrate, membership in these groups can place individuals at risk of multiple negative outcomes in at least two ways.

First, the particular characteristics of many vulnerable populations, such as psychiatric symptoms and learning, developmental, sensory, communicative, and mobility limitations, can interfere with acquiring and/or using relevant knowledge and skills for achieving empowerment-related goals. Second, compared with dominant groups, vulnerable populations are more likely to experience a variety of social factors that place them at risk for adverse outcomes. Vulnerable populations are more likely to face discrimination, stigmatization, rejection, and high stress levels. They frequently are denied opportunities to learn and use relevant knowledge and skills to achieve their social, educational, work, and recreational/leisure goals, to make and communicate their own choices, and to participate in the macro decisions that affect many areas of their lives. These personal and societal factors, in turn, can result in a variety of negative outcomes for vulnerable groups. The outcomes include social isolation and exclusion, feelings of powerlessness and alienation, mental health problems (or exacerbation of mental health problems), inadequate economic resources, denial of legal and personal rights, and social policies and community and organizational practices that are unresponsive to their needs.

As the following chapters suggest, practitioners can use CB interventions to empower vulnerable groups by assisting them in improving these negative outcomes and/or in decreasing the risk of their occurrence. The CB interventions teach vulnerable clients the knowledge and skills for increasing social and economic resources, enhancing self-determination, and increasing involvement and influence in macro decision making. In many cases, the interventions for specific vulnerable groups, such as children and adults with disabilities, involve nondisabled peers. Such strategies not only can increase social interactions between peers with and without disabilities but can promote social integration of individuals with disabilities into work, school, and community settings. The CB interventions also include multiple strategies to accommodate the special needs and circumstances of vulnerable clients, including psychiatric symptoms, and developmental, learning, and communicative difficulties, which allow clients to take advantage of resources and opportunities when they are available.

Despite the multiple interventions presented in this book and the different vulnerable groups to which they are applied, the interventions for achieving particular intervention goals are not inclusive of every group identified as vulnerable for two reasons. First, research-based relevant CB interventions could not be located for every vulnerable group. For these cases, the end-of-chapter summaries, "Analysis and Critique for Practice and Research," provide suggestions for additional applications. Second, some of the identified vulnerable populations would not be considered at risk of failing to achieve particular goals. For example, racial/ethnic minorities would not necessarily be at a disadvantage to learn and use social skills for increasing their social interactions and friendships. However, because of factors such as segregation and discrimination, they might be at a disadvantage to learn and use social skills for recruiting mentors to assist them in achieving personal goals or in securing employment.

Before the CB interventions that empower vulnerable populations are described, certain groundwork needs to be explored. Chapter 2 discusses CB theories, assessment procedures, and common strategies used in the interventions described in subsequent chapters of this book.

ADDITIONAL READINGS AND RESOURCES

Beebe, D. W., & Risi, S. (2003). Treatment of adolescents and young adults with high-functioning autism or Asperger syndrome. In M. A. Reinecke, F. M. Dattilio, & A. Freeman (Eds.), *Cognitive therapy with children and adolescents: A casebook for clinical practice* (2nd ed., pp. 569–401). New York: Guilford.

Donohue, B., Acierno, R., Hersen, M., & Van Hasselt, V. B. (1995). Social skills training for depressed, visually impaired older adults: A treatment manual. *Behavior Modification, 19*, 379–424.

Granholm, E., McQuaid, J. R., Auslander, L. A., & McClure, F. S. (2004). Group cognitive-behavioral social skills training for older outpatients with chronic schizophrenia. *Journal of Cognitive Psychotherapy: An International Quarterly, 18*, 265–279.

McClannahan, L. E., & Krantz, P. J. (2004). Some guidelines for selecting behavioral intervention programs for children with autism. In H. E. Briggs & T. L. Rzepnicki (Eds.), *Using evidence in social work practice: Behavioral perspectives* (pp. 92–103). Chicago: Lyceum.

Mennuti, R. B., Freeman, A., & Christner, R. W. (Eds.). *Cognitive-behavioral interventions in educational settings: A handbook for practice.* New York: Routledge.

Safren, S. A., Hollander, G., Hart, T. A., & Heimberg, R. G. (2001). Cognitive-behavioral therapy with lesbian, gay, and bisexual youth. *Cognitive and Behavioral Practice, 8*, 215–223.

Safren, S. A., & Rogers, T. (2001). Cognitive-behavioral therapy with gay, lesbian, and bisexual clients. *Psychotherapy in Practice, 57*, 629–643.

Sweetland, J. D. (1990). Cognitive-behavior therapy and physical disability. *Journal of Rational-Emotive and Cognitive-Behavior Therapy, 8*, 71–78.

Thurston, L. P. (1990). Women surviving: An alternative approach to "helping" low-income urban women. *Women & Therapy, 8*, 109–127.

Westwood, M. J., Mak, A., Barker, M., & Ishiyama, F. I. (2000). Group procedures and applications for developing sociocultural competencies among immigrants. *International Journal for the Advancement of Counseling, 22*, 317–330.

Williamson, P. N., & Ascione, F. R. (1983). Behavioral treatment of the elderly: Implications for theory and therapy. *Behavior Modification, 7*, 583–610.

Wong, S. E., Wilder, D. A., Schock, K., & Clay, C. (2004). Behavioral interventions for severe and persistent mental disorders. In H. E. Briggs & T. L. Rzepnicki (Eds.), *Using evidence in social work practice: Behavioral perspectives* (pp. 210–230). Chicago: Lyceum.

Wood, P. S., & Mallinckrodt, B. (1990). Culturally sensitive assertiveness training for ethnic minority clients. *Professional Psychology—Research & Practice, 21*, 5–11.

2 Cognitive-Behavioral Theory and Methods

Behavior therapy was introduced into the social work profession about four decades ago (Reid, 2004). Although not all social workers have embraced the use of these methods, social work scholars and practitioners have used behavioral and later CB interventions to address a variety of client problems (Gambrill, 1995b; Gold, 1981; Granvold, 1994; Rose, 1989; Rose & Edleson, 1987; Thomas, 1967). Problems include depression, anxiety, phobias, child and adolescent behavioral and emotional disorders, pregnancy prevention, child maltreatment, addictions, marital discord, and multiple issues related to mental retardation, severe mental illness, health, and aging.

This chapter begins by defining CB terms and discussing common characteristics of the interventions. A brief discussion of theory and conducting a CB assessment follows. The chapter ends with a description of commonly used interventions included in the treatment packages and multicomponent programs presented in part II through chapter 13 in part V, which are referred to as intervention chapters.

DEFINITION OF TERMS AND COGNITIVE-BEHAVIORAL THERAPIES

Definition of Terms

Researchers who have designed and evaluated the CB interventions included in this book, as well as authors of texts and articles on CB theories and therapies (e.g., Dobson & Khatri, 2000; Gambrill, 1994; Latimer & Sweet, 1984; Spiegler & Guevremont, 2003), give various definitions of *behavior modification, behavior therapy, applied behavior analysis, CB therapy*, and *cognitive therapy*. Some of the terms are used interchangeably. Scholars who define and distinguish among the various terms and provide examples of representative interventions are frequently inconsistent with one another.

Even so, behavior therapy, behavior modification, and applied behavior analysis broadly refer to a process of analyzing the functional relationship between behavior and the environment. This analysis is followed by developing and implementing interventions to change the environmental events (referred to as maintaining antecedents and consequences) in order to change an identified behavior, frequently referred to as the *target behavior*. Behavior can be overt. That is, it can be directly observed, such as speech. Behavior also can be covert. That is, it can only be indirectly observed, such as an emotion. Common behavioral interventions have been drawn from various learning theories, such as operant and respondent conditioning, which have evolved over time (see Gambrill, 1994; Latimer & Sweet, 1984, for a discussion of these issues). Although interventions referred to as cognitive or CB therapies frequently incorporate behavioral interventions, the belief that cognitive processes, such as perceptions, thoughts, beliefs, and expectations, mediate behavioral change is a basic premise of these therapies. Therefore, cognitive and CB therapies attempt to change cognitions directly to assist clients in coping with a life problem or changing an identified overt or covert behavior.

In this book, *behavioral interventions* are actions carried out by a practitioner, client, or others that change the maintaining conditions of an identified behavior but do not directly attempt to change cognitions or cognitive processes. *CB interventions* are those that can be used alone or in conjunction with behavioral interventions, but the interventions attempt to directly change cognitions or cognitive processes to achieve a specified goal. The term *CB* also is used as a generic term encompassing both behavioral and cognitive interventions.

Defining Characteristics

Interventions labeled as *behavioral* or *CB* share certain common characteristics and values, some of which are shared with other types of therapies (Evans, 1997; Spiegler & Guevremont, 2003). Shared characteristics and values include the goal of assisting individuals and significant others in resolving problems that are important to or valued by them. Selection of the problems, goals, and interventions is a collaborative process involving the practitioner and others participating in the interventions. The practitioner-client relationship is valued and considered a necessary component of successful treatment. Assessment and treatment procedures are individualized, and treatment frequently involves multiple interventions to resolve a presenting problem. Combining multiple CB interventions is commonly referred to as a *treatment package*.

Other characteristics and values, when considered as a group, distinguish CB interventions from other therapies (Evans, 1997; Gambrill, 1994; Spiegler & Guevremont, 2003). They include the commitment to a scientific approach, valuing transparent sources of information on which to base treatment decisions, and focusing on present circumstances. Problems, assessment procedures, goals, and interventions are clearly defined, and the behaviors or problems targeted for change are monitored before, during, and after intervention. Interventions are selected based on empirically tested theories and intervention research. CB therapies de-emphasize diagnoses and labels and reject hypothetical underlying causes of behavior. Instead, the interventions emphasize the importance that learning plays in the development, maintenance, and change of behavior, even if the behavior is influenced by biological or genetic factors. CB interventions also de-emphasize past events and actively involve individuals, groups, and significant others in the assessment and intervention process to change current circumstances.

COGNITIVE-BEHAVIORAL THEORIES

This section provides a brief overview of the theories that support many of the interventions described in the intervention chapters of this book. It is not a comprehensive explication of CB theories. Operant and respondent learning, which provide the theoretical basis for many of the behavioral interventions, are discussed first. A brief discussion of social learning and cognitive theories, which serve as an underlying rationale for many cognitive or CB interventions, follows.

Behavioral Theories

Operant conditioning. *Operant conditioning* is a process in which events that occur or are presented after a behavior is performed increase or decrease the likelihood that the behavior will be performed again. Three main principles of operant conditioning are *reinforcement, punishment,* and *extinction.*

Reinforcement occurs when a behavior is followed by an event (*consequence*) resulting in a strengthening of the behavior; that is, the behavior is more likely to be repeated. Reinforcement can be *positive* or *negative.* For example, a child with a disability asks an able-bodied peer to play, and the peer plays with the child. If in the future the child asks the same or other able-bodied peers to play more frequently, *positive reinforcement* has taken place. The peer's playing with the child is the likely consequence that strengthened the play initiating behavior and is referred to as a *positive reinforcer.*

Negative reinforcement occurs when an event (usually something unpleasant) is removed, decreased, or avoided after a behavior is performed, and the behavior subsequently increases. For example, a child with a disability is teased by able-bodied peers after she attempts to join them at a lunch table, and the teasing stops after she withdraws to a table by herself. If the child with a disability subsequently increases eating alone in the lunch room, negative reinforcement has occurred. The teasing that she avoids is referred to as an *aversive stimulus*.

Punishment occurs when an event is presented or removed after a person performs a behavior, and the frequency of the behavior decreases. Punishment can be positive or negative. *Positive punishment* is a process in which a behavior is followed by an aversive event, and the behavior is less likely to be performed again. For example, an African American adolescent recruits assistance from a community member to achieve her goal of entering a prestigious university, and the person discourages her. If the adolescent subsequently asks fewer or no community members for assistance, positive punishment has taken place. When a behavior is followed by removal of a desirable event and the behavior subsequently decreases, *negative punishment* has occurred. For example, a child with a learning disability acts inappropriately in the classroom (e.g., speaks out without raising his hand), and the teacher removes the privilege of recess. If the inappropriate behavior subsequently decreases, negative punishment has taken place.

Extinction is a process whereby a reinforcer is withdrawn from a previously reinforced behavior, and the behavior subsequently decreases or is eliminated. An example of extinction is group home staff withdrawing attention (a reinforcer) after an adult with mental retardation complains about participating in a recreational activity, and the complaining subsequently stops.

While principles of reinforcement, punishment, and extinction explain ways in which consequences can affect behavior, *stimulus control* applies to antecedent conditions. Stimulus control occurs when individuals learn that performing certain behaviors in the presence of particular stimuli or events in particular situations either is likely to be punished or is likely to be reinforced. For example, an employee with mental retardation learns through instruction, experience, or observation that when a supervisor signals it is time to work, if the employee refuses, talks, or is disruptive, an aversive event (punishment) likely will follow. Aversive events might include a reprimand, a request to leave the work area, or even job loss. On the other hand, if the employee begins to work, a desirable event (reinforcer), such as praise, money, and continued employment, likely will follow. A behavior (e.g., begin working) is under stimulus control when the presence of an event (e.g., the supervisor signals it is time to work) increases the chance that a specific behavior will occur in a specific situation.

Respondent conditioning. Unlike operant conditioning, which applies to behaviors that operate on or affect the environment in some way (e.g., talking, working, playing), *respondent conditioning* applies to behaviors or responses that are automatic and frequently involve the autonomic nervous system. For example, when someone is threatened with bodily or psychological harm, common responses are increased heart rate, respiration, and muscle tension.

Respondent conditioning is a process in which a previously neutral event or stimulus is paired with an event, the *unconditioned stimulus (US)*, that automatically elicits a response, the *unconditioned response (UR)*. After the neutral stimulus is paired with the US, the neutral stimulus becomes a *conditioned stimulus (CS)* that elicits a response similar to the UR. This similar response is referred to as a *conditioned response (CR)*.

Respondent conditioning is frequently used to explain anxiety disorders (e.g., phobias and social anxiety). For example, before a male high school student disclosed that he was gay to his classmates, he experienced no anxiety when participating in social activity with his peers (neutral stimulus). After his disclosure, his engaging in social activity was frequently met with ridicule, rejection, and avoidance by his peers (US), which automatically elicited anxiety (UR). Over time, the pairing of the previous neutral event (participating in social activity with peers) with the US (ridicule, rejection, and avoidance) resulted in engaging in social activity becoming a CS, which elicits anxiety (CR). Even though the adolescent is socially skilled, he discontinues engaging in social activities with his peers because these situations now elicit a high level of anxiety.

Social Learning and Cognitive Theory

Albert Bandura (1969, 1977) developed *social learning theory*. While acknowledging the importance of both operant and respondent conditioning, his theory also emphasizes a cognitive mediational process. Bandura argued that learning takes place through observation, imitation, and cognitive processes, such as expectations, beliefs, and thoughts, which directly influence behavior. An example of this type of learning is *observational learning*, which involves learning a behavior simply by observing the actions of models (e.g., parents, siblings, therapists, peers, teachers). This focus on internal events as initiating causes of behavior departed from "radical behaviorism," which acknowledged the importance of internal events, such as cognitions, but did not attribute a direct causal or explanatory role to such events (see Gambrill, 1994, for a comprehensive discussion of these issues).

A number of distinctive cognitive or CB therapies are derived from the basic assumption that cognitive processes mediate behavioral change. Spiegler and Guevremont (2003) conceptualize these therapies into two basic intervention models. The first is *cognitive restructuring therapy*, which includes *cognitive therapy* (A. T. Beck, 1976; J. S. Beck, 1995) and *rational emotive behavior therapy* (REBT; Ellis, 1998). The second model, *CB coping skills therapy*, teaches clients cognitive and behavioral responses to cope more effectively with difficult life situations. *Problem-solving therapy* (D'Zurilla & Nezu, 1999), *self-instructional training* (Meichenbaum & Goodman, 1971), and *stress inoculation therapy* (Meichenbaum, 1993) are commonly used interventions in this model.

Although Ellis's REBT and Beck's cognitive therapy incorporate other CB methods into the treatment process, both therapies are based on an underlying theory that explains the way in which cognitions influence psychological problems. Basically, Ellis's (1998) "A-iBs-C" model contends that an activating event (A) triggers an individual's irrational beliefs (iBs), which results in a consequence (C), such as an undesirable emotion, behavior, or physiological response. For example, if a client diagnosed with schizophrenia recently lost his employment in a competitive work setting because he was unable to handle the stress (activating event) and was experiencing depressive symptoms (consequence), Ellis would contend that the employment loss was not the reason for his depression. Instead, an irrational belief, such as "I *must* be employed in a competitive work setting in order to be a worthwhile and happy person," is initiating the depressive symptoms.

J. S. Beck's current theoretical model (1995) is more complex. The model postulates that the underlying core belief (cognitive schema) individuals hold about themselves, others, and the world influences a set of intermediate beliefs (rules, attitudes, and assumptions) that affect their perception of a particular situation. These core and intermediate beliefs are expressed by automatic thoughts, which, in turn, can result in an undesirable emotion, behavior, and/or physiological response. For example, through childhood experiences and interactions, the client diagnosed with schizophrenia developed the core belief that he is incompetent. The client would then interpret life events that were relevant to such a belief in terms of this schema. The core belief also influences a set of intermediate beliefs. For example, the client might have the rule that "I should succeed in activities that are important to me," the attitude that "it's awful not to succeed in activities that are important to me," and the assumption that "if I am not successful in such activities, I must continue trying until I am." When a specific situation occurs, such as the client's losing his job, his core and intermediate beliefs are activated and influence his perception of the event, which is reflected in his automatic thoughts (e.g., "I am a loser"). The automatic thoughts trigger the depressive symptoms.

Regardless of their differences, both Ellis's and Beck's models make the assumption that a client's cognitions (perceptions, beliefs, thoughts, expectations, images, etc.) are at least partially responsible for the problems they experience. The goals of both therapies are to identify these irrational or dysfunctional cognitions, confront or more gently evaluate them, then substitute a more functional or rational belief, thought, or image.

COGNITIVE-BEHAVIORAL ASSESSMENT

CB assessment involves defining and measuring the behavior that is targeted for change, establishing treatment goals, and conducting a functional assessment. When one defines a target behavior, as described in many of the interventions in this book, a *task analysis* is frequently conducted. A task analysis breaks down a more complex behavior into the subtasks necessary to perform the behavior competently. For example, a practitioner might teach a client with mental retardation to successfully eat at a fast-food restaurant. To do this, the practitioner breaks down the complex behavior into subtasks, such as entering the restaurant, deciding what to order, ordering, paying for the food, taking the tray to the table, eating, and cleaning the eating area. The behavior also is measured before (referred to as a baseline), during, and after intervention. Common measures include frequency, duration, and intensity of the behavior. Depending on the protocol design, the data are frequently graphed for analysis. Baseline measures assist practitioners in determining whether intervention is necessary. If intervention is needed, the baseline measures are compared with measures during and after intervention to provide feedback on the effectiveness of the intervention.

A *functional assessment* is an individualized assessment method in which information on the antecedents and consequences (environmental events) of the target behavior is gathered to determine which events reliably predict and maintain the behavior. In other words, the behavior is considered a function of the environmental events. The assumption is that if the maintaining conditions are identified and interventions are used to change them, the behavior will change in the desired direction.

Maintaining antecedents are stimuli or events that precede or are present when a behavior is performed and increase the probability that the behavior will be performed. A functional assessment determines when, where, with whom, and under what conditions the behavior is least and most likely to occur. Maintaining antecedents can be divided into the two broad categories of *stimulus control* and *prerequisites* (Spiegler & Guevremont, 2003). Stimulus control involves *prompts* and broader, complex *setting events*. Prompts are specific cues, such as a practitioner suggesting to a student with a disability, "You could ask the children at that lunch table if you can sit with them." Setting events are much broader and include the time, place, and environmental circumstances that are appropriate for performing a particular behavior. For example, because of setting events, we behave much differently when attending a church service versus attending a party. Setting events include both social and physical environments. Students with an attention deficit, for example, might increase their on-task behavior in a smaller classroom or in a classroom in which other students do not provide distractions. Prerequisites, the second main type of maintaining antecedents, include the skills, resources, knowledge, and opportunities necessary to perform an identified behavior. For example, if clients with a disability learn their legal rights and self-advocacy skills, they will be more likely to advocate for their legal rights.

Cognitions, such as thoughts, beliefs, expectations, perceptions, and images, also can be maintaining antecedents. A functional assessment can assess cognitions when appropriate, such as when clients' developmental age suggests that their cognitions can be assessed and modified. The assessment determines which cognitions precede an identified covert (e.g., depression) or overt (e.g., withdrawal) behavior.

Maintaining consequences are events or stimuli that occur as a result of the behavior being performed. Generally, when an event is perceived as positive or favorable, the behavior is more likely to be repeated. Thus, the behavior is reinforced. When an event that follows is perceived as aversive or negative, the probability of the behavior being repeated usually decreases. Therefore, the behavior is punished. A functional assessment identifies the maintaining consequences by answering questions such as: "What occurs as a result of the behavior being performed?" "What do the client and others do?" "In which ways does the client benefit?" and "What does the client avoid?" Finally, a functional assessment identifies behaviors that must be learned and desirable behaviors the client already has learned that can be reinforced to compete with an existing problem.

A variety of methods, such as asking relevant questions during the interview, self-recording (i.e., the client observes and records the occurrence of the target behavior and its antecedents and consequences), asking others to do the recording, role playing, and naturalistic observations, are used to identify the maintaining conditions of the identified behavior. Assessment procedures for identifying irrational or dysfunctional cognitions frequently involve recording forms that assist clients in assessing their cognitions, which are in response to specific situations and trigger the overt or covert behavior targeted for change (see J. S. Beck, 1995; Blankstein & Segal, 2001; Ellis, 1998, for examples of these methods). Frequently, practitioners use more than one assessment method.

Readers interested in obtaining more detailed information on conducting a functional assessment are referred to "Additional Readings and Resources" at the end of this chapter. The references also contain CB assessments specifically designed for vulnerable clients, including sexual minorities and clients from different cultural backgrounds and with a variety of disabilities. Readers also might be interested in broader social work assessment frameworks that integrate traditional behavioral assessment procedures (see Gambrill, 1997; Mattaini, 1997, for excellent examples).

COMMON INTERVENTIONS

The intervention chapters of this book describe multiple CB interventions, which are combined in various ways into intervention packages or multicomponent programs. My focus in this section is on behavioral and CB interventions that are used frequently in these treatment packages or programs, thus avoiding the repetition of the details of the interventions in subsequent chapters. For example, when reinforcement or social skills training is implemented, these interventions are not described in detail, because they are described here. Interventions that are not described in this section are presented in more detail in the intervention chapters.

Behavioral Interventions

Changing antecedent conditions based on operant conditioning. Introducing a stimulus or an event to cue appropriate behavior at the appropriate time and in the appropriate context (establishing stimulus control) is frequently referred to as *prompting*. Prompts and interventions to change setting events, including physical and social environments, are discussed first. A description of interventions to change the antecedent condition of lacking prerequisites, such as skills, knowledge, resources, and opportunities, follows.

Prompts are instructions or reminders to perform an identified behavior. They can take many forms. Prompts can be verbal (e.g., "What do you do next?"), auditory (e.g., a recorded messsage), pictures (e.g., an employee performing a job task), gestures (e.g., pointing), and "social scripts" or other written instructions (e.g., reminder cards). Physical guidance, in which the practitioner physically assists the client in performing the desired behavior, also can prompt behavior. Examples of practitioners, teachers, peers, staff, caregivers, and clients themselves using a variety of prompts to initiate many types of behaviors are provided in the intervention chapters. The behaviors include initiating and sustaining social interactions, engaging in recreational/leisure activity, performing job tasks, recruiting assistance, evaluating choices, and engaging in advocacy and political activity.

As examples in this book demonstrate, practitioners also can use a *prompt hierarchy* to teach new behaviors, such as job tasks or purchasing food in a community restaurant. When using a prompt hierarchy, the client is given an opportunity to perform the behavior first, and a prompt follows only if the behavior is not performed or is performed inappropriately. When prompts are necessary, a lesser controlling prompt is provided first. For example, a verbal prompt ("What do you do next?"), might be followed by a gesture (a nod), a minimal physical prompt (touching the client's hand), then a total physical prompt in which the practitioner physically guides the client in performing the behavior.

Fading is gradually withdrawing a prompt, including the gradual use of less physical assistance when physical guidance is used, as the client performs the identified behavior more frequently or appropriately. Fading also can involve a time delay procedure in which practitioners increase the amount of time that they wait for the client to perform the relevant behavior. For example, a practitioner teaching a recreational game might verbally prompt the client to move the game piece then immediately follow this with verbal instruction. The practitioner would then increase the length of time (e.g., two seconds, four seconds) between the verbal prompt and verbal instruction (or other type of prompt), until the client can perform the behavior without being prompted.

In many cases, broader setting events, such as the physical and social environments, must be modified to change an identified behavior. Examples of interventions in this book that change physical environments to increase social interactions include installing exterior ramps to home entrances for wheelchair users, switching from institutionalized meal service to serving meals family-style, rearranging furniture in institutionalizing settings, and providing recreational/leisure activities in school and residential settings. Distractions of workers with mental retardation can be reduced by the use of partitions to divide production tables. CB interventions also can modify social environments. In educational settings, practitioners can teach and motivate peers with no disabilities to engage in recreation, play, and other social activity with students with disabilities and to become members of their social networks. The peers also can facilitate changes in the attitudes of other able-bodied students toward and increase their interactions with students with learning and developmental problems. A final example is recruiting a co-worker advocate to assist employees with disabilities in integrating into their work environment. The co-worker uses a variety of actions, such as sitting with the employees at lunch and break times and encouraging other workers to do so.

As previously discussed, prerequisites, which include having the required skills, knowledge, resources, and opportunities, also determine whether clients will perform a particular behavior. Thus, clients' lack of knowledge of particular skills and a skills deficit can be maintaining antecedents of their failing to engage in an identified behavior. *Skills training* is a common behavioral intervention that can teach basic skills, such as those required to do a job. *Social skills training* (SST) focuses specifically on skills that enhance interpersonal or social competency in multiple situations. These skills include engaging in conversation and initiating social interactions; requesting information about medications; recruiting assistance for performing routine activities, handling emergencies, and attaining personal goals;

job interviewing; accessing public and private sources of assistance; participating in educational conferences; and choice-making, self-advocacy, negotiation, political, and leadership behaviors.

Regardless of whether the skill is basic or social, similar components are used to teach it. The components include defining the target skill, providing a rationale for and instruction on the skill, modeling, prompting, behavioral rehearsal, and assigning homework to practice the skill in natural settings.

Modeling involves learning a behavior by observing someone else (the model) perform it. Models can be live; practitioners, peers, teachers, and parents and other caregivers can serve as models. For example, an adolescent female can learn to appropriately negotiate safe sexual behavior by watching another female engage in such a negotiation. Models performing the identified skills also can be viewed on video, can be depicted in storybooks and folk tales, and can involve puppets. Prompting is used in a similar manner, as previously discussed.

During *behavior rehearsal* clients practice the modeled behavior (frequently in role-play situations). Based on the clients' performance, practitioners either provide corrective feedback (coaching) or provide reinforcement. In *role playing*, clients are asked to respond to an artificially contrived situation as if they were in the actual situation. Practitioners can use preconstructed situations from manualized interventions, and practitioners, clients, and group members also can construct the situations. Role plays can be used to assess competence of social skills and to practice the skills. Finally, *homework assignments*, which involve practicing the acquired skills in the settings (e.g., school, community, work, home) and situations in which they are expected to be performed, are given to clients. These settings and contexts are frequently referred to as the *natural environment*.

Assertion or *assertiveness training* is a type of SST that teaches clients how and when to engage in assertive behavior. After determining which types of situations and with whom the assertive behaviors are to be performed, the procedures commonly involve teaching clients to distinguish between assertive responses and aggressive or passive responses. This procedure is followed by using SST to teach the assertive responses. Methods such as reinforcing the assertive responses instead of the outcome (which is not under a client's control) as well as modeling successful coping strategies when the desired outcome is not achieved are also used. Examples in this book of situations for which assertiveness training can be used include obtaining information about wheelchair accessibility, requesting assistance, obtaining community resources and services, and asserting one's right to refuse to engage in unwanted or unprotected sexual behavior.

The interventions described in this book also recognize the importance of providing other types of knowledge, as well as the necessary resources and opportunities, if clients are to perform the identified behaviors. In addition to teaching knowledge on appropriate social responses, numerous other examples of providing relevant knowledge and information are evident. Examples include knowledge and information on methods to seek employment; on Western values for recent immigrants preparing for job interviews; on availability of community resources and public benefits; on legal rights (e.g., work and educational accommodations and civil rights) and appeals processes; on contraceptive methods, risks of unprotected sex, and safe sex practices; and on political processes, social policy, and social change strategies for issues related to disabilities, mental illness, aging, and women's health.

The intervention chapters also provide multiple examples of providing the resources necessary for clients to perform the identified behaviors. Examples include specially designed communication and picture books, choice charts, and augmentative communication systems for clients unable to communicate effectively. Providing emergency telephone books adapted for clients with cognitive limitations and the necessary facilities, supplies, and other resources needed to seek and obtain employment is yet another example.

Also provided are examples of interventions that open up opportunities for clients to perform the identified behaviors. For example, co-workers teach work skills to employees with multiple disabilities, which increases opportunities for social interactions to occur between the co-workers and workers with disabilities. Staff supervision of group homes increases opportunities for clients with disabilities to engage in social and recreational activity by providing choices, activities, and transportation. During intervention, job coaches provide multiple opportunities for clients who have low income, minority racial/ethnic backgrounds, and severe mental illness to practice job-seeking and interviewing skills. Teachers provide opportunities in classrooms for students with disabilities to achieve their own goals (e.g., contributing to the class). A final example is staff in group homes, institutions, and employment settings ensuring that clients with disabilities have opportunities to make choices in recreational/leisure activity, food, job tasks, and community residence.

Changing antecedent conditions based on respondent conditioning. Exposure therapies are designed to change the antecedent condition of an overt behavior (e.g., withdrawing) or covert behavior (e.g., feelings of anxiety). In this case, the CS (e.g., the social situation) is the antecedent condition that elicits behaviors such as withdrawing and feeling anxious. Various types of exposure therapies have been developed, including brief, graduated exposure, such as *systematic desensitization*, and prolonged, intensive exposure, such as *flooding* (Spiegler & Guevremont, 2003). All of the examples in this book involve graduated exposure.

When using graduated exposure, the practitioner assists the client in constructing a hierarchy of situations that elicit the anxiety/withdrawal behaviors. Then beginning with the situation that causes the least amount of anxiety, the client is repeatedly exposed to the situation (either covertly or in vivo) until it no longer evokes the anxiety/withdrawal. Only then does the practitioner expose the client to the next situation in the hierarchy, and the client ascends the hierarchy in a similar manner. In brief, graduated exposure, such as systematic desensitization, the client is frequently taught a competing response to the anxiety (e.g., deep muscle relaxation). This book provides examples of using brief, graduated exposure to assist gay men in reducing their social anxiety, thus increasing their personal interactions and relationships with other gay men.

Changing consequences based on operant conditioning. Practitioners, clients, and others can change the consequences of an identified behavior by using positive and negative reinforcement, positive punishment (e.g., scolding a student with an emotional/behavioral disability for not completing class work) and negative punishment (e.g., removing a privilege such as attending a school outing for disruptive class behavior), and extinction. Negative reinforcement is rarely used as an intervention, and because almost all of the intervention packages described in this book use positive reinforcement, this is my focus here. Although punishment (particularly negative punishment) is commonly used, only one of the treatment packages described in the intervention chapters uses this type of intervention. One treatment package also uses a time-out procedure, which can be used to extinguish a particular behavior.

When using positive reinforcement, the practitioner first must identify potential reinforcers for each client. Providing the reinforcer is then made contingent on the client's performing the identified behavior (i.e., the reinforcer is given only after the behavior is performed). The practitioner must then determine whether the behavior increases. Positive reinforcers can be social, activities, and tangibles (both edibles and concrete objects). Examples of social reinforcers are praise, acknowledgment, approval, hugs, pats on the back, and thank-you letters. Activities include games, going out for lunch, and attending a party. Tangible reinforcers include edibles, such as food and soda, and objects, such as clothing, toys, money, and tokens.

Tokens, which can be points, check marks, stickers, fake money, and the like, are used in establishing a *token economy*. A token economy is a program in which individuals earn tokens contingent on performing desired behaviors or achieving specific goals. Practitioners assign a specific number of tokens that can be earned for each behavior that is performed and the token cost of the predetermined reinforcers, referred to as *backup reinforcers*. The predetermined number of tokens is given immediately after the behavior is performed, and the earned tokens are later exchanged for the backup reinforcers. Token economies also can be established in which clients lose tokens for undesirable behaviors (negative punishment), in addition to earning tokens for desirable behaviors. This book contains no examples of removing tokens to decrease unwanted behaviors.

As the interventions described in the following chapters demonstrate, practitioners, parents, teachers, staff, and peers can reinforce students and clients after exhibiting a wide range of desirable behaviors, such as engaging in social interactions and leisure/recreational activity and attending self-help meetings. Clients also can *self-reinforce*, which is a *self-management strategy* involving clients providing themselves with a reinforcer after performing the desired behavior. For example, clients can be taught to give themselves tokens after socially interacting with others, which can be exchanged for candy and soda.

Thinning (or *fading*) reinforcers involve gradually increasing the criteria for performance of the identified behavior before a reinforcer is provided. For example, a student with a disability might have to initiate a conversation one time before receiving a token. After this occurs without effort, the frequency is gradually increased before a token is given. The tokens are eventually discontinued entirely. Because social reinforcers are naturally occurring, they are more successful in maintaining behavior after formal intervention ends. Social reinforcers, therefore, are frequently paired with artificial reinforcers, such as tokens, and can continue after artificial reinforcers are discontinued.

Time-out procedures are used after an individual performs an undesirable behavior. For example, a preschooler with a developmental delay inappropriately takes a toy from another child and does not respond to the teacher's prompt to perform a related desirable behavior (e.g., return the toy). The child is then taken from the immediate environment and placed into a brief time-out. This procedure can be considered "time-limited" extinction (Spiegler & Guevremont, 2003), because the child is temporarily denied access to potential reinforcers (e.g., the toy and playing with other children). When a time-out procedure is used, the reason for the time-out is given, and the child is placed in a location free of reinforcers for a brief period of time (generally 1 minute for each year of age, with a maximum of five minutes).

Although identifying and removing a positive reinforcer that is maintaining an identified behavior can extinguish the behavior, no such example of extinction appears in the interventions described in this book. The use of negative and positive punishment also can decrease an undesirable behavior, but punishment is rarely used in the interventions presented in this book.

An exception is sending an employee with mental retardation home after he refuses to fulfill his job duties.

Cognitive-Behavioral Interventions

The most commonly used CB interventions described in subsequent chapters are problem-solving therapy or training, cognitive restructuring, and self-instructional training.

The goal of *problem-solving training (PST)* is to teach clients cognitive skills to assist them in solving common problems for which they are unable to find a satisfactory solution (D'Zurilla & Nezu, 1999). When clients cannot find a satisfactory solution to common problems, they can experience undesirable emotions and overt behaviors, as well as other negative outcomes, such as the inability to achieve personal goals. PST begins by assisting the client in recognizing that a problem exists, perceiving problems as an expected, normal part of life, and approaching problem solving in a careful, deliberate way. The practitioner then assists the client in identifying and defining the problem and goal. After alternative solutions to the problem are generated through brainstorming, the most reasonable of the possible solutions are chosen for further evaluation. Evaluation is accomplished by methods such as listing and comparing the advantages and disadvantages or the benefits and costs of each solution. Based on the evaluation, an alternative is selected.

Before the client implements the chosen solution, the practitioner determines whether the client has the necessary knowledge, resources, skills, and opportunity to implement the selected option. If the client has the prerequisites, the selected option is implemented. Of course, if the client does not have the prerequisites, the practitioner must assist the client in learning the knowledge and skills, obtaining the needed resources, and ensuring that opportunities to carry out the identified solution exist, or another solution must be chosen. After implementation, an evaluation is conducted to determine whether the solution resolved the problem. If the problem is resolved, problem solving ends. If the problem is unresolved, problem solving continues, with the client returning to the relevant step in the problem-solving process.

As the interventions described in this book demonstrate, variations of PST can be used to assist children, adolescents, and adults with physical, sensory, and/or psychiatric disabilities in attaining a variety of goals. The goals include enhancing appropriate social interactions, increasing friendships, improving job performance and job-related social skills, managing symptoms and medications at the workplace, coping with stressors, recruiting social support, obtaining public and private sources of assistance, and establishing and attaining personal goals. PST also can assist residents in resolving community problems in low-income neighborhoods and assist women with low income and racial/ethnic minority youths in developing strategies to cope with antecedent conditions that increase the probability of engaging in high-risk sexual behavior.

Cognitive restructuring is a process of identifying, evaluating or challenging, then altering a client's dysfunctional, maladaptive, or irrational thoughts, beliefs, or images that are maintaining an overt or a covert behavior. Although the basic steps of cognitive restructuring are similar across various therapy models, the therapies use different processes. For example, Beck's cognitive therapy is a collaborative process, which uses gentle Socratic questioning (e.g., "Where is the evidence? Could there be an alternative explanation?") to assist clients in examining the evidence for their own beliefs. On the other hand, Ellis's REBT is more didactic and employs verbal persuasion to rationally dispute the irrational or illogical thinking.

Several examples of cognitive restructuring appear in the intervention chapters. A gay client is assisted in learning to recognize and challenge the maladaptive thoughts (e.g., "I'd like to talk to him . . . but he might not like me") maintaining his social anxiety and preventing him from meeting other gay men. The therapist then teaches him to compose more functional thoughts to replace the dysfunctional ones. A lesbian client is taught to identify and change several negative beliefs she holds about lesbians and about herself as a lesbian, which are causing anxiety and interfering with building a social support network. A final example is group facilitators teaching youths to recognize and dispute beliefs leading to high-risk sexual behaviors and to replace the beliefs with statements more consistent with safer behaviors, for example, "If he won't use a condom, then he doesn't really care about me."

Self-instructional training involves teaching clients to talk to themselves for the purpose of learning new behavior, or self-control, or performing an already learned behavior. After identifying the situation and desirable behavior(s), the practitioner develops a set of self-instructions. While performing the behavior, the practitioner states the self-instructions out loud, followed by the client's performance of the behavior while the practitioner verbalizes the instructions out loud. Clients then perform the behavior while verbalizing the instructions out loud themselves, perform the behavior while whispering the instructions to themselves, and perform the behavior while saying the instructions silently. Clients are encouraged to develop their own self-instructions. Practitioners frequently teach the procedures using SST techniques, including having clients practice the self-instructions in role plays and then in natural settings. Using self-instructional training to assist clients with a variety of disabilities in increasing their social interactions with peers, increasing their leisure/recreational activity, and performing job tasks are examples in this book.

The next and final introductory chapter discusses the consistency of CB methods with empowerment and social work practice.

ADDITIONAL READINGS AND RESOURCES

Cowick, B., & Storey, K. (2000). An analysis of functional assessment in relation to students with serious emotional and behaviour disorders. *International Journal of Disability, Development and Education, 47,* 55–75.

Groden, G. (1989). A guide for conducting a comprehensive behavioral analysis of a target behavior. *Journal of Behavior Therapy and Experimental Psychiatry, 20,* 163–169.

Haynes, S. N., & O'Brien, W. H. (2000). *Principles and practice of behavioral assessment.* New York: Kluwer Academic/Plenum.

Horner, R. H., & Carr, E. G. (1997). Behavioral support for students with severe disabilities: Functional assessment and comprehensive intervention. *Journal of Special Education, 31,* 84–104.

Kazdin, A. E. (2001). *Behavior modification in applied settings* (6th ed.). Pacific Grove, CA: Brooks/Cole.

Martell, C. R., Safren, S. A., & Prince, S. E. (2004). *Cognitive behavioral assessment.* In C. R. Martell, S. A. Safren, & S. E. Prince (Eds.), *Cognitive-behavioral therapies with lesbian, gay, and bisexual clients* (pp. 18–37). New York: Guilford.

Murphy, V. B., & Christner, R. W. (2006). A cognitive-behavioral case conceptualization approach for working with children and adolescents. In R. B. Mennuti, A. Freeman, & R. W. Christner (Eds.), *Cognitive-behavioral interventions in educational settings: A handbook for practice* (pp. 37–62). New York: Routledge.

Okazaki, S. M., & Tanaka-Matsumi, J. (2006). Cultural considerations in cognitive-behavioral assessment. In P. A. Hays & G. Y. Iwamasa (Eds.), *Culturally responsive cognitive-behavioral therapy: Assessment, practice, and supervision* (pp. 247–266). Washington, DC: American Psychological Association.

Spiegler, M. D., & Guevremont, D. C. (2003). *Contemporary behavior therapy* (4th ed.). Belmont, CA: Wadsworth & Thomson.

Sundel, M., & Sundel, S. S. (2004). *Behavior modification in the human services: A systematic introduction to concepts and applications* (5th ed.). Newbury Park, CA: Sage.

Tanaka-Matsumi, J., Seiden, D. Y., & Lam, K. N. (1996). The Culturally Informed Functional Assessment (CIFA) Interview: A strategy for cross-cultural behavioral practice. *Cognitive and Behavioral Practice, 3,* 215–233.

Wehmeyer, M. L., Baker, D. J., Blumberg, R., & Harrison, R. (2004). Self-determination and student involvement in functional assessment: Innovative practices. *Journal of Positive Behavior Interventions, 6,* 29–35.

3 Empowerment and Cognitive-Behavioral Methods

This chapter discusses the concept of empowerment, defines empowerment for the purposes of this book, and provides a context for understanding the selection of the four broad intervention goals. The goals are to enhance social resources, to acquire economic resources, to increase self-determined behavior, and to influence macro decision making. Common criticisms of CB methods are considered, and consistency of these methods with empowerment and social work practice is discussed.

EMPOWERMENT AND SELECTION OF INTERVENTION GOALS

Empowerment is one of the most frequently used, yet variously and ambiguously defined, concepts in the social work and related literature. Empowerment has been referred to as a practice, a set of strategies, a process, a goal, a product, a feeling, a capacity, a life force, a reflective activity, a potentially unifying approach to practice, and the central task of the profession. The concept of empowerment has been applied to both micro and macro levels of practice and to multiple client groups. Vulnerable populations, such as the poor, women, elderly, lesbians, gays and bisexuals, racial/ethnic and cultural minorities, and individuals with mental, developmental, and physical disabilities, have been the main target groups of empowerment practice (Browne, 1995; Carr, 2003; East, 2000; Hasenfeld, 1987; Kondrat, 1995; Lee, 1996; Saleebey, 2002; Simon, 1994; Staples, 1990).

Definitions of the term *empowerment* also vary. Solomon (1976), credited with introducing empowerment practice to social work in her book *Black Empowerment: Social Work in Oppressed Communities* (Browne, 1995; Lee, 1996), defined empowerment as a "process whereby persons who belong to a stigmatized social category throughout their lives can be assisted to develop and increase skills in the exercise of interpersonal influence and the performance of valued social roles" (p. 6). Solomon also believed that empowerment can be an "appropriate goal" (p. 21). Gutiérrez (1990) described empowerment as "a process of increasing personal, interpersonal, or political power so that individuals can take action to improve their life situations" (p. 149).

From a social work strengths perspective, Saleebey (2002) defined empowerment as "the intent to, and the process of, assisting individuals, groups, families, and communities to discover and expend the resources and tools within and around them" (p. 9). From a behavioral perspective applied to intervening with clients diagnosed with severe mental illness, Corrigan (1997) defined empowerment as "individuals making decisions about their treatment, work, recreation, and living arrangements" (p. 49). Community psychologists have defined empowerment as a process "by which people, organizations, and communities gain mastery over their lives" (Rappaport, 1984, p. 3) and "of gaining some control over events, outcomes, and resources of importance to an individual or group" (Fawcett et al., 1994, p. 472). Lee (1996) provides still more definitions of empowerment. A central theme in all of these definitions is that individuals or groups develop a sense of power, control, or mastery over important aspects of their lives.

So as not to add to the ambiguity and confusion by providing yet another definition of empowerment, Yeheskel Hasenfeld's (1987) definition is adopted for use in this book. Hasenfeld defines empowerment as "a process through which clients obtain resources—personal, organizational, and community—that enable them to gain greater control over their environment and to attain their aspirations" (pp. 478–479). This definition is appropriate because it emphasizes accessing a variety of resources that assist individuals in increasing control over their lives and in attaining their own goals, outcomes that are consistent with social work values.

It can also be assumed that empowerment is more than a process or the acquisition of empowering skills. Research must provide some evidence that the process or acquired skills result in vulnerable individuals or groups enhancing their power. This is indicated by increases in social and economic resources, personal decision making, and input into the macro decisions that affect the lives of vulnerable populations. This latter assumption is related to what Rosen and Proctor (1981) define as instrumental versus ultimate outcomes or goals. Instrumental goals, such as enhanced social, employment, or self-advocacy skills, are designed to achieve clients' ultimate goals, such as forming friendships, finding employment, and securing legal rights. This book focuses on CB interventions for which research has provided some evidence that the interventions can assist vulnerable populations in achieving their ultimate goals.

Consistent with other scholars, Hasenfeld also argues that empowerment must occur on at least three levels: the practitioner-client, organizational, and social policy. At the practitioner-client level, social workers should increase clients' power resources by providing information on community resources and by teaching self-advocacy and other skills for assisting clients in securing their rights, obtaining social and economic resources, and achieving personal goals. At the organizational level, practitioners should use the power of their agency to address client needs. At the policy level, social workers should ensure that clients directly affected by social policy decisions have opportunities to influence the formation and implementation of those decisions. The evaluations of the CB interventions presented in this book suggest that the interventions can assist vulnerable populations in increasing their power resources and in influencing organizational and policy decisions that affect their lives.

CRITICISMS OF COGNITIVE-BEHAVIORAL METHODS AND THEIR CONSISTENCY WITH EMPOWERMENT AND SOCIAL WORK PRACTICE

The use of CB methods in social work practice has been directly criticized, or criticized for particular procedures that are shared with other approaches, such as focusing on clients' problems instead of their strengths. Criticisms have come primarily from scholars and practitioners who share a humanistic philosophy or orientation. These include feminism, empowerment, and the related strengths perspective. Criticisms of the use of these methods also have come from CB researchers and practitioners themselves. Among the most frequent criticisms of CB methods is that they are expert driven and controlled and thus constrain individual freedom. Second, CB methods identify and change individual deficits and assist clients in adapting to current unjust or unfavorable environments. Thus, the interventions are inconsistent with a social justice perspective. Third, CB methods assess and change narrowly defined behaviors, establish quantitative intervention goals, and use standardized procedures, all of which lack social relevance. The next three sections address each of these criticisms in turn and discuss the consistency of CB methods with empowerment and social work practice.

Do Cognitive-Behavioral Methods Constrain Individual Freedom through Expert Control?

CB interventions are expert driven in the sense that they are derived from experimentally tested theory and intervention research. Opposition to expert control of the intervention process has been voiced by empowerment, feminist, and strengths-based scholars (e.g., Hurst & Genest, 1995; Rappaport, 1981; Saleebey, 1996). Scholars and practitioners have argued that expert-driven methods constrain individual freedom in two main ways. First, practitioners or other experts in charge use the techniques to control individual behavior. Second, the practitioner, not the individual or group, defines the target behavior and chooses the assessment, intervention, and evaluation procedures. Using such practices only reinforces the client's sense of powerlessness.

Many social work scholars and practitioners acknowledge that the profession frequently serves a social control function (e.g., Gambrill, 1997; Rothman, 1989), regardless of the approach (e.g., feminist, strengths-based, or CB) used by social workers. That is, social workers frequently intervene to decrease or eliminate certain problems and to assist individuals or groups in conforming to social norms. This is particularly the case with problems such as child and spouse abuse, other forms of violence, substance abuse, and a variety of other illegal behavior. Assisting individuals in controlling such behavior, however, does not necessarily decrease but can enhance individual freedom. Decreasing or controlling certain behaviors, such as substance abuse, can increase choices, such as in employment and interpersonal relationships. Having alternatives to choose from is an important element of freedom. Thus, even this type of behavioral change can be consistent with empowerment.

Despite this argument, multiple examples of "experts" misusing behavioral techniques to control behavior, particularly the behavior of vulnerable populations, certainly exist. Examples include using inappropriate and unnecessary aversive techniques, establishing reinforcing or punishing consequences that encourage submissiveness and discourage independent decision making, and requiring clients to earn reinforcers to which they are legally entitled for engaging in identified behavior, such as working for meals (Corrigan, 1997). Although behavioral interventions have been misused to inappropriately deny individual freedom, this book demonstrates ways in which such applications can be used to enhance individual choice and freedom.

In response to early criticism that behavior therapy was undermining clients' autonomy and freedom of choice through external control, even in circumstances in which clients set their own intervention goals, CB scholars developed a variety of self-control assessment and intervention methods (Browder & Shapiro, 1985; Goldfried & Castonguay, 1993; Rasing, Coninx, Duker, & Van den Hurk, 1994). Self-recording, in which clients observe, record, and assess changes in their own behavior, is the main assessment method. Examples of self-control interventions include self-instruction, using other personalized prompts, self-reinforcement, problem solving, and cognitive restructuring. In addition, as this book suggests, CB interventions can assist vulnerable clients in increasing and accessing resources from their environment, enhancing self-determination, and influencing macro decision making and practices affecting the services they receive and other important aspects of their lives. Thus, CB interventions can be used to empower people, rather than control them.

A related criticism of CB methods is that the practitioner, not the client, is in control of defining the behavior to change and selecting the assessment, intervention, and evaluation procedures. Regardless of the practitioner's philosophy or theoretical orientation to social work practice, selection of the client's problem and goals and the assessment, treatment, and evaluation procedures are constrained in some way (Rothman, 1989). Society (e.g., social norms and funding sources), characteristics of practitioners (e.g., ethics, beliefs, knowledge and training, personal biases), and organizational or agency mandates, policies, and resources all constrain these aspects of practice. Admittedly, even when clients are offered a choice among ways to define problems and goals and assessment and intervention procedures, CB applications can be more constraining than other approaches. For example, problems and behaviors are precisely defined, assessment methods consist of a limited range of options, interventions are frequently technical and directive, and because interventions are based on empirical research, they frequently are standardized. These aspects of CB applications clearly place much of the control of the assessment and intervention process in the hands of the expert, which can be inconsistent with an empowerment approach.

Fawcett and his colleagues (Fawcett, Seekins, Wang, Muiu, & Suarez de Balcazar, 1984) recognized the apparent contradiction in using social technologies (defined as a replicable set of procedures designed to change participants' socially relevant behaviors under a variety of real-life circumstances) to empower individuals. They acknowledged that by choosing to use and participate in standardized interventions, the practitioner and participants must give up some freedom or control. However, if using standardized interventions gives participants increased options and more control over their lives, then the use of such interventions can increase personal freedom and empowerment. For example, if a practitioner chose to use social skills training to teach clients with disabilities self-advocacy skills, the practitioner would necessarily give up some control of the intervention process to teach the skills. If the clients agreed to this intervention, they also would give up some control over the choice of methods to learn the skills. But, if by using the standardized intervention the clients acquire the self-advocacy skills, the clients would have increased options to obtain resources and influence decisions made about their lives. Moreover, if using the skills resulted in clients' increasing their social or economic resources, participating in decision making that affects their lives, or securing individual rights, these outcomes would be consistent with empowerment. As this book demonstrates, CB applications can be used to assist vulnerable populations in achieving such outcomes.

In addition to the argument that CB interventions can empower clients by assisting them in achieving their goals (or by making it more likely that clients will achieve the goals or achieve them in a shorter period of time, compared with other interventions), these methods are consistent with an empowerment perspective and social work practice in other ways. First, the defining characteristics and values of CB approaches include a commitment to empirically evaluating interventions, to offering clients research-based therapies, and to evaluating the effectiveness of the interventions when used with individuals or groups. These characteristics are consistent with the educational policy and accreditation standards for social work programs (CSWE, 2001), as well as with the NASW (1999) Code of Ethics. CB interventions are well represented among effective interventions for a wide range of client problems in the social work and related literature (e.g., Kazdin & Weisz, 2003; MacDonald, Sheldon, & Gillespie, 1992; O'Hare, 2005; Reid, Kenaley, & Colvin, 2004).

Second, as the intervention chapters suggest, CB applications also can assist vulnerable groups in achieving outcomes for which traditional psychotherapies might be inappropriate or not particularly helpful. Examples include assisting clients with mental retardation in increasing social interactions, clients with severe mental illness in actively participating in the medication decisions made about their psychiatric condition, and students with learning disabilities in defining and achieving their own goals. CB techniques also are particularly relevant to vulnerable populations because they can be implemented in settings, such as school and work, where traditional psychotherapy might be difficult to use.

Third, problem and goal selection, assessment and intervention procedures, and tracking progress are individualized, described, negotiated, and agreed upon with the client. Prior to treatment for a particular problem, the practitioner can describe the viable alternative interventions to the client and/or others involved in the intervention procedures. The description can include the underlying rationale, details of the interventions, the expected activity of the client and significant others, an estimate of the duration and success rate of the interventions, and the advantages and disadvantages of the intervention options. This transparent process puts the clients and/or significant others in control, because it provides them with the opportunity to ask informed questions and to make informed choices. This process is unlike other therapies or approaches that use deceptive interventions (e.g., paradoxical interventions); cannot or do not adequately describe their assessment and intervention procedures; establish vague goals that the client and practitioner would find extremely difficult to determine if they were achieved; provide no clear intervention options with information on their advantages, disadvantages, and estimate of duration and effectiveness; and use CB interventions without even realizing or informing their clients (Hudson & Macdonald, 1986; Spiegler & Guevremont, 2003; Thyer, 1991).

Thyer (1991), for example, argued that social workers who are trained in and use behavioral techniques are guided by learning theory and use interventions, such as positive reinforcement, in a deliberate and professional manner. Social workers use reinforcers to motivate clients to remain committed to the therapeutic process, to actively work on their problems during the sessions, and to complete homework assignments related to their goals. Thyer also cited research suggesting that positive reinforcement is commonly used in psychodynamic and client-centered therapy, such as that practiced by Carl Rogers. However, as Truax (1966) demonstrated, Rogers was unaware that during treatment he used verbal and other forms of reinforcers (e.g., eye contact) contingent on the client's self-disclosures and displayed emotions. Principles of learning also likely apply to the activities of practitioners who engage in traditional empowerment or strengths-based approaches. That is, social workers withdraw attention from (extinguish) client statements of problems or deficits and pay attention to (reinforce) behaviors that the "expert" practitioner defines as strengths or as legitimate means to resolve problems. Perhaps traditional empowerment and strengths-based approaches are not as client-based versus expert-based as some scholars and practitioners might believe.

Are Cognitive-Behavioral Methods Inconsistent with a Social Justice Perspective?

Promoting social justice, particularly with and on behalf of vulnerable and oppressed populations, is a core value of the social work profession. Interventions aimed at ensuring that all people have equality of opportunity, access to needed information, resources and services, and meaningful participation in decision making are consistent with the pursuit of social justice (NASW, 1999). Some social work scholars and practitioners contend that CB interventions, or practice methods that focus on individual problems or deficits, are inconsistent with a social justice and/or a person-environment perspective. That is, practitioners using such interventions frequently identify and focus on changing individual deficits, thereby assisting individuals in adapting to, instead of changing, unfavorable or unjust environments that cause the problem.

Representing a strengths-based perspective, Cowger (1994) argued that assessment, evaluation, and intervention procedures that focus on individual problems or deficiencies inappropriately place the cause of the problem on the client. Such practices can reinforce the powerlessness that the individual is already experiencing, thus placing additional obstacles to the client's exercising personal and social power. In addition, such practices do not change the inequitable social and economic structures that are the cause of the problem. Cowger also agreed with Goroff (1983), who argued that social work practice itself is a political activity, and that attributing individual deficiencies as a cause of human problems is politically conservative and supports the status quo.

CB methods are problem focused, and they identify and track individual behavior before, during, and after intervention to determine if goals are met. However, during assessment and intervention, client strengths and adaptive behavior, not just deficiencies, are identified and frequently reinforced. In addition, diagnosing or labeling individuals is not the primary focus of CB assessment. Reinhard (2000) objected to labeling cognitive therapy "victim-blaming" because it locates the need to change within the individual. He argued that cognitive therapy can empower clients by teaching them that they frequently can choose how to respond to situations. Thus, clients do not have to be victims of their past or current situations. In addition, accepting responsibility for one's problem can be appropriate and even therapeutic for many problems, such as sexual abuse and addictions.

Other CB therapists and researchers (e.g., Goldfried & Castonguay, 1993) acknowledge that assisting clients with a history of frequent invalidating reactions from others in changing their own behavior can send the message that the clients are indeed deficient. Goldfried and Castonguay suggest that establishing a therapeutic relationship based on unconditional regard prior to intervention might avoid such a reaction. CB interventions then can assist clients in perceiving that they do have choices, and they do not have to accept others' definitions of themselves. Feminist scholars also suggest that victim blaming can be avoided by CB practitioners validating clients' experiences and interpreting their problems as the result of adapting to negative situations, not as pathology (Hurst & Genest, 1995). Finally, empowerment and feminist scholars frequently distinguish between the inappropriateness of accepting responsibility for the cause of the problem and the appropriateness of accepting responsibility for attempting to change the problem, which frequently involves learning new knowledge and skills (Gutiérrez, 1990; Gutiérrez & Ortega, 1991; Hurst & Genest, 1995; Lee, 1996; Lewis, 1994; Wolfe, 1995).

As some empowerment and feminist scholars advocate, and as this book suggests, assisting vulnerable populations in gaining knowledge (e.g., about their legal rights and political processes) and in learning skills (e.g., self-advocacy, job seeking, interpersonal, political) can result in their making informed decisions, achieving personal goals, and influencing the macro decisions and practices that affect their lives. Balcazar's (1993) observation concerning traditional community organizing strategies, such as those used and advocated by Alinsky (1971) and Kahn (1970), also is applicable to interventions described in this book. The successes achieved by these well-known organizers appeared to be the result of their own skills, abilities, and personalities. Because they failed to use a systematic method to train community members in the skills for continuing their work after withdrawing, community members alone rarely were able to continue the activities.

Learning and using relevant skills to attain personal or group goals after professionals withdraw are essential to empowerment.

Despite the previous arguments that CB methods are not necessarily in conflict with social justice values, other scholars have presented contrasting views. Social work researchers (Gorey, Thyer, & Pawluck, 1998) contrasted "personal" social work methods (including CB interventions), which assist clients in adapting to their environments by emphasizing the need for individuals to change, with "systemic-structural" or more "progressive" social work interventions (e.g., feminist and person-in-environment approaches), which target the environment. Other social work scholars (Berlin, 2002; Wodarski & Horme, 1981), as well as feminist and Marxist scholars (Hunter & Kelso, 1985; Kantrowitz & Ballou, 1992; Ulman, 1995), also have observed that the goal of most CB interventions is to assist clients in adapting to current environments, leaving untouched the socio-political environments that are the source of many problems. CB interventions frequently are used to change covert behavior (e.g., using exposure therapy to decrease fear of public speaking and cognitive restructuring to decrease depression) and overt behavior (e.g., using child management training to increase child compliance). Even when the environment is changed, for example, when parents are taught to prompt their children to obey, then reinforcing the children when they comply, the goal still is for the client to adapt to social norms or to cope with situations more effectively within certain social contexts.

Of course, goals related to improved adaptation and coping can be appropriate and consistent with social work values and the goals of clients, significant others, and society. This is particularly the case for illegal and harmful behavior and for situations that cannot be changed (e.g., a family death or terminal illness), that cannot reasonably be expected to conform to the unique problems of each client (e.g., giving public testimony for an individual who suffers from extreme anxiety), or that involve the actions of others over whom clients have little or no control (e.g., being rejected because of an individual characteristic, such as a disability). In many cases, especially for vulnerable populations who frequently lack social and economic resources, face discrimination and denial of their legal rights, and have constrained opportunities to set and achieve personal goals and to influence macro decision making, establishing other or additional intervention goals is appropriate.

As Berlin (1980) noted almost three decades ago, and summaries of other behavioral applications demonstrate (e.g., Fawcett et al., 1984, 1994; Mattaini, 1993; Thyer, Himle, & Santa, 1986), the fact that CB interventions have been used most frequently to assist clients in adapting to current sociopolitical environments does not mean that the interventions must be limited to these types of goals. As the many examples in this book demonstrate, CB interventions are not necessarily politically conservative or inconsistent with a social justice or empowerment perspective. Social workers and other professionals can use CB interventions to assist clients, especially vulnerable clients, in achieving other types of goals. Goals include accessing and increasing social and economic resources; enhancing self-determination by increasing personal control and input into decision making, increasing choice making, and securing legal and personal rights; and influencing the macro decisions that affect the lives of vulnerable groups.

CB models of practice are value laden, as are all practice models and approaches. However, scholars, particularly feminists (e.g., Kantrowitz & Ballou, 1992; Van Den Bergh, 2002), have critiqued CB approaches and their underlying theories because they are not explicit regarding the practitioner's or societal values that are embedded in defining when a problem exists and in selecting the problem, intervention, and goals. Even though the problem and assessment and intervention procedures are precisely defined in CB applications, because of the social power differential between practitioners and clients, this transparency does not prevent societal and practitioner values from unduly influencing the treatment process (Leslie, 1997). Such undue influence is particularly applicable to vulnerable populations. For example, using aversive techniques to change a client's sexual orientation. Feminists (e.g., Fodor, 1988) also have pointed out that given the instructional nature of CB therapies, practitioners are in a powerful position (e.g., in using cognitive restructuring) to impose their values and worldviews on clients. But imposing personal values and views on clients is a risk regardless of practitioners' theoretical orientation or chosen methods. Indeed, as Hurst and Genest (1995) cautioned, feminist practitioners must themselves be careful not to impose their views on women who choose traditional goals in therapy.

Contemporary CB therapists and researchers recognize that using rigorous research methods, good intentions and motives, and transparency of process cannot answer the value-laden questions inherent in clinical applications and social policy decisions (Evans, 1997; Peterson, 1997). Applying CB strategies to assist any client, particularly the vulnerable populations identified in this book, involves the perspectives and values of the clients, significant others, society, and professionals. A further examination of values follows.

Do Cognitive-Behavioral Methods Lack Social Relevance?

Feminist scholars have critiqued CB assessments, interventions, and outcome measures and the traditional scientific methods used to determine treatment effectiveness because they reduce complex human processes to narrowly defined behaviors that can be observed and measured (Kantrowitz & Ballou, 1992; Van Den Bergh, 2002). Feminist scholars further argue that those practices fail to consider the interpersonal sociocultural context in which behaviors are performed and individual differences as a result of gender, sexual orientation, culture, race/ethnicity, socioeconomic class, developmental status, and personal experiences. Similar views have been shared by CB researchers and practitioners, some of whom also are feminists (Casas, 1988; Delamater & McNarma, 1986; Iwamasa, 1997; Mathur & Rutherford, 1996; McNair, 1996; Norman, 1996; Olmeda & Kauffman, 2003; Purcell, Campos, & Perilla, 1996). Two main strengths of CB approaches partially address these criticisms. First, the treatment procedures are grounded in theory that should have application across populations. Second, CB therapies are based on a functional analysis in which the practitioner identifies the relationship between a presenting problem and events in the individual's sociocultural environment (Hansen, Zamboanga, & Sedlar, 2000).

Based on studies of applications of CB methods (Clarke, Dunlap, & Stichter, 2002; Van Acker, Boreson, Gable, & Potterton, 2005), and as the interventions described in this book demonstrate, individual functional assessments, unfortunately, are infrequently completed and standardized interventions are commonly used. Although precise definitions of behaviors, goals, and assessment and intervention procedures can contribute to an accurate assessment, evaluation, and replication of the results, scholars also acknowledge problems with such procedures. Failing to assess and to incorporate factors such as cultural influences, past experiences, and socioeconomic contexts can affect treatment in at least three main ways. First, such factors might influence the acceptability of CB methods. The explanation of the cause of the problem and the assessment and intervention procedures might not be congruent with clients' worldviews, their life experiences (e.g., poverty, discrimination, rejection), and their current situation.

Second, when identifying a behavior or skill for change, particular sociocultural contexts and individual characteristics define what is considered a skill deficit or a functional skill. Third, intervention or instructional materials might be inconsistent with the cultural or socioeconomic context in which the skills or behaviors are to be performed. In such circumstances, the behaviors might meet with unexpected adverse consequences. This is particularly the case for vulnerable populations, many of whom lack economic and social power and are dependent on others for their care. For example, teaching assertiveness or self-advocacy skills might elicit unfavorable evaluations from others, threaten or damage interpersonal relationships, or risk other social or economic benefits.

CB researchers frequently refer to the relevance of the identified behavior or skill, assessment and intervention procedures, and intervention goals and results as issues of social validity. Three decades ago, Wolf (1978) acknowledged that behavioral therapists and researchers cannot simply assume that their behaviors targeted for change, intervention procedures, and intervention goals and results are important and socially appropriate. Since social importance and appropriateness are subjective value judgments, such judgments must be made by clients, caregivers, and other individuals involved in or affected by the intervention process. Wolf and others (Baer, Wolf, & Risley, 1987; Foster & Mash, 1999; Kennedy, 2002; Meyer & Evans, 1993) have articulated five main areas in which CB procedures must demonstrate social validity.

First, the social significance of the intervention goal must be determined. That is, the goal must be important, desirable, acceptable, and viable from the perspective of the client and others involved in or affected by the intervention. Second, the effects or results of the intervention (including both negative and positive ones) must be satisfactory. That is, the extent of change must be meaningful, relevant, or sufficient for clients and significant others to conclude that a difference has been made in an important aspect of clients' lives. Third, the intervention procedures must be socially appropriate. That is, the treatment procedures must be acceptable and feasible to those involved in the intervention process. This includes taking into account culture and values, costs, special resources and training, ease of administration, and compliance with the intervention procedures. More recently some researchers have argued that two additional areas that have caused concern among CB practitioners and researchers are related to or are important components of socially relevant interventions (Hansen et al., 2000; Kennedy, 2002; Meyer & Evans, 1993). These two areas are maintaining intervention gains after formal intervention and transferring the gains to other settings, contexts, materials, and individuals different from the intervention conditions.

Baer et al. (1987) challenged researchers and practitioners to develop methods for consumers of CB therapies to provide feedback after intervention, as well as for actively involving consumers in program development, thus increasing the chance that the interventions will be accepted and will achieve their goals. As the evaluations of the CB interventions discussed in the next ten chapters demonstrate, many methods for evaluating the social validity of intervention goals, results, and procedures have departed from traditional scientific methods. Instead, they rely more on subjective and qualitative evaluations. Evaluations of the interventions examined in this book provide multiple examples of using such methods with clients, caregivers, family members, educators, peers, and others involved in the intervention process before, during, and after intervention. A variety of strategies for maintaining and transferring intervention gains also are discussed in subsequent chapters of this book.

Summary

CB applications are consistent with empowerment and social work practice in important ways. Practitioners establish a collaborative relationship with clients in which clients are active participants in selecting problems, goals, interventions, and evaluation procedures. The assessment and intervention processes are individualized, transparent, and informed by research and emphasize the individual, environmental processes, and client strengths. Finally, CB interventions can be used to assist vulnerable individuals and groups in attaining goals consistent with social justice and empowerment perspectives. Many such applications are demonstrated in the next ten chapters.

This is not to say that CB methods cannot or have not been misused or applied inappropriately. As is the case with other types of interventions, CB strategies have been used to control behavior unnecessarily, constrain freedom, and assist individuals in adapting to adverse social and economic environments. Practitioners and researchers sometimes have ignored individual characteristics and the context in which behaviors are performed, and they simply have made assumptions regarding the social significance of their goals, interventions, and treatment results. Some of the interventions described in this book exemplify some of the latter problems. However, in this book a distinction is made between how CB methods have sometimes been used and how they *can* be used. As this book demonstrates, socially relevant CB interventions can be developed and can assist vulnerable clients in achieving goals that are consistent with an empowerment perspective and with social work values.

In addition to issues of social validity, which are addressed in the subsequent chapters of this book, two aspects of CB methods are considered that may be thought to contradict some definitions of empowerment. First, practitioners serve in the role of "expert" in the sense that they offer and use interventions that have empirical support. Second, many of the interventions are directive and didactic in nature. If, however, the interventions are explained to clients (and to others involved in the interventions) in enough detail for them to make informed decisions, and they choose the interventions to meet their own goals, there is no inconsistency between the use of the interventions and an empowerment perspective. Indeed, only when practitioners explain and provide intervention options to individuals and groups from which they can choose to meet their goals is empowerment possible. Presuming to know what is best for clients based on a particular ideology or philosophy, then declining to offer clients certain types of interventions that conflict with that ideology or philosophy (e.g., interventions that are based on research, relatively directive, or problem focused) is the antithesis of empowerment. As Cowger (1994) argued, social work practice based on empowerment assumes that individuals must have available options and must make their own choices.

OVERVIEW OF PARTS II THROUGH V

The next four parts of this book describe and critically review CB interventions that assist vulnerable populations in achieving four main types of goals consistent with an empowerment perspective. In part II, the goals are related to accessing and increasing social resources. The target goals include increasing the number and quality of social interactions; increasing leisure, recreational, and other community activity; and recruiting assistance to enhance social support, meet medical and emergency needs, perform routine activities, and attain individually defined goals. In part III, empowerment goals are related to increasing economic resources. The specific outcomes include obtaining employment by learning job-seeking skills; maintaining and advancing in employment by increasing on-the-job productivity, work quality, and related social skills; and acquiring economic assistance from members of social support networks, social benefits programs, and other community sources.

In part IV, empowerment goals are related to increasing self-determination. More specifically, the outcomes include enhancing personal control and input into decision making in academic, home, and work settings; increasing choice making in daily activities and longer-term decisions; and securing legal and personal rights. The final intervention chapter in part V focuses on CB interventions that assist vulnerable populations in influencing macro decision making and the community and organizational practices that affect their lives.

Finally, chapter 14 in part V reviews the effectiveness of the CB applications discussed in the previous ten chapters. This chapter returns to a discussion of the consistency between CB methods and empowerment, including issues of personal freedom and control, social justice, and social validity. Suggestions for practitioners and recommended directions are provided for future research on CB interventions that empower vulnerable populations.

ADDITIONAL READINGS AND RESOURCES

Balcazar, F. E. (1993). Intervention research and the empowerment of African-American men. *Journal of Men's Studies, 1*, 277–286.

Balcazar, F. E., Keys, C. B., & Suarez-Balcazar, Y. (2001). Empowering Latinos with disabilities to address issues of independent living and disability rights: A capacity-building approach. *Journal of Prevention & Intervention in the Community, 21*, 53–70.

Corrigan, P. W. (1997). Behavior therapy empowers persons with severe mental illness. *Behavior Modification, 21*, 45–61.

Dickerson, F. B. (1998). Strategies that foster empowerment. *Cognitive and Behavioral Practice, 5,* 255–275.

Fawcett, S. B., Seekins, T., Wang, P. L., Muiu, C., & Suarez de Balcazar, Y. (1984). Creating and using social technologies for community empowerment. *Prevention in Human Services, 3,* 145–171.

Hess, R. E., Clapper, C. R., Hoekstra, K., & Gibison, F. P., Jr. (2001). Empowerment effects of teaching leadership skills to adults with a severe mental illness and their families. *Psychiatric Rehabilitation Journal, 24,* 257–265.

Zirpoli, T. J., Hancox, D., Wieck, C., & Skarnulis, E. R. (1989). Partners in policymaking: Empowering people. *Journal of the Association for Persons with Severe Handicaps, 14,* 163–167.

PART

TWO

Accessing and Increasing Social Resources

4 Enhancing Social Interactions

The NASW (1999) Code of Ethics recognizes the importance of human relationships as a basic social work value. Establishing and strengthening relationships among individuals and groups is considered central to the well-being of all individuals. Unfortunately, vulnerable populations often are unsuccessful in developing interpersonal relationships, as well as in accessing other types of social resources in residential, school, work, and other community settings. The CB interventions described in the three chapters of part II assist vulnerable populations in achieving three main goals related to enhancing social resources. They include initiating and engaging in social interactions, including establishing meaningful relationships, participating in leisure and recreational activity, and recruiting assistance to perform routine activities and to enhance personal well-being. The interventions empower vulnerable populations by assisting them in accessing and increasing social resources in the settings in which they learn, work, and engage in daily activity.

This chapter focuses on CB strategies that increase the number and quality of social interactions of children, youths, and adults with a variety of disabilities (i.e., physical, sensory, learning/developmental, emotional/behavioral, and severe mental illness), the elderly, and sexual minorities. The chapter begins by briefly discussing the importance of acquiring basic communication and other social skills. Examples of CB interventions that enhance the social interactions of vulnerable children and youths are described first, followed by CB interventions for vulnerable adults. The chapter concludes with a closer examination of the interventions, including their effectiveness and additional applications, as well as issues of personal freedom, control, and social justice, and social validity.

ACQUIRING BASIC COMMUNICATION AND OTHER SOCIAL SKILLS

The ability to communicate effectively is essential to empowerment and to a meaningful life. Individuals who are skilled in communicating with others are more likely to obtain relevant information, make and convey their choices and desires to other persons, engage in social interactions, develop and maintain meaningful interpersonal, romantic, and sexual relationships, and attain personal goals (Chadsey-Rusch, Drasgow, Reinoehl, Halle, & Collet-Klingenberg, 1993; Schloss & Wood, 1990). Acquiring basic communication skills also can be the first step for noncommunicative clients to engage in more meaningful social interactions and relationships (Wong & Woolsey, 1989). Individuals who lack the appropriate social skills to initiate and maintain social interactions are less likely to establish reinforcing interpersonal relationships. Instead, their inappropriate attempts to communicate will frequently face rejection, resulting in fewer subsequent attempts to initiate social interactions and social isolation (Kelly, Urey, & Patterson, 1980).

Multiple studies have evaluated CB interventions that assist vulnerable populations in increasing basic verbal and nonverbal conversational, dating, and related social skills. The strategies include SST and PST for children and adolescents with hearing impairments (Van Hasselt, Hersen, Kazdin, Simon, & Mastanuono, 1983), mental retardation (Downing, 1987), and multiple disabilities (Taras, Matson, & Leary, 1988); for adults with mental retardation (Hall, Schlesinger, & Dineen, 1997; Valenti-Hein, Yarnold, & Mueser, 1994) and severe mental illness (Wong & Woolsey, 1989); and for the elderly (Berger, 1981). Evaluations of these SST and PST interventions suggest that they are generally effective in increasing a variety of conversational and other social skills, as measured by role plays, ratings of conversational ability, and observations in treatment settings. Although practitioners might find these interventions useful, the evaluations failed to determine whether improvements in conversational and other social skills resulted in participants' increasing their social resources (e.g., initiating and sustaining conversations and forming relationships). If such outcomes were measured, they were assessed only in treatment settings or in other artificial environments. The definition of empowerment guiding the selection of interventions presented in this book assumes that research must provide some evidence that the interventions result in more than skill development. That is, vulnerable individuals must use the acquired skills to access some type of social resource in the environments in which they work, play, learn, and engage in routine activity. This and the next two chapters focus on interventions for which research has provided such evidence.

INTERVENTIONS FOR VULNERABLE CHILDREN AND YOUTHS

Educators, policy makers, and helping professionals often assume that placing children and youths with disabilities into integrated classrooms, competitive work sites, and other community settings will result in increased social interactions with and acceptance by their able-bodied peers. Unfortunately these outcomes have not always been realized. Instead, children and youths with disabilities are frequently rejected and avoided and experience loneliness and few positive social interactions with their able-bodied peers (Gresham, Sugai, & Horner, 2001; Hepler, 1997; King et al., 1997; Storey & Garff, 1999).

The inability of many children and youths with disabilities to access social resources and to socially integrate into school, work, and other community settings occurs for many reasons. Physical, cognitive, and neurocognitive limitations and psychiatric symptoms can deter these children and adolescents from learning and exhibiting what able-bodied peers and others consider to be appropriate social behavior. When children and adolescents with disabilities engage in inappropriate or unresponsive social behavior, the interpersonal interactions can be unrewarding for their able-bodied peers. Children and youths with disabilities also can have limited opportunities to use acquired social skills with their nondisabled peers, or they lack access to the specialized equipment or necessary communication adaptations to communicate effectively. Negative and prejudicial attitudes of others, and lack of knowledge about the special problems and communicative behaviors of children and youths with disabilities, also can result in few social interactions between them and their able-bodied peers (Hepler, 1997; King et al., 1997).

Because of stigmatization of minority sexual orientation, lesbian, gay, and bisexual (LGB) youths frequently experience multiple stressors, low levels of social support, and difficulties establishing dating and other relationships (Hart & Heimberg, 2001). They also have limited opportunities for meeting and interacting with one another in casual social settings. This social isolation, in turn, can result in LGB youths having few opportunities to observe social and personal interactions of other sexual minorities and to practice the appropriate social skills needed to establish and maintain personal relationships (Safren, Hollander, Hart, & Heimberg, 2001; St. Lawrence, Bradlyn, & Kelly, 1983).

This section examines CB interventions that assist children and youths with physical disabilities, sensory impairments, developmental and learning problems (i.e., learning disabilities, mental retardation, and autism), behavioral/emotional disorders, and multiple disabilities in increasing the quality and frequency of their social interactions. An example of a CB intervention that assists LGB youths in enhancing their social interactions also is described. These interventions address many of the factors that deter children and youths with disabilities and LGB youths from increasing and accessing social resources.

Children and Youths with Physical Disabilities and Sensory Impairments

Intervention frequently is necessary to assist children and youths with physical disabilities and sensory impairments in enhancing social interactions.

The physical limitations of children and adolescents with a physical disability can restrict their social activity with others. Such restrictions likely lead to fewer opportunities to learn and practice appropriate social skills and to form interpersonal relationships. Children and youths with sensory impairments also are at a social disadvantage. They are less likely to gain knowledge (e.g., on fashionable clothing or current topics of conversations) that others acquire visually or through hearing, or to learn appropriate social skills by observing and listening to appropriate models (Erin, Dignan, & Brown, 1991). Children and youths with hearing impairments also frequently have difficulties communicating orally with others. These problems place children and youths with physical disabilities and sensory impairments at risk of engaging in few social interactions and establishing few meaningful relationships with peers. These observations are consistent with descriptions of the participants involved in the interventions presented in this section. The children and adolescents were described as unpopular, socially withdrawn, and displaying few age-appropriate social skills.

The three treatment packages discussed now use various combinations of CB interventions to enhance the social interactions of children and youths with physical disabilities and hearing impairments. The programs apply SST strategies (i.e., instruction, modeling, prompting, practice, reinforcement, and feedback) in unique ways. Other interventions, such as PST, additional self-management strategies, and reinforcement, also are used. All of the interventions were evaluated using multiple-baseline designs.

Physical disabilities. "Joining in" is a group SST intervention designed to increase the social resources of 8- to 15-year-old students with physical disabilities, such as cerebral palsy and spina bifida (King et al., 1997). The group intervention targets five basic social skills chosen from a survey of teachers and therapists. The skills include interpersonal problem solving, verbal and nonverbal communication, initiating interactions with peers, conversational skills, and coping with difficult others.

The group facilitator begins the intervention by involving group members in defining the components that constitute each skill and initiating discussions on specific questions, for example, "What are the social and personal advantages of using problem solving?" and "What are the common difficulties in applying problem solving in real life and how do we cope with them?" The group members then watch videos in which children with disabilities model the skills as they interact with able-bodied peers both appropriately and inappropriately. Appropriate interactions are followed by a positive consequence, such as peer approval, while inappropriate interactions are followed by a negative consequence, such as peer rejection. The group facilitator then uses other SST techniques to teach the skills that group members observe in the videos. Because individuals can never control the reactions of others, a "reality check" is incorporated into the intervention. The group facilitator cautions the group members that even when they perform the skills appropriately they cannot always expect positive consequences. This warning is followed by presentation and discussion of examples of these types of situations, such as experiencing rejection. Group members also are given homework assignments, referred to as "missions," which involve observing and evaluating the interactions of others, practicing the social skills, and evaluating their own performance.

Eleven students participated in the evaluation of joining in. Baseline self-report measures of self-worth, social acceptance, close friend and classmate support, loneliness, and dissatisfaction with their relationships were compared with measures taken after intervention and six months later. Of the five measures, only the students' reports of social acceptance improved after intervention, but that improvement was not maintained at the six-month follow-up. However, self-reports of loneliness and dissatisfaction with relationships decreased at follow-up. The decrease in loneliness was considered to be socially relevant, as it was similar to the mean in a normative sample of children with no disabilities.

Hearing impairments. The first of the two CB interventions for children and youths with hearing impairments discussed here is designed to increase the social interactions of preschool children with moderate to severe hearing impairments who primarily communicate orally (Ducharme & Holborn, 1997). The skills targeted for change, which were selected through a survey of teachers and parents, include play organizing (i.e., the child initiates or maintains a play activity), sharing or cooperating, and assisting another child in response to a request or through an offer to help (e.g., "Can I hold the mirror for you?"). Socially skilled peers, chosen as "play partners," also are involved in the intervention.

The practitioner begins by using SST to explicitly teach the skills, after which the skills are taught within the context of a play activity. During the sessions, the practitioner sets out play materials then prompts the child to select an activity and ask a play partner to play. If the child complies, the practitioner praises the child. If the child is not successful in obtaining a play partner, the practitioner provides a second prompt. If the child continues to be unsuccessful, the practitioner takes the child to one of the play partners, models how to organize play (e.g., if face painting was chosen, the practitioner might say "I want you to make me a clown, put red on my nose"), and instructs the child to imitate what he or she observed. If the play partner declines to play, the practitioner prompts the child to repeat the request. If the play partner once again declines, the practitioner coaches the play partner to play with the child. The practitioner then uses the same techniques to teach the children to share or cooperate and to assist each other.

The children participating in the evaluation (N = 5) exhibited increased and continuous social interactions in the training setting after intervention. Only after generalization strategies were implemented, which included multiple instructors, peers, and play activities, and gradually withdrawing prompts and praise, did the intervention gains transfer to a second classroom setting (containing other peers, teachers, and play materials) without additional prompting and reinforcement. After intervention, teachers and parents continued to support the selected skills and the continued use of the intervention. Their ratings of the effectiveness of the intervention and transfer of the skills to natural settings also were favorable. Problems included the instructional time involved and the structured training that conflicted with some teachers' philosophy of "entirely child-directed play."

This intervention, which was developed for adolescents residing in a residential facility for the hearing impaired, incorporates self-management strategies into a group SST program (Rasing, Coninx, Duker, & Van den Hurk, 1994). The behaviors targeted for intervention, and appropriate and inappropriate examples of those behaviors, were selected by teachers and residential staff. The target skills include initiating interactions (e.g., calling a hearing person's name once and tapping a hearing or deaf person on the arm once or twice), turn waiting, staying on the subject, communicating orally, and using appropriate sentences.

The group facilitator begins the intervention by prompting the adolescents to demonstrate appropriate and inappropriate instances of the identified behaviors (which are posted on the wall and floor) and to discuss the rationale for performing the appropriate behaviors. The group facilitator teaches a self-management strategy (which also is posted on the wall and floor) by asking the adolescents to read a script of a situation in which the identified behavior has to occur. Consistent with PST, the group facilitator prompts the adolescents to analyze and discuss the situation using the following questions.

What is the problem?
How can I handle it?
What are the consequences of the responses for the previous question?
How should I respond to it?
Did I choose a correct response? (Rasing et al., 1994, p. 418)

After the adolescents role play their responses to the fourth question on how to respond, the group discusses the appropriateness of the responses then selects the most appropriate response. The group facilitator individualizes the intervention by asking group members to discuss their own experiences related to the target skill. To facilitate transfer of the skills to natural settings, teachers and staff members use verbal prompts (which are eventually faded) to remind the adolescents to carry out the self-management procedure. Adolescents also monitor their own target behaviors, record their own performance, and provide themselves with their earned tokens and backup reinforcers.

The intervention was evaluated on two groups of four adolescents. For the group of adolescents with a hearing impairment and language disability, improved social interactions were observed in the classroom and during dinner in the residential facility after intervention. Gains were maintained nineteen to thirty-four weeks after the program was discontinued. Interventions for the group of adolescents with hearing impairments and severe language disabilities were identical, except that "finger spelling" was used as a form of communication. Improvement in the interaction skills of those adolescents was not considered to be clinically significant.

Children and Youths with Learning, Cognitive, and Developmental Disabilities

CB strategies designed to enhance the social interactions of children and youths diagnosed with learning disabilities (LD), mental retardation/developmental delay, and autism are discussed now. Children and youths with LD have neurological problems that can negatively affect auditory processing, attention, memory, spacial and visual perception, and motor and verbal skills, all of which can affect social functioning. Following conversations and remembering group norms, for example, would be more difficult for children and adolescents with a short-term memory problem. Failing to observe or misreading important cues in assessing social situations also can result in inappropriate social behavior (Hepler, 1997).

Children and youths with mental retardation or developmental delays have cognitive and language limitations, frequently resulting in difficulties with learning social skills, communicating, and establishing interpersonal relationships (Hall, Dineen, Schlesinger, & Stanton, 2000). Individuals with autism exhibit a variety of behaviors (e.g., disinterest in and unresponsiveness to others, echolalia, insistence on sameness, focusing on irrelevant objects or topics) that interfere with developing and using adequate social skills (Pollard, 1998).

Having few social skills can result in peer rejection, social isolation, and developing few meaningful social relationships. The descriptions of the vulnerable children and youths who participated in the evaluations of the interventions discussed in this section reflect these problems. Participants had limited social skills, rarely or inappropriately interacted with others, established no friendships with their nondisabled peers, and experienced little or no social integration into work, school, and community settings, even when opportunities for social integration were available.

Ten CB programs that enhance the social interactions of children and youths with learning and developmental problems are discussed. The various applications of SST incorporate games, videos, and affection activities. PST, other self-management strategies, homework assignments, and a variety of prompting and reinforcement interventions also are common. Seven of the programs involve able-bodied peers. In one intervention, peers are sensitized to the special behaviors and communication styles of the children with disabilities. Peers serve as models, partners, and members of support networks. Peer involvement appears to facilitate changes in the attitudes of able-bodied children and adolescents toward, and can increase their interactions with, children and youths with learning and developmental problems. With one exception (Hepler, 1997), the interventions were evaluated using multiple-baseline designs.

Learning disabilities. Hepler (1997) developed a group CB program to increase the social interactions and friendships between fifth graders with LD and their peers with no learning disability (NLD). The program focuses on five social skills: initiating conversations, maintaining conversations, entering an ongoing activity, including others, and responding appropriately to negative comments. The small groups (4 to 5 members) include students with LD and students with NLD who are well liked by their peers. After introducing a social situation focusing on one of the social skills, the group facilitator leads the students through the problem-solving process to identify the most effective responses. Modeling and role playing are used to teach the identified social skills. During the week, the students complete written homework assignments, which include a checklist of the specific steps in various social interactions. The following week, the group facilitator discusses the homework assignments with group members, as well as any problems the students experienced. To increase motivation and participation in the program, students receive tokens for participating in the group and completing homework assignments. Tokens are pooled for a group pizza party (SST manual providing details of each session is available from the author).

To assess the effectiveness of the program, four classrooms were randomly assigned to one of five small groups or to a control group (N = 41). Peer sociometric ratings (indicating how much each student liked playing with other students) of the students with LD in the treatment group increased after intervention; ratings for the students with LD in the control group declined. Although the sociometric ratings of the children with LD in the treatment group decreased slightly by the end of the school year, they were still above baseline levels. The majority of the participating students reported enjoying the program, making new friends, and experiencing more positive feelings about classmates. Evaluations of participating teachers were very positive. Observations of free play also indicated that students with LD in the treatment group were more integrated with their peers with NLD compared with students in the control group.

Mental retardation/developmental delays. The two behavioral treatment packages discussed here assist children with mental retardation or developmental delays in becoming more socially integrated into their school settings. Peers participate in both sets of interventions. The first, the "buddy skills-training program," is designed to increase social interactions and friendships between children with developmental delays and their peers developing within normal ranges in integrated preschools (English, Goldstein, Shafer, & Kaczmarek, 1997). The intervention for the peers has two major components. First, the practitioner shows and discusses videotapes that sensitize the peers to the types of attention-getting and requesting behaviors that children with developmental delays might use to communicate. Second, the practitioner uses a training sequence, referred to as "STAY-PLAY-TALK," in which three buddy strategies are instructed, modeled, and practiced. The strategies are as follows.

1 Stay close to an assigned child when verbally reminded.
2 Say the child's name, gain attention, and suggest a play activity or talk about the current activity.
3 Stay close and continue to play and talk with the child.

During sessions involving the child with a developmental delay and his or her peer, the practitioner uses similar interventions (instruction, modeling, and practice) to teach the child to "stay and play" with the peer buddy. Peers are then assigned to buddy days on a rotating basis and instructed to stay with their assigned child and to use the learned strategies. Later in the program, the practitioner tells each buddy pair to use their buddy strategies at any time during the day. Stickers, which are later faded, and praise by teachers and classroom aids serve as reinforcers.

The evaluation suggested that the increase in the number of social interactions directed by the four peer buddies and other classmates to the five preschoolers with developmental delays occurred as a result of the program. The children with developmental delays also increased their social interactions directed to their classmates. After intervention, individuals working in early childhood intervention rated improvements in the social and communicative interactions between the children with developmental delays and their peers. However, the children's sociometric rankings changed little after intervention, suggesting that the intervention did not enhance friendship development.

This second intervention designed for children with mental retardation involves a peer trainer and incorporates children's games into the procedures (McMahon, Wacker, Sasso, Berg, & Newton, 1996). The goals of the intervention are to increase the frequency and type of interactions between grade-school students with mild to moderate mental retardation and their able-bodied peers within an integrated public school. Sessions are conducted with a student and a peer. During the sessions, the practitioner instructs the peer to teach the student seven game-playing skills while playing a board game (e.g., *Candyland* and *Trouble*). The skills are asking the peer to play, waiting for a response, setting up the game with the peer, deciding who will move first, appropriately taking turns, deciding when the game is over, and jointly putting the game away. The practitioner instructs the peer to prompt, praise, and correct the student's play behaviors. As the student's skills improve, the practitioner instructs the peer to fade the feedback.

All four students with mental retardation who participated in the evaluation learned the game-playing skills and increased overall frequencies of their interactions with their peers. After the intervention was terminated, interactions between three of the pairs were primarily social, and the skills generalized to a play situation in which no one instructed the pair to play. When a group of five students (two of the students with mental retardation and three of the peers) played freely in an after-school day-care room, the interactions between the students with developmental delays and their able-bodied peers were less consistent.

Autism. Perhaps because of the pervasive communication and social interaction problems characteristic of children and youths diagnosed with autism, numerous studies evaluating primarily behavioral techniques have been conducted with this population. Seven multicomponent CB interventions are discussed here, four of which involve peers in the intervention procedures.

The first of the programs involves group "affection activities" designed to increase the social interactions of young children with autism in an integrated early childhood educational setting (McEvoy et al., 1988). The intervention involves bringing the children with autism into a kindergarten classroom attended by six peer volunteers and the regular classroom children, none of whom have a disability. In a corner of the classroom, but in view of all the children, each child with autism separately joins the six peers. Using SST techniques, the classroom instructor, who is trained in the procedures, teaches the children affection activities to use while singing various children's songs. For example, when the children sing the song "You're Happy and You Know It," they are asked to "hug your friend," "give your neighbor a high-five," or "pat your friend on the back." The three children with autism who participated in the intervention increased their reciprocal verbal and nonverbal peer interactions after affection activities were taught. The social interactions transferred to free play situations, which included the children with autism and all of the classroom children.

Video modeling also can assist high functioning children with autism in initiating and engaging others in conversation (Charlop & Milstein, 1989). In the first step of the intervention, the practitioner develops five scripted conversations on the topic of the child's preferred toys. Videotapes are then created depicting two familiar adults engaging in the conversations while holding the preferred toys. After viewing a video three times, the practitioner prompts the child to engage in a similar conversation. Praise is given for appropriate responses, and the steps are repeated until the child masters each conversation. After intervention, all three boys (ages 6 and 7 years) participating in the evaluation met the criteria established for appropriately engaging in the conversations. The conversational skills generalized to untrained topics of conversation, and to other materials, individuals, and natural settings, including the home. The skills were maintained 15 months later. Parents of children without disabilities who rated tapes of the participants' conversations before and after intervention also observed positive changes in the children's conversations. For example, the speech sounded natural and other children showed an interest in the conversation.

Self-management procedures are incorporated into this intervention, which can be implemented in a clinical setting, to improve the social responsiveness of children diagnosed with autism (Koegel, Koegel, Hurley, & Frea, 1992). The self-management training begins with the clinician generating questions for the child based on his or her interests and cognitive abilities, for example, "Who is your best friend?" and "What is your favorite TV program?" The clinician then uses the questions and modeling to teach the child to discriminate between a correct and incorrect response and to record an appropriate response on a wrist counter (an inexpensive golf counter). The child then practices making appropriate responses and the self-recording procedures. Prompting is used as needed, and small edible reinforcers are provided after appropriate responses. As the child acquires the skills, prompts are faded and reinforcers gradually thinned. When the child masters the self-management technique, the clinician informs the child that he or she can now earn points (which are traded for backup reinforcers) by responding appropriately to individuals in home, school, and community settings.

At the end of treatment, the four male children (6–11 years) involved in the evaluation appropriately responded to social situations 90–100% of the time in the clinic setting (35–61% at baseline). The treatment gains were maintained after formal intervention was discontinued. Performance levels in home and community settings, which were even lower at baseline, increased to similar levels. As assessed by informal observations, two of the four children increased their verbal initiations, and three of the children began to initiate conversations in natural environments without the wrist counter.

Researchers at the Princeton Child Development Institute, a private nonprofit educational and treatment program for autistic children, developed a behavioral procedure called script-fading to initiate and sustain conversations of 4- to 5-year-old (Krantz & McClannahan, 1998) and 10- to 15-year-old (Stevenson, Krantz, & McClannahan, 2000) children and youths with autism. Both evaluations demonstrated increases in the participants' initiating and sustaining conversations after intervention. A description of the unique intervention for young adolescents with autism who are unable to read (evaluated in the second study) follows.

The training materials include five social activities and twenty-five nonsocial activities. The nonsocial activities are represented by photographs of leisure (e.g., a puzzle) and academic (e.g., a worksheet) materials available in the training room (only 5 are available in any one session). The social activities are represented by five photographs of "Language Master Cards," which play previously recorded scripts of various statements or questions when placed in the "Language Master." The photographs prompt the youth to approach a familiar teacher and initiate an interaction. During the training, the instructor stands behind the youth and uses a graduated prompting strategy that provides only the amount of manual guidance needed to accomplish the following tasks.

1 Open an activity schedule book.
2 Select a photograph from a display board.
3 Mount the photograph on the relevant page.
4 Obtain the depicted materials.
5 Complete the activity, involving either approaching the teacher who has the Language Master and cards on her lap, running the card through the Language Master, and repeating the verbalization most recently played on the Language Master, or saying the words to engage in a nonsocial activity.
6 Return the materials to their original location.
7 Return to the schedule book and turn the page.

If the youth chooses to use the Language Master Cards and speaks to his or her teacher, the teacher appropriately responds. Eventually the instructor fades the scripts by deleting words and fades the pictures representing social activities by cutting off sections of the photographs of the Language Master cards.

The evaluation indicated that the script fading intervention increased the social interactions of the four male participants. The youths mastered the scripts, increased unscripted responses, and maintained the social skills for ten to ninety-two sessions (for more information on the Princeton Child Development Institute and CB resources for treating individuals with autism, refer to the "Additional Readings and Resources" at the end of this chapter).

The next two behavioral interventions involve peers and establish peer support within the school to enhance the social integration of students with autism. This first intervention, involving SST and a peer network strategy, is designed to increase the social interactions of moderate- to high-functioning elementary school students with autism (Kamps, Potucek, Lopez, Kravits, & Kemmerer, 1997). For each student, the practitioner sequentially applies an individualized peer network intervention that is appropriate to multiple naturally occurring school settings. Classroom, center/game, lunch, and recess are examples of such settings. Although the intervention varies to some degree by setting and student, it basically involves a group of two to five peers rotating as peer support group members. The practitioner uses SST to teach the peers relevant social skills and interaction strategies for the respective setting. For example, for recess the skills include turn taking, helping, giving compliments, and following game rules. The interaction strategies include prompting the students with autism to participate and praising the students after participating. During the sessions, the peers practice the skills with the students with autism, and the practitioner provides the peers with task and social scripts to use as prompts. A reinforcement system, such as star charts, is established for peer interactions. School staff also provide peers with intermittent prompts and praise them after interacting with the students with autism in the different settings.

After the peer network intervention, the duration of social interaction for all three students with autism (ages 6–8 years) involved in the study increased, and the improvements generalized for two of the students to nonintervention settings. More casual observations indicated that when interactions occurred in untrained settings, they were initiated by peers both involved and uninvolved in the intervention. The students with autism also were more responsive to the social initiations of all their peers.

This second peer support intervention, which includes multiple behavioral strategies, was developed to enhance the social interactions and interpersonal relationships of early adolescent students diagnosed with autism (Haring & Breen, 1992). In this intervention, four or five able-bodied students serve as members of each student's peer support network. The respective social network members meet once a week with the student and an adult facilitator. During the meetings, the facilitator encourages peer control and maximum input into the peer network intervention but prompts, supports, reinforces, and focuses the discussion when necessary. Themes routinely discussed and reinforced include normalizing interactions, building friendships rather than helping relationships, respecting the students' abilities, and peer ownership of the network. Behavioral strategies include the following.

1. Scheduling interactions between the peers and students; peers record and rate the appropriateness of the interactions
2. Discussing strategies for initiating contact with the students, such as identifying initiating topics of conversations and methods for establishing eye contact, and for including the students in larger group activities
3. Using SST to teach the students frequently used peer initiations
4. Developing strategies for the peers to facilitate students' responses, such as persistence and modeling appropriate responses

The evaluation of this social network intervention reported an increase in the number and quality of the social interactions between the two students with autism (age 13 years) and their able-bodied peers after intervention. Friendships also appeared to have developed between the students with autism and their peers as a result of the intervention, and treatment gains generalized to the community. For example, community social interactions with peers involved going to the beach, eating dinner at a friend's home, and shopping trips to the mall. One of the student's mothers reported that this was the first time same-age friends involved her child in community activities. This same student's peer network recruited five of their friends to provide him with a social network before leaving for high school the following academic year. Peers and students were highly satisfied with the intervention, and the majority of the peers described their relationships with the students as friendships. Other anecdotal evidence from peers, parents, and teachers also suggests that the intervention assisted the students with autism in becoming socially integrated into the school.

Peers without disabilities also are involved in this SST program designed to increase the social interactions during coffee breaks at the job sites of high school students with severe autism (Breen, Haring, Pitts-Conway, & Gaylord-Ross, 1989). The peers serve as "training co-workers" during training that is conducted in the students' job break rooms. The practitioner first provides the training co-workers with a script containing examples of responses to the students' conversation initiators (e.g., the student might say, "Hi, how are you?" and the co-worker might respond, "Fine," "Great," or "I'm doing OK.") and with examples of follow-up questions. The practitioner uses the script to train the co-workers to respond to the students but instructs them to respond naturally.

In the second part of training, which involves a co-worker and a student with autism, the practitioner uses a previously developed task analysis of a break time social sequence for each student. Examples of a student's tasks are leaving the work area, getting coffee, and initiating and maintaining a conversation with a co-worker. During the training, the practitioner verbally praises the student with autism if he or she independently conducts any of the relevant steps. If the student fails to appropriately conduct a step, the practitioner uses a sequence of prompts from the least to the most intrusive. An example follows.

Indirect verbal (e.g., "what do you do next?")
Direct verbal (e.g., "go make coffee")
Gestural (e.g., point to coffee)
Partial physical (e.g., guide hand to spoon)
Full physical (e.g., guide hand to spoon, place on spoon, and push fingers to grasp spoon)

As the student practices with the training co-worker, the practitioner uses both indirect (e.g., "What do you say") and direct (e.g., "Say, 'Want coffee?'") modeling to teach verbal social responses. As the student masters the skills, the prompts and praise are gradually withdrawn.

The four male students involved in the evaluation of the peer intervention learned to initiate and carry on conversations with the co-workers during intervention. For two of the students, the skills did not transfer to natural settings until they practiced the skills with additional co-workers. After intervention, two of the students made spontaneous social remarks, and when students initiated social interactions, the co-workers continued the interaction in the majority of cases.

Children and Youths with Behavioral/Emotional Disorders

Children and youths with emotional or behavioral disorders also are at risk of having few positive social interactions with their peers. Psychiatric symptoms and related behavior of these children and adolescents can interfere with their learning appropriate social skills, resulting in poor social functioning. Peers and community members frequently perceive the social behavior of these children and youths negatively, which can lead to rejection and social isolation in integrated educational, community, and work settings (Plienis et al., 1987).

The two CB programs discussed here were designed to be implemented in school settings. Despite being routinely integrated into regular classes, the students with emotional/behavioral disorders who participated in the evaluations of these interventions had few social skills, were socially isolated, and were ignored, teased, or called names by their peers. Both interventions use group SST techniques. The first intervention incorporates peers with no disabilities into "friendship circles" to enhance the social interactions and social integration of students with emotional/behavioral disorders into the school setting. The second intervention also uses PST. Both programs were evaluated using multiple-baseline designs.

In the first intervention, peers are included in friendship circles to enhance the social interactions between young adolescent students receiving special education services for an emotional/behavioral disorder and their nondisabled peers (Miller, Cooke, Test, & White, 2003). The friendship circles, which include four able-bodied peers and one student with an emotional/behavioral disorder, meet weekly. During the first session, the group facilitator uses some ice-breaking activities then engages the group in discussing the main responsibilities of friendship circle members. The responsibilities involve sitting together during lunch and practicing friendship behaviors during the week. The members name their circle and generate a written list of characteristics that define friendship, which are posted and referenced during future meeting. Finally, the members discuss situations in the past in which they have exhibited friendship behaviors. In subsequent meetings, the main activities include discussing strengths, problems, and suggestions related to interactions between the peers and the students with an emotional/behavioral disorder during the previous week. Friendship circle members role-play situations in which they, the group facilitator, or the general education teacher observed inappropriate social interactions. During role plays, the group members reenact the situations, demonstrating friendship behaviors. After playing a cooperative game, the group facilitator prompts the students to practice friendship behaviors during the week.

All three 11-year-old students with disabilities (two had an emotional/behavioral disorder; one had a hearing impairment) participating in the evaluation of the friendship circles increased percentages of their appropriate social interactions during lunch time. The treatment gains generalized to recess for two of the students. The positive social interactions were maintained for approximately five weeks after intervention, and interaction levels approached those of a comparison peer group. Teachers reported improved social interactions for two of the three students throughout the day. Information gathered from sociograms also demonstrated that after intervention the students with disabilities more frequently listed members of their friendship circles as their friends. However, very few peers listed the students as their friends.

The goal of the second group intervention, which uses SST and PST, is to enhance the social interactions of adolescent students with emotional/behavioral disorders, including depression and schizophrenia (Plienis et al., 1987). The conversational skills that the intervention targets for assessment and change were selected based on research establishing a relation between the skills and social likeability or distinguishing lonely versus nonlonely youths. High-interest conversational topics among adolescents, which are used in the SST, were identified through a survey of adolescents in the students' high schools.

During the conversational skills phase, the practitioner uses SST to teach group members to ask appropriate questions in conversations, convey verbal and nonverbal interest and attention, disclose appropriate personal information, discuss high-interest topics, and appropriately pace the flow of conversation. The practitioner individualizes the intervention by asking the students to identify personal situations in the school and community that provide opportunities to talk with other people. The practitioner reinforces students' reports of their successful use of the skills and leads a group discussion when a student reports problems applying the skills. Finally, the practitioner encourages the students to discuss difficult life problems they encounter and then teaches the group members to apply basic problem-solving skills (which are taught using SST techniques) to those situations.

The effectiveness of the intervention varied across the three students involved in the evaluation and by outcome measure. However, all of the students enhanced the quality of their social conversations during unstructured practice conversations, including conversations with novel individuals. All but one student increased the quality of their social initiations, responses to initiations, and conversations during informal class parties after intervention. Teacher ratings of social interactions in the classroom indicated improvement for all but one student. A six-week follow-up demonstrated maintenance of the treatment gains. After the study ended, school officials requested that the program be continued for other students with emotional/behavioral problems.

Children and Youths with Multiple Disabilities

Six CB interventions designed to increase the social resources of children and youths with multiple types of disabilities are discussed here. The disabilities include combinations of physical, sensory, learning, and developmental disabilities, as well as emotional/behavioral disorders. If having one type of disability can impede the learning and use of appropriate social skills and development and maintenance of interpersonal relationships, children and youths with multiple disabilities are likely to encounter even more problems in these areas. Consistent with that assumption, the children and adolescents involved in the evaluations of these interventions were extremely socially isolated, exhibited problems in initiating and maintaining social interactions, including playing with other children, and rarely engaged in social interactions in the school or community.

The CB programs discussed here include variations of SST, a time-out procedure, graduated prompting strategies, high-probability requests, self-management training, and reinforcement. All of the interventions incorporate peers either with or without disabilities into the treatment procedures. Peers serve as practice partners, initiators of social interactions, role models, and job-task coaches. In two of the programs, peers are sensitized to the unique social initiations of and problems confronted by children with multiple disabilities. All but one of the interventions (LeBlanc & Matson, 1995) were evaluated using multiple-baseline designs.

LeBlanc and Matson (1995) developed this first multicomponent intervention discussed here for preschoolers with mild to moderate developmental delays and a physical and/or sensory disability. The intervention targets the social behaviors of appropriate greetings, requesting or showing a toy, and initiating play. To accommodate the young ages and developmental level of the children, the therapist and an assistant use puppets to model the social skills. Each child practices the behaviors with the puppet, then with another child. The children then engage in free play in the classroom, while the therapist prompts the children to engage in the target skills. The therapist provides praise and edibles after a child performs the social interaction skills. If a child exhibits inappropriate behavior, such as taking a toy from another child, the child is prompted to perform a related prosocial behavior (e.g., returning the toy). If the child does not comply, he or she is placed into a brief time-out.

To evaluate the intervention, African American and white children ($N = 32$) were assigned to either a treatment or control group after being matched for levels of appropriateness of social behaviors. Only children in the experimental group increased their social interaction skills, and the skills generalized to interactions with novel children in a classroom setting. However, teachers evaluating videotapes of the children's interactions detected no changes in their social behaviors after intervention.

This behavioral intervention uses high-probability requests to increase the social interactions of young children with severe, multiple disabilities (including combinations of mental retardation, autism, and speech impairments) with their able-bodied peers (Davis, Brady, Hamilton, McEvoy, & Williams, 1994). For each child, the practitioner selects eight peers with no disability to participate in two natural play settings where the interventions are implemented (e.g., an integrated play setting in the school and an after-school day care). For each child, the practitioner also identifies both low-probability requests to initiate social interactions and high-probability social requests. Low-probability requests are those to which a child has a history of not responding. An example of a low-probability request to initiate a social interaction with an able-bodied peer is "Max, give the ball to Ryan." High-probability requests are instructions or requests to which a child has a history of responding (e.g., "Give me five").

To ensure that the peers recognize the social initiations of the child with disabilities, the peers listen as the practitioner describes a play situation specific to the child's setting and available toys, then identifies the child's initiation behavior. The peers then describe how they might respond to the initiation and role-play their social responses. During the high-probability intervention (in which peers are present), the practitioner quickly gives three to five high-probability requests to the child then provides a social reinforcer for each behavior the child performs. A low-probability request is given five seconds after reinforcement for performing the last high-probability request. If the child does not respond to a high-probability request, the practitioner continues to give the request until the child responds three consecutive times. When the child learns to appropriately respond, the prompts (the high- and low-probability requests) are removed. After intervention, the three 5- and 6-year-old boys participating in the evaluation increased their unprompted social initiations and durations of their social interactions with their training peers and with peers uninvolved in the intervention. These results also were observed in a nonintervention setting, and the gains in social interactions were maintained for up to twelve weeks.

The goal of this behavioral program is to increase the social interactions in a school setting between children with no disabilities (companions) and children who are legally blind, in addition to having multiple other learning, hearing, and/or physical disabilities (Sisson, Van Hasselt, Hersen, & Strain, 1985). In the first phase of the intervention, the practitioner holds sessions with each companion (there is one companion for two children). During the sessions, the practitioner discusses the children's disabilities with the companion then enhances the companion's appreciation of the disabilities. This is accomplished by engaging the companion in activities, such as wearing blindfolds and glasses that simulate visual disabilities and ear muffs that distort hearing, while playing with various toys. Using SST strategies, the practitioner then teaches the companion four skills to facilitate play. The skills include suggesting play, showing the child how to play, sharing toys, and offering assistance. Companions also are taught to cope with inappropriate behavior by interrupting the child with play initiators, and to handle nonresponse by tapping the child on the arm and waiting for the child to direct his or her attention toward the companion. During the role plays, the practitioner models typical behavior of the children with disabilities. The children with disabilities and the companions are then placed into a classroom at the children's school, and the companion is prompted to initiate play with one of the two children.

The evaluation of the intervention (including two companions and four children ages 9–11 years with multiple disabilities) indicated that the companions increased their social initiations with the children with disabilities in unstructured free play. The children with disabilities also increased their appropriate social responses and social initiations. The treatment gains transferred to a play situation in which companions did not initiate play, and the rate of interactions remained high at the follow-up four months later. Reports from observers also suggested qualitative changes in the interactions between the companions and children with disabilities. Informal comments of the children with disabilities, companions, and supervising staff regarding their involvement in the intervention also were positive.

In this intervention, peers with and without disabilities teach high school students with moderate mental retardation and multiple physical and behavior problems a self-instructional strategy to increase their social interactions (Hughes, Harmer, Killian, & Niarhos, 1995). The identified social skills include initiating a conversation in which the partner responds and making eye contact with the partner. The skills were chosen based on the importance of the skills to the students and on information obtained from surveys conducted with general education students and teachers. The researchers also observed conversations of diverse high school students to identify a range of acceptable performance for student conversations, and student questionnaires provided examples of appropriate conversation initiators.

To teach the components of the self-instructional SST, the peer tutors are given a script (available from the authors). During the training sessions, the peer tutors, who are rotated randomly across the students, verbalize the self-instructional statements while modeling appropriate conversation. The procedures include the following steps.

1 The peer gazes at the student and asks questions he or she chooses from a list of conversational openers.
2 The student looks at the peer and asks an appropriate question while the peer verbalizes aloud the self-instruction.
3 The student practices the social initiation while verbalizing the self-instruction himself or herself.

The self-instructional sequence and corresponding statements include the following.

First, identify the problem (e.g., "I want to talk").
Second, state the response (e.g., "I need to look and talk").
Third, self-evaluate (e.g., "I did it, I talked").
Fourth, self-reinforce (e.g., "I did a good job"). (Hughes et al., 1995, p. 207)

The students develop their own adaptations of the statements, and the peers provide prompts, praise for appropriate responses, and corrective feedback for a nonresponse or inappropriate responses. Feedback consists of modeling appropriate responses and asking the students to practice them.

The evaluation of this program suggests that peers can successfully teach the self-instruction. After intervention, the four female high school seniors participating in the study (three whites, one African American) increased their initiating conversations and making eye contact with the training peers, with other peers, and in multiple school settings. The enhanced performance approached the performance of general education students. For the two students who remained in high school, a follow-up nine to eleven months later found that one student maintained her rate of initiating conversations within the range of general education students, and the other student's rate was slightly below the range. Questionnaires and interviews with students, peers, teachers, and family members demonstrated socially valid interventions and changes in the students' social interactions. For example, the students enjoyed the program, reported greater ease in talking with others, and spoke up more frequently. Family members reported that the students were more assertive and confident and initiated more conversations.

This behavioral intervention involves peers and a unique accommodation—a "communication book." The communication book is designed to assist high school students with articulation problems and other severe and multiple disabilities (e.g., mental retardation and a seizure disorder) in increasing their social initiations and length of conversations with their able-bodied peers (Hunt, Alwell, Goetz, & Sailor, 1990; for the instructional handbook, see Hunt, Alwell, & Goetz, 1990, in "Additional Readings and Resources" at the end of this chapter).

Developing the student's communication book is the first step. The practitioner interviews the student and significant others to identify activities, materials, and individuals the student enjoys and/or likes. Using this information, menus of topic areas are created in the student's communication book. The communication book, which serves as the medium for conversation, includes relevant photographs and drawings of objects, places, activities, and individuals associated with the topic areas. To assist conversational partners (regular education students) in interpreting the pictures, many are labeled with short phrases identifying the activities or individuals. The pictures are grouped by the environment (the home, school, and community) in which the activities, individuals, places, or objects are present or occurred and also by special events (e.g., a birthday party). The photographs are updated at least weekly to maintain the students' and conversational partners' interest.

The intervention is conducted with the conversational partners in various classroom, school, and job settings. The practitioner teaches the students to initiate conversations by removing their communication books from the pouches they carry with them and pairing their verbalizations with pointing to the relevant pictures. A "prompt-fade teaching strategy," which involves physical, gestural, and verbal prompts, depending on the students' performance and need, is used to teach the students the procedures. Appropriate responses are followed by social reinforcers. The practitioner uses SST to teach the conversational partners to reply to the student's initiation. That is, the conversational partners are taught to refer to the pictures in the student's communication book, to ask a question related to one of the pictures, and to pause after the student answers the question to provide another opportunity for the student to continue the conversation. All three students who participated in the evaluation demonstrated increases in their conversational initiations and reciprocal turn taking after intervention. The gains were generalized to untrained conversational partners in other school settings and job sites when conversational opportunities were provided (i.e., a conversational partner was seated next to the student and was not participating in other activities). The students' teachers also provided feedback about the richness of the exchanges between the students and conversational partners.

This final behavioral intervention uses "natural supports" to assist transition-aged high school students with multiple disabilities (combinations of LD, language delays, and emotional/behavioral disorders) in socially integrating into their competitive employment settings (Storey & Garff, 1999). This intervention does not directly teach social skills to students with disabilities. Instead, practitioners teach co-workers without disabilities methods to instruct the students on a new job task, which provides opportunities for social interaction. In the first phase of the intervention, the practitioner uses a skills training manual (see Curl & Hall, 1990, in "Additional Readings and Resources" at the end of this chapter) to teach the co-workers the instructional skills necessary to teach the students a new job task (e.g., putting together social service client packets). The instructional skills involve traditional skills training techniques (instruction, modeling, practice, feedback, and reinforcement), which are referred to as Tell-Show-Watch-Coach. In the second phase, the co-workers teach the job skills to the students. This takes place after the co-workers master the instructional skills, which is judged by their ability to use the skills to teach the job skills to the practitioner.

As judged by normative comparisons, increases in appropriate social interactions between the students with disabilities and their co-workers and job coach were observed after intervention. Conversations included work topics as well as social topics. The job coach's ratings also indicated that the students increased their social interactions, discussions of nonwork-related topics, overall social skills, and integration with co-workers on the job site. Interestingly, the evaluation also suggested that by previously providing job training himself, the job coach actually hindered the students' integration into the workplace.

LGB Youths

LGB youths frequently have few opportunities to observe interpersonal interactions of other sexual minorities and to practice the appropriate social skills needed to establish and maintain social relationships. In recent years, practitioners and researchers have begun to use and evaluate CB applications to resolve these unique problems encountered by LGB populations (Martell, Safren, & Prince, 2004). An example is a group CB intervention that assists LGB youths in the process of coming out (Safren et al., 2001). Although the intervention was not described in detail, the group facilitator's creation of a safe environment and assistance to the adolescents in self-disclosing are the underlying themes. The group facilitator also encourages group members to discuss and role-play strategies for meeting others and for introducing themselves in a way that highlights their positive attributes. After intervention, the eight youths participating in the evaluation reported reduced social anxiety and an increased use of the acquired social skills to maintain friendships and initiate social interactions.

INTERVENTIONS FOR VULNERABLE ADULTS

CB interventions designed to enhance the social interactions of vulnerable adults, including adults with physical disabilities, mental retardation, severe mental illness, and multiple disabilities, the elderly, and gay men, are discussed in this section. As is the case with placing children and youths with disabilities into integrated school placements without appropriate social skills and support, attempting to integrate adults with cognitive, psychiatric, and physical disabilities into the community without adequate social skills and support also can lead to negative social consequences. The consequences include limited participation in community, work, and residential social activity, few supportive ties with community members, social isolation, and reinstitutionalization (Griffiths, Feldman, & Tough, 1997; Hall et al., 2000).

The intervention programs described here assist adults with physical, cognitive, and psychiatric disabilities in enhancing their social interactions by using various combinations of CB interventions. The strategies include SST, PST, other self-management techniques, homework assignments, changing the physical environment, providing opportunities for social interactions and social integration, and involving others to prompt and reinforce social behavior and to advocate for the clients. Some of the interventions involve peers and co-workers and make appropriate accommodations for the unique needs of these vulnerable clients.

For many elderly persons, the aging process involves physical, social, and/or residential changes, which can result in social isolation. The CB interventions described in this section are designed to assist the elderly in enhancing their social interactions. The strategies include prompting appropriate letter writing and social interactions, rearranging and enriching the physical environment, and SST. The final two case studies demonstrate multiple CB interventions that increase the social interactions and enhance the interpersonal relationships of gay men. The interventions include SST, cognitive restructuring, exposure therapy, and homework assignments.

Adults with Physical Disabilities

Dattilo and Camarata (1991) developed a behavioral intervention to increase the social initiations and interactions of adults with severe motor and speech impairments resulting from cerebral palsy. An augmentative communication system ("Touch Talker") is integrated into the intervention. The Touch Talker is comprised of a keyboard, display monitor, and software used to program personal messages for each client. The messages appear on the monitor and also are produced as synthetic speech. Message inventories can be adjusted for the client's cognitive ability. For example, one client's message inventory might include only five sentences, all of which are related to one topic—requesting participation in preferred recreational activities (e.g., playing cards and listening to music). Another client's message inventory might include sentences grouped into a number of main topics, such as dining out, music discussion, school, leisure activities, and general conversation. Each topical area includes multiple preprogrammed sentences, which facilitate the client's ability to make requests and engage in a conversation on the particular topic. For example, for dining out, the relevant sentences might include "I want a tossed salad," "This tastes really good," and "I am ready to leave."

Skills training techniques, including instruction, prompting, and practice, are used to teach the clients to independently use the Touch Talker. Although skills training can teach the clients to activate the device, an additional intervention might be necessary to increase the clients' initiation of conversations, rather than simply reacting to others' conversations. This is accomplished by the practitioner's placing recreational materials in view of each client and instructing the client that the practitioner will respond to requests that he or she produces with the Touch Talker. After the client makes such a request, the practitioner responds immediately. After the second intervention, the percentage of self-initiated conversations of the two men participating in the evaluation increased markedly in the treatment setting as well as in their residences (a multiple-baseline design across the two men was used). The improvements were validated by friends and caretakers, who reported positive changes in both men's social behaviors and interactions in a variety of community settings.

In many circumstances, communication difficulties or a lack of social skills is not the reason adults with physical disabilities experience difficulties engaging in social interactions and forming relationships. Physical environmental antecedents, such as barriers that prohibit wheelchair users from independently entering and leaving their homes, likely inhibit some individuals with disabilities from developing and accessing social resources. One study suggests that simply installing exterior ramps to the home entrances of wheelchair users can enhance the social interactions of individuals with physical disabilities (White, Paine-Andrews, Matthews, & Fawcett, 1995). In this intervention, community development block grant funds were used to install exterior ramps to the homes of six low-income wheelchair users. After intervention, the number of weekly community visits and home visitors and the size of the social networks of the participants all increased.

Adults with Mental Retardation

Three CB programs and one intervention that changes the physical environment to enhance the social interactions of adults with mental retardation are discussed now. The interventions include traditional SST and specific strategies, such as providing opportunities for, prompting, and reinforcing social interactions. The programs also include PST and a variety of other self-management techniques (self-monitoring, self-reinforcement, and self-instruction). The final intervention discussed in this section enhances social interactions among institutionalized residents simply by changing the method of serving meals. With the exception of the evaluation conducted by Griffiths et al. (1997), multiple-baseline designs were used to evaluate all of the interventions.

The "social life" program is a unique group intervention designed to increase the social competence of adults with mild to moderate mental retardation (Griffiths et al., 1997). The program involves a card game, SST, PST, and six generalization strategies to enhance transfer of the treatment gains to natural settings. The generalization strategies include (1) using multiple examples of situations requiring clients to demonstrate a variety of appropriate social skills; (2) providing opportunities during intervention to practice individually selected social skills; (3) conducting the training in natural settings (e.g., in a group home and sheltered workshop); (4) teaching the problem-solving process; (5) creating situations and providing opportunities for clients to perform the identified social skills in natural settings, followed by feedback or social reinforcement; and (6) varying the antecedent conditions.

Social skills targeted by the intervention were selected individually by the group home residents and their group home staff assistants based on criteria such as relative importance and the residents' desire to learn the skills. The common themes that emerged from the selections include relationships (e.g., making and keeping friends), problem solving (e.g., conflict resolution), interactions (conversational skills), and appropriate expression of feelings. The skills are taught through a total of seventy-two game cards in four different categories, with each card designating a certain amount of game money that clients can win or lose. The four categories and examples of each follow.

> First, "give and take" cards describe appropriate or inappropriate social situations but do not require a player to respond, for example, "You shook hands when introduced to someone the first time. Win $5," or "You gave a hug to a stranger. Lose $5."
> Second, "right or wrong" cards require players to judge a statement as right or wrong, for example, "You should never let a stranger in the house. Win or lose $10," based on the response.
> Third, "fill-in" cards require players to fill in a blank, for example, "If I was lost, I would _____. Win $15," for an appropriate answer.
> Fourth, "play a role" cards require players to interact appropriately with others, for example, "Show how you would answer the door to talk to a stranger. Win $20," for an appropriate interaction.

When playing the game, a group member throws a die, moves the applicable spaces, picks up a game card, and responds to the card. The group leader then facilitates a group problem-solving process. The other group members assess the player's response, evaluate alternatives and their consequences, and decide whether the response is the most appropriate one for that particular situation. If the player's response is appropriate, the group facilitator reinforces the response with praise and the allotted game money. If the response is inappropriate, the group facilitator models the correct response. On the client's next turn, he or she has a choice of responding to the same card or drawing a new card. After the game, the group facilitator provides tangible reinforcers based on the amount of game money each participant wins. To enhance transfer of the social skills to natural settings, residential and vocational staff are instructed to set up situations and provide opportunities in several natural settings for the clients to exhibit the identified skills. As appropriate, staff provide the clients with social reinforcement or corrective feedback and modeling. In addition, staff vary other antecedent events (e.g., use a variety of prompts), and they provide social reinforcement after the clients spontaneously perform their identified social skills.

The social life program was evaluated through the random assignment of adults with mild or moderate mental retardation (N = 43) to the "social life" group, a "game" group with only three generalization strategies, or a "no-training" control group. Compared with the control group, clients in the social life group performed the target skills more frequently in their residential and work environments. In addition, based on observations of interactions with peers, family, and other community members, ratings of the likeability and quality of the relationships of the social life group participants were higher than the control group. On the other hand, the game group was significantly better than the control group on only one generalization measure (an evaluation of a conversation with a stranger). On almost all measures participants in the social life group maintained their improvement over a three-month follow-up.

This CB intervention, which was developed by Matson and Andrasik (1982), uses self-management strategies to enhance and generalize social interaction skills to the natural environments of adult clients with mild to moderate mental retardation. The intervention is designed for clients who are living in a residential facility and preparing for community living. The intervention begins with the practitioner teaching the client a variety of social skills, including introducing oneself to or greeting another person, asking another person a question or for a favor, offering to share an activity with another person, and requesting the use of an item. The practitioner teaches the skills by describing a scene for role play, which incorporates the identified social skills, followed by a resident assistant (who is previously trained using the same procedures) prompting the client to respond. Depending on the quality of the response, the resident assistant provides social reinforcement or instruction, feedback, and/or modeling. If the client exhibits inappropriate social skills, they are identified as inappropriate, and examples of alternative appropriate social responses are provided. The practitioner also uses SST techniques to teach self-management procedures. The procedures involve the clients recording in a natural setting (e.g., during leisure time in the residential facility) when they use the identified social skills and giving themselves tokens (exchangeable for candy and soda) when they judge their social interactions as appropriate. When discrepancies exist between staff observations and the residents' recordings, the practitioner provides corrective feedback.

The results of the evaluation (N = 8) suggest that the program is effective in increasing appropriate verbal interactions that generalize to the natural setting of a leisure room for adults with mild to moderate mental retardation. The evaluation also found that a combination of SST, self-monitoring, and self-reinforcement was more effective than SST alone in increasing social interactions.

Matson and a colleague (Matson & Adkins, 1980) also designed an SST program, which involves self-instruction and audiotape recordings, for moderately mentally retarded adults who lack basic social interaction skills. The skills identified for intervention include initiating conversations, complimenting others, making appropriate requests, and responding appropriately to requests. The audiotapes present ten different scenes depicting appropriate use of the identified skills. The following is an example of the audio recording of a therapist presenting a situation to teach the skill of complimenting others:

"You can get along better with people if you say nice things. You might say something nice about their appearance." This statement is followed by a prompt, "Can you say something nice about someone," followed by 10 seconds of silence to allow the subject time to respond. For the tape with answers on it a response is then provided, "If you said I like your hair, that would be something nice. Did you make a comment that would make the person feel good about their appearance?" (Matson & Adkins, 1980, p. 246)

Following the self-instruction, the therapist reviews the scenes with the client. If needed, additional SST techniques (e.g., instruction, modeling, role playing, and performance feedback) are used. After intervention, the two adults with mental retardation who participated in the evaluation substantially increased their appropriate verbal interactions during leisure time in their residential facility.

As White et al. (1995) demonstrated by providing ramp access to the homes of wheelchair users, vulnerable clients do not always need SST to assist them in increasing their social interactions. Social interactions among institutionalized young adults with mental retardation, for example, can be increased simply by switching from an institutionalized style of serving meals that places food on individual trays to serving meals family style (Van-Biervliet, Spangler, & Marshall, 1981).

Adults with Severe Mental Illness

Although definitions of severe mental illness include a variety of mental disorders (e.g., bipolar, major depression, schizophrenia), the majority of interventions developed to enhance the social interactions of clients diagnosed with severe mental illness focus on schizophrenia. Schizophrenia is a biopsychological, genetically based disorder that is characterized by psychotic (e.g., delusions, hallucinations) and other symptoms (e.g., disordered thinking), severe problems in social functioning, and deterioration in interpersonal relationships. A combination of biopsychological vulnerability, related symptoms, and social-environmental factors (e.g., institutionalization, social isolation, rejection from others) appears to contribute to the inability of many clients diagnosed with schizophrenia to learn and use adaptive social skills. Although neuroleptic medications can control symptoms and reduce relapse rates for clients diagnosed with schizophrenia, the medications contribute little to enhancing social functioning. This inability to effectively cope in the social environment can be a significant source of stress for many of these clients, frequently resulting in an unsatisfactory lifestyle and relapse (Halford & Hayes, 1991; Hampton, James, Wrigley, & Fullwood, 1980; Liberman et al., 1993).

With the exception of the two interventions discussed at the end of this section—a social skills group intervention to increase male social interactions with females and an SST peer intervention to increase the social interactions of a psychiatric inpatient—the interventions described here were developed by Robert Liberman, Charles Wallace, and their colleagues. These researchers have developed social and independent living skills modules at the UCLA Center for Research on Treatment and Rehabilitation of Psychosis (CRTRP) to increase the social and independent living skills of clients with severe mental illness. This section presents an overview of the rationale for and description of the modules (Liberman & Corrigan, 1993; Liberman et al., 1993; Liberman, Glynn, Blair, Ross, & Marder, 2002), followed by a discussion of the research that has evaluated the effectiveness of the modules (see "Additional Readings and Resources" at the end of this chapter for availability of the modules, including a module on friendship and intimacy).

The training modules are based on the belief that effective intervention for increasing the social and independent living skills of clients with severe mental illness must be based on three main assumptions. Intervention must be consistent with a "vulnerability-stress-coping-competence model" of severe mental illness, must incorporate principles of learning, and must focus on specific elements of socially skilled behavior. The competence model assumes that interactions among biopsychological vulnerability, socio-environmental stressors (e.g., family conflict, work stress), and protective factors (e.g., social support, appropriate social skills, neuroleptic medication) are related to psychiatric symptoms and psychosocial well-being. The main goal of the SST and PST incorporated into the modules is to increase the protective factors that can buffer the effects of the biopsychological vulnerability and socio-environmental stress, thus enhancing social functioning.

Each module provides a curriculum for teaching particular skill areas required for effective community functioning. For example, modules include skill areas for medication management, symptom management, recreation for leisure, conversational skills, and community re-entry. Although all of these modules might enhance a client's ability to access social resources, only the skill areas for basic conversational skills are discussed in detail in this section. The skill areas for recreation for leisure and medication and symptom management are discussed in chapter 5 and chapter 6, respectively.

General areas for basic conversational skills include active listening (effective verbal and nonverbal listening techniques), initiating conversations (identifying likely places to meet others and whether another is willing to converse), maintaining and ending conversations, and integrating all skill areas into natural and spontaneous conversations. Seven CB strategies, which are consistent with SST and PST and frequently implemented in groups, are used to teach the skills. First, the therapist provides basic instruction on and rationales for the skills, which are then discussed with group members. Second, the skills are demonstrated by video modeling, followed by group discussion. Third, role plays are used. In the role plays, the client's receiving, processing (assessing various alternatives to address the situation), and sending skills (incorporating the verbal and nonverbal skills) are evaluated by the therapist and group members. An example of receiving, processing, and sending skills relevant to initiating social interactions is given in table 4.1.

Fourth, the therapist begins to prepare the clients to use the skills in natural settings. To accomplish this, the therapist uses prompting, coaching, and feedback to teach the clients a problem-solving process to identify the resources needed to perform the skills. Fifth, the therapist teaches the clients to apply a problem-solving process to overcome unexpected barriers or obstacles to performing the skills. The therapist assists the clients in identifying aspects of the obstacle (receiving skills) and in brainstorming methods to remove the obstacle (processing skills). After selecting a solution to resolve the barrier, the clients practice verbal and nonverbal sending skills by role playing the solution. Sixth, the therapist supervises the clients as they perform agreed on tasks in natural settings. Finally, the clients complete homework assignments that require independent performance of the skills, and they provide evidence of completion of the assignments.

The modules also incorporate a variety of strategies to address the thought disorder, hyperarousal, and distractibility frequently experienced by clients with severe mental illness that can interfere with their acquisition of the social skills. Strategies include reducing external distractions; keeping training tasks brief, focused, and slow paced; providing frequent prompts and incentives; posting charts that explain skill areas; and, for distractions caused by hallucinations and other thought disorders, teaching thought stopping. When using thought stopping, practitioners teach clients to disrupt

Table 4.1. Example of Receiving, Processing, and Sending Skills

Receiving Skills	Processing Skills	Sending Skills
I see a girl sitting alone in the dance hall.	The girl staring at me in the corner may want me to ask her to dance.	
I hear the music in the dance hall.	My alternatives at the dance are: ask the girl to dance, ask someone else to dance, go to the refreshment table instead.	I asked the girl to dance by approaching her, making eye contact, and saying in a pleasant voice, "I'd like to have the next dance with you."

Note. From "Designing New Psychosocial Treatments for Schizophrenia," by R. P. Liberman and P. W. Corrigan, 1993, *Psychiatry, 56*, p. 241. Copyright 1993 by Guilford. Reprinted with permission.

an unwanted or disturbing thought by silently saying, "Stop!"; clients then substitute a pleasant or more functional thought for the unwanted thought. Self-monitoring and other techniques to avoid stressors that might exacerbate symptoms also are used. For clients who experience difficulties with acquiring and/or using the skills, practitioners can provide additional environmental assistance. Examples include conducting the interventions in natural settings, recruiting and teaching significant others to prompt and reinforce newly learned skills, and constructing specialized, supportive environments requiring a more limited set of skills. Practitioners also can conduct booster sessions to maintain and/or transfer the treatment gains to natural settings.

Marder et al. (1996) evaluated the effectiveness of four of the modules by randomly assigning outpatient clients diagnosed with schizophrenia (eighty males; majority were nonwhite) to an SST group or supportive group therapy group. The clients all received maintenance doses of neuroleptic medication. Clients in the SST group participated in the Medication Self-Management and Symptom Self-Management modules during the first six months, and a Social Problem-Solving module during the second six months. The latter module taught clients to recognize social barriers to attaining community life goals and to identify, select, and implement appropriate solutions. The final training, a Successful Living Skills module, taught clients to identify and pursue their own goals. SST was determined to be more effective than the supportive group therapy as indicated by the personal well-being scale (e.g., attention to personal appearance, loneliness, and global satisfaction) and the total adjustment scale that involved clients' rating their functioning in areas such as work, household, external family roles, social and leisure activities, and personal well-being. The SST advantage over the supportive group therapy was greatest when combined with active drug supplementation given to clients exhibiting increases of symptoms related to relapse. Specifically, those differences were found in social and leisure activities (including amount and quality of interactions with friends and romantic relationships), clients' interactions with and reactions to family members, and a measure of total adjustment. However, the SST appeared to be more effective than the supportive group therapy only for clients with a relatively early onset of schizophrenia (24 years and younger) and optimally effective for those clients who remained stable or, if unstable, received effective drug intervention.

In a subsequent evaluation of the modules, participants included 80 outpatient clients (white, African American, Latino, and Asian) with persistent schizophrenia and currently on neuroleptic medication (Liberman et al., 1998). The clients were randomly assigned to an intensive SST program or to a psychosocial occupational therapy group. The SST program incorporated the basic conversation, recreation for leisure, medication management, and symptom management modules. At the end of the six-month intervention, clients were assigned to community case managers for eighteen months. The primary responsibilities of the case managers were to encourage the clients to use their acquired social skills in natural settings and to coordinate and facilitate their successful adjustment into the community. At a two-year follow-up, clients receiving the SST scored significantly higher on an independent living skills survey that measured specific activities in which they had engaged during the preceding six months. The activities included involvement in social relationships.

In summary, the modules developed at the UCLA CRTRP for individuals with severe mental illness provide multiple comprehensive CB programs that enhance social skills, build social relationships, and facilitate integration into the community. The final two SST interventions that follow also were designed to enhance the social interactions of individuals diagnosed with schizophrenia. They were both evaluated using multiple-baseline designs.

This group SST intervention focuses specifically on difficulties male clients diagnosed with schizophrenia can have in initiating conversations with unfamiliar women (Kelly et al., 1980). The intervention targets three social skills, which research has identified as predicting favorable evaluations of conversations. The skills include eliciting information, appropriate self-disclosure, and using complimentary statements. After identifying and providing a rationale for the conversational skill, the therapist shows a modeling video in which males and females interact with one another using the relevant skill. The therapist occasionally stops the tape and asks the group members to pay attention to when and the ways in which the models use the identified skill. The therapist then prompts the group members to provide examples of ways in which they could use the skill in their own interactions, after which group members rehearse the skill. During the sessions, the therapist emphasizes the *general class* of skills being taught, not parroting specific behaviors viewed on the videos or performed by other group members.

Three young adult males diagnosed with schizophrenia and attending a community after-care program participated in the evaluation of the group SST intervention. After intervention, all three men improved their performance in the three skill areas. In addition, global ratings in other areas, such as demonstrating active interest in the female and sincerity and authenticity in their responses and emotions, increased after intervention. The skill gains were generally maintained ten weeks later. After intervention, the men also reported increased social contacts in the community and increased comfort levels when approaching unfamiliar females. Finally, the program staff observed an increase in the frequency and appropriateness of the men's social interactions.

In this final intervention, meal-time peers are incorporated into SST procedures to increase the social interactions of isolated clients diagnosed with schizophrenia and residing in a community-based residential facility (Hampton et al., 1980). The target social skills are appropriately attending, appropriate body gestures, and verbally responding to or initiating social interactions with a peer. During group sessions, the therapist uses SST to teach the skills to the socially isolated resident and to his or her meal-time peers. Group members then practice the behaviors outside of the group. In additional sessions including only the meal-time peers, the therapist also uses SST to teach the peers to prompt the three social skills and to reinforce the resident's performance of the skills. An example for the attending behavior is referring to the resident by name, followed by verbal reinforcement, such as "I like it when you seem interested in what I'm telling you." After intervention, the adult male client participating in the evaluation demonstrated marked improvements in the three social skills, including increases in interactions between him and his five meal-time peers. The treatment gains were maintained for up to six months. Staff and residents also reported the client engaging in more social activity in the residential facility after intervention.

Adults with Multiple Disabilities

These two case studies provide examples of using SST and a co-worker intervention to increase the social integration of two employees with multiple disabilities into their competitive work settings (Gaylord-Ross, Park, Johnston, Lee, & Goetz, 1995). The clients were Terry and Tootsie. They both were diagnosed with severe mental retardation and had visual and hearing impairments. Although the women were in a supported work program, they rarely interacted with other employees. In order to facilitate social integration, the SST was implemented in naturally occurring situations at the two women's work sites. For Terry, the situations were checking in, and in the break room of a Pizza Hut restaurant. For Tootsie, the situations involved responding to initiations made by co-workers in the four departments of a Whole Earth Access department store.

The first step in the intervention involved identifying the social routines for each client. For example, Terry's checking in routine involved ten tasks: going to the counter/register; activating a switch that played, "Hello"; waiting for a co-worker to say, "Hello"; signing, "Hello" back; giving a co-worker a card that stated, "Please sign me in"; waiting for the co-worker to punch in for her; receiving the card from the co-worker; putting the card away; waiting for the co-worker to turn off the switch; and signing, "Thank you." For Tootsie, the social routine involved orienting her head and body to greet a co-worker, who extends a hand and says hello, and extending her hand to shake the co-worker's hand.

The SST was similar for each client and her co-worker. For example, for Terry's checking-in routine, the practitioner modeled the social routine for the co-worker then assisted the co-worker through the exchange using verbal cues. The practitioner then physically guided Terry through the routine, which was gradually faded, and provided social reinforcement when Terry correctly performed the sequence. The second part of the intervention involved recruiting a "co-worker advocate" to assist in each woman's program. During the six-week intervention sessions, the advocates identified one or more activities that could facilitate the women's integration into their workplace (e.g., sitting with co-workers during break time). The strategies were discussed, written down, and carried out with each woman at her job site. During subsequent meetings, the practitioner and co-worker advocates discussed any problems with implementing the activities, made any necessary changes, and generated additional activities.

Compared with baselines, the number and duration of social interactions between the women and their co-workers increased after each of the interventions was implemented. The co-workers' social validity ratings indicated significant changes in Tootsie's, but not Terry's, overall social competence and social acceptance. However, the ratings of Terry's advocate (who also was her supervisor) indicated steady increases in both social outcomes.

The Elderly

Elderly persons can experience social isolation for many reasons. Chronic illness; visual, hearing, or cognitive impairment; reduced mobility and opportunities to meet others; death of significant others; relocation after retirement; and placement in institutionalized settings, such as nursing homes, are among the reasons. Because of these changes, elderly individuals might need to learn or reactivate previously acquired social skills in order to establish friendships and to successfully cope with new or increased interactions with medical personnel, social workers, and caregivers. In addition, placement into nursing homes frequently is sudden, providing little time for the resident to develop the social skills necessary to cope with and interact successfully in the new physical and social environments. Nursing home staff and physical environments also can inadvertently extinguish adaptive behavior, such as engaging in social interactions and meaningful activity, and can reinforce maladaptive behavior, such as passivity and social isolation. After nursing home placement, interactions with family and friends frequently become less frequent, contributing to social isolation, inactivity, and loneliness (Berger, 1981; Engelman, Altus, & Mathews, 1999; Fernandez-Ballesteros, Izal, Diaz, Gonzalez, & Souto, 1988; Goldstein & Baer, 1976).

With one exception, the behavioral interventions discussed here were implemented in nursing homes or in other institutional settings. Evaluations of the interventions, some of which involved experimental designs, suggest that simply changing the physical and social environments can increase the social interactions among elderly residents in such settings. The final case study uses SST to enhance the social interactions of an older woman with a visual impairment.

More than three decades ago, Goldstein and Baer (1976) developed the "RSVP" procedure to increase the mail correspondence of elderly nursing home residents who receive few visitors. The behavioral intervention consists of prompting the residents to write letters to others (or to dictate the letters if they are unable to write) and to quickly respond to received letters. The residents also are prompted to include a stamped, self-addressed envelope with each letter and to include content that would likely result in a reply. Examples include a question, a request for a reply, refraining from reprimanding individuals for not writing (e.g., "Why don't you ever write to me?"), and a thank-you to correspondents who do write. The multiple-baseline design indicated that the three elderly residents participating in the evaluation increased their letter writing, number of correspondents, and return rates after intervention.

Interventions that change the physical environment, such as rearranging the chairs from along a wall or around a television set and placing them in circular patterns or around tables, adding a kitchenette, and switching to family-style meals, can increase both verbal and tactile interactions among elderly residents in institutional settings (Bakos, Bozic, Chapin, & Neuman, 1980; Melin & Götestam, 1981; Peterson, Knapp, Rosen, & Pither, 1977). Increases in interactions with other residents can be particularly high for residents involved in decision making about the design changes (Bakos et al., 1980).

Other interventions conducted in institutional settings for the elderly demonstrate that enriching the physical environment and adding prompts can increase social interactions among residents. For example, providing coffee and cookies in a lounge area (Quattrochi-Tubin & Jason, 1980) and beverages in a common area before breakfast (Blackman, Howe, & Pinkston, 1976) can increase the residents' social interactions. In an evaluation of the former intervention, increases in social interactions generalized to other times and other locations within the institution. In the latter intervention, staff also prompt the residents to attend the activity by announcing the refreshments in advance, individually reminding the residents of the event, and assisting residents who wish to participate but require assistance.

Linsk, Howe, and Pinkston (1975) also describe successful prompting interventions that can increase attendance and social interactions in three group activities among female nursing home residents. The group activities involve a newspaper discussion, folktale reading, and a resident's meeting.

Before each meeting, the social worker spends time inviting, encouraging, and requesting residents to attend, as well as physically assisting some residents to the group activity. The reversal design indicated that the social worker increased participation and interactions in the group discussion by increasing the number of questions that she directed to the elderly participants.

This final case example demonstrates a therapist using SST with a 65-year-old widowed woman with a diagnosis of major depression and macular degeneration, a progressive eye disease that had resulted in almost total blindness (Donohue, Acierno, Van Hasselt, & Hersen, 1995). The woman self-referred to a clinic for older adults, where the therapist determined that the onset of her depression had occurred two years before, after she received the macular degeneration diagnosis. Before she became visually impaired, the client had an active and satisfying social life. After the visual impairment, she felt uncomfortable when requesting others to join her in social activities. The therapist assessed the client's social skills using relevant role-play scenarios from social situations generated by clients at a center for the blind. Asking others to be involved in social activities was one of the three main areas in which the client needed assistance. The therapist taught the skills using traditional SST techniques (see Donohue, Acierno, Hersen, & Van Hasselt, 1995, in "Additional Readings and Resources" for a detailed manual of the training procedures). An example of a scenario in the area of social involvement that the therapist used in the SST follows: "You are walking to your apartment. You are bored and wish you could find someone that you could spend time with in the future, suddenly you hear an old friend say to you 'Hi.'"

The multiple-baseline design across behaviors indicated progressive improvement in the client's use of the social skills in natural settings. The client's assertiveness scores and happiness ratings also increased, and her depression decreased to a nonclinical level. The interpersonal skills and depression scores were maintained at a seven-month follow-up. However, at the 6-month assessment the therapist conducted a telephone booster session. At the time, the client had experienced an increase in her depression after a recent surgery failed to improve her vision.

Gay Men

The following two case studies demonstrate the use of multiple CB interventions, including SST, cognitive restructuring, and exposure therapy, to assist gay men who have difficulties establishing interpersonal relationships.

This first case study involved a 35-year-old gay man who exhibited long-term problems with interacting and establishing personal relationships with other gay men (St. Lawrence et al., 1983). Because of his fear of rejection and increased anxiety when interacting with others, the client rarely initiated conversations at gay bars. The client's goals were to increase his ability to meet others with less discomfort, initiate conversations more easily, appropriately respond to the social initiations of others, and assert his own feelings and opinions, especially with other gay men. Based on information gathered from several interviews with the client, the therapist constructed role-play scenarios of problematic situations for the client. One-half of the scenarios involved positive interactions with others, such as initiating conversations, giving and receiving compliments, and expressing affection. The remaining scenarios involved problematic situations in which the client was required to assert himself, such as responding to unreasonable requests from others, expressing displeasure, and expressing justified anger.

The therapist used SST with the constructed scenarios to teach the client the identified verbal (e.g., greetings and asking conversational questions) and nonverbal (e.g., eye contact and controlling extraneous movements, such as rocking in his chair) skills. The therapist also taught the client to use cognitive restructuring to change the negative cognitions that triggered his anxiety and reticence in initiating social contacts. During this process, the client described occasions when he felt anxious and identified self-statements that contributed to his anxiety. For example, the client identified a sequence of self-statements that began with "I'd like to talk to him" and led to ". . . but he might reject me and then I'd feel devastated and my night would be ruined." The practitioner taught the client to stop the self-statements early in the sequence, evaluate the self-statement, and substitute a more functional thought. An example follows.

> I'd like to talk to him . . . but he might not like me (CUE to STOP). But then not everyone I talk to is going to like me and the more people I talk with, the more doors I open where friendships might develop later on. Besides, he looks interesting and I might enjoy talking to him for a few minutes. (St. Lawrence et al., 1983, p. 47)

The client practiced modifying his self-talk in a hierarchy of increasingly anxiety-provoking situations. Finally, the practitioner gave homework assignments relevant to the settings and interactions in which the client had experienced a great deal of discomfort. For example, because the client was initially hesitant to accept the importance of making eye contact during social interactions, the therapist asked the client to go to a gay bar, identify a popular man and a socially isolated man, then observe whether each of them made eye contact with their companions. The homework assignments also began with the least anxiety-producing situation and gradually progressed to situations that triggered more anxiety.

Self-surveys, self-monitoring, and ratings by trained observers of the client's performance in the role-play scenarios used for generalization suggested that the intervention resulted in enhanced social skills, decreased anxiety, and increased social contacts and meaningful relationships. At the one- and six-month follow-ups, the client reported continued satisfaction with his interpersonal skills and relationships. He also reported feeling less shy and anxious when initiating conversations, continuing use of his acquired skills, and spending more time with his new gay friends in a variety of social settings.

This second case study used CB interventions with Michael, a 25-year-old gay white male who was experiencing symptoms of social anxiety (Safren & Rogers, 2001). The client reported few friendships, loneliness, social isolation, and never experiencing a significant relationship with another man. The client traced his social anxiety back to junior high school, when he began to "feel different from other boys his age." During college his social anxiety only heightened as he began to realize that he was attracted sexually and emotionally primarily toward men. Michael's few friends at the time ridiculed students who attended the LGB student union, resulting in Michael's avoidance of this opportunity to meet other gay men.

The therapist's initial assessment determined that Michael's social anxiety, such as his fears that others would dislike him, find him uninteresting, or notice his anxiety, not a lack of social skills, was responsible for his social avoidance. Treatment included cognitive-restructuring, in-session role plays of a hierarchy of anxiety-producing situations, and real-life exposure to the identified anxiety-producing situations (refer to the article for extensive client-therapist dialogue demonstrating the interventions). Compared with baselines, Michael reported decreased anxiety and substantial increases in his social contacts and social activities after intervention.

ANALYSIS AND CRITIQUE FOR PRACTICE AND RESEARCH

This chapter presented examples of CB interventions that can enhance the social interactions of vulnerable populations. Vulnerable populations include children, youths, and adults with physical, sensory, learning/developmental, emotional/behavioral, and multiple disabilities; the elderly; and sexual minorities. Specific measures of enhancing social interactions are initiating, increasing, and sustaining interpersonal interactions (e.g., playing; conversing with peers, co-workers, and significant others; and corresponding through mail); increasing the number of community visits and home visitors; developing friendships and personal relationships; increasing social acceptance; and decreasing loneliness.

SST is the most commonly used intervention to achieve the goal of enhancing the social interactions of vulnerable clients. SST is combined with additional CB strategies, such as PST, cognitive restructuring, and other self-management interventions (i.e., self-monitoring, self-reinforcement, and self-instruction). Other interventions, used alone or in combination with SST, include prompting strategies, reinforcement, time-out procedures, exposure therapy, high-probability requests, and enriching and changing the physical environment. Interventions can be administered individually or in groups. Peers, including students with and without disabilities, co-residents in residential facilities, and able-bodied co-workers, frequently are involved in the interventions. The peers serve as play and conversational partners, buddies, companions, tutors, coaches, models, and members of support networks. The peers provide instruction, prompts, feedback, and reinforcement and assist children, youths, and adults with disabilities in integrating into school, work, and community settings.

These interventions suggest that practitioners can draw on and present to vulnerable clients a variety of options for enhancing their social interactions. A more critical, detailed evaluation of the interventions discussed in this chapter follows. Effectiveness and additional applications of the interventions and issues involving personal freedom, control, and social justice and social validity are examined.

Effectiveness and Additional Applications

Despite the overall positive results of the CB interventions, the evaluations are far from conclusive. Participants were usually volunteers (not randomly selected), and few studies randomly assigned participants into control or experimental groups, making it difficult to rule out alternative explanations for the positive outcomes. In addition to the small number of participants in most of the studies, the unique characteristics of the clients and settings suggest the results might not apply to other clients and settings. For example, unique characteristics of the school systems, the students with disabilities, or their able-bodied peers might have accounted for the positive outcomes for interventions involving peers within particular schools. Many of the evaluations failed to establish relations between skill development and other outcome measures, such as establishing friendships and decreased loneliness. The majority of the studies also reported inconsistent or no improvement for some participants. These findings indicate the need for practitioners to track the target skill and other outcome measures, and to continuously assess relevant symptoms (e.g., those related to schizophrenia) and make any necessary adjustments in treatment.

Gresham, Sugai, and Horler's (2001) review of studies conducted with children and youths with disabilities (e.g., LD, mental retardation, emotional/behavioral problems) concluded that CB interventions have variable but overall modest effects on enhancing socially competent behavior. The review also suggests that combinations of modeling, coaching, and reinforcement tend to be more effective in increasing social skills and related outcomes than are interventions such as PST and self-instructional training. Which intervention, or combination of interventions, is most effective for which client and goal, however, is far from settled. The use of multiple interventions, while failing to determine which intervention or combination of interventions results in a particular outcome, is one of the reasons for this uncertainty.

Kavale and Mostert's (2004) more recent meta-analysis of research examining the impact of CB interventions (primarily SST) on various social behaviors of children and youths with disabilities also indicated variable but generally modest effects. The reasons the reviewers suggested for these modest findings can inform both practice and future research. Among the reasons are failing to use more intensive, lengthy treatment programs; failing to conduct individual assessments, thus not matching specific social skills problems with intervention procedures; failing to conduct interventions in natural settings; failing to ensure the accuracy and consistency of the treatment procedures; and failing to adequately program for transfer and maintenance of skills.

Dilk and Bond's (1996), meta-analysis of studies evaluating SST for clients with severe mental illness concluded that the interventions are moderately to strongly effective in increasing social skills and reducing psychiatric symptoms. However, they observed that SST appears to be less effective in enhancing more socially relevant measures, such as appropriate social functioning in a variety of contexts. Dilk and Bond's critique of SST for clients with severe mental illness is similar to the two previous reviews of research conducted with children and youths with disabilities. Techniques, however, that might facilitate learning in one group of vulnerable clients might not be applicable to another group. For example, Liberman et al. (1993) recommended lengthier, more intensive sessions (one to one-and-a-half hours each, two or three times per week, for approximately four months) for individuals diagnosed with schizophrenia. However, after lengthening the SST sessions for elderly nursing home residents, Berger (1981) observed an increase in dropouts. When determining treatment issues, such as the intensity and length of sessions, practitioners and researchers must consider the special problems of vulnerable clients. Becoming easily tired, the inability to maintain focus for long periods of time, and the added inconvenience, such as for wheelchair users (Glueckauf & Quittner, 1992), are among the problems.

Research also has not determined under what circumstances group (versus individual) treatment or including peers without disabilities in the treatment process enhances treatment outcomes. Still, the interventions discussed in this chapter can inform practice in these areas. For example, conducting treatment in groups appears to have a number of advantages. These include providing group members with a safe environment to work on common problems, with available peers to rehearse skills and receive additional feedback, and with a forum for discussing specific applications of the skills and homework assignments. These advantages might be particularly relevant for enhancing the social interactions of vulnerable clients, who might have few opportunities for interacting with peers sharing similar problems. Including peers (both able-bodied and with disabilities) in the intervention process can have additional advantages, such as enhancing the maintenance and transfer of the social skills, interactions, and relationships to natural settings. Involving able-bodied peers also could promote positive attitudes toward their peers with disabilities, resulting in friendships and increased integration of individuals with disabilities into work, school, and community environments.

The evaluations of the CB interventions designed to enhance the social interactions of vulnerable clients did not involve all of the vulnerable populations identified in chapter 1. The interventions also were not evaluated in other settings in which they might be applicable. Although examining additional applications is an area of future research, practitioners could adopt the interventions for use with other vulnerable clients or in other settings. The CB strategies that integrate peers into the intervention process might apply to other children, youths, or adults who are more likely to be excluded from social interactions and peer groups within school, work, residential, or community settings. Examples include racial/ethnic minorities, recent immigrants, and individuals with other types of emotional/behavioral problems (e.g., social anxiety), or any chronic physical disability or illness that might result in social isolation (e.g., HIV-infected children, youths, and adults) or compromise a client's ability to learn or use appropriate social skills. The CB strategies used in the final two case studies that assisted gay men in enhancing their social relationships likely are applicable to lesbian, bisexual, and transgender clients and to other vulnerable clients.

Practitioners also might find that some of the interventions can be applied in other settings. For example, some of the group SST programs that were conducted in school settings could be implemented in outpatient mental health clinics, inpatient and residential facilities, and medical and rehabilitation settings. Peer-mediated programs also might be applicable to vulnerable groups in after-school community programs, day-care centers, group homes, and other residential facilities (e.g., nursing homes).

Freedom, Control, and Social Justice

The interventions discussed in this chapter incorporate a variety of methods to enhance participants' input into and control over the intervention procedures. Group facilitators involve group members with physical disabilities in identifying specific behaviors that define the social skills targeted for change. The case studies using CB applications to assist gay men in enhancing their interpersonal relationships illustrate methods to incorporate individual goals and unique situations into standardized cognitive restructuring and exposure therapies. The modules developed for individuals with severe mental illness also assist clients in establishing their own goals and providing opportunities for clients to have input into the intervention process. Self-management strategies such as self-instruction, self-recording, self-reinforcement, and problem solving are yet other examples of CB interventions that enhance clients' control and freedom. The "Social Validity" section that follows also describes additional methods to individualize interventions, which can increase clients' freedom and control.

Several of the interventions also address a legitimate criticism of CB interventions, such as SST, from an empowerment perspective. That is, the trainer frequently uses methods such as instruction, modeling, and prompting without first determining whether such methods are even required. These types of practices can send a message to clients that they possess no social skills and also can inhibit the practitioner from building on the skills clients already possess. Practitioners could address these concerns by providing an opportunity for clients to exhibit the skills, then using more intrusive or comprehensive interventions only if needed. Finally, after clients learn the relevant skills, decrease their anxiety, and/or change their negative cognitions, their freedom is enhanced. They now have a choice whether to engage in social interactions and to develop relationships with others.

The goals of the previously discussed CB interventions are consistent with a social justice perspective. Increasing the ability of vulnerable children, youths, and adults to access social resources, such as engaging others in play, conversation, and other social activity, forming relationships with others, and increasing social integration into school, work, and community settings, all are consistent with the value of social justice. In addition, some of the interventions sensitize individuals with no disabilities to the unique problems and communicative behaviors of their peers with disabilities. If these interventions enhance the positive perceptions of able-bodied persons toward and increase their social initiations with their peers with disabilities, these activities and outcomes also are consistent with a social justice perspective.

Social Validity

Socially relevant goals and results. Designers of the interventions discussed in this chapter frequently established the social validity of their intervention goals by citing the shared social value of the goals. Society values vulnerable groups acquiring basic social skills, engaging in social interactions, forming relationships, and becoming socially integrated. However, the majority of the intervention goals were related to increasing conversations, other types of social interactions, or the quality of the social interactions (e.g., staying on the conversational topic). More meaningful goals, such as forming friendships or romantic relationships, were less frequently established. Of course, for some clients (e.g., those with severe autism) a goal such as forming romantic relationships is likely to be unrealistic. Only in rare circumstances do the interventions accommodate individual goal setting, which would be particularly important from a social validity and empowerment perspective. These observations suggest the need for researchers to develop and evaluate CB interventions that achieve more socially relevant goals related to enhancing social interactions. Practitioners also must ensure that the goals established with clients are socially valid. That is, the goals are individualized, meaningful, and take into consideration the clients' unique characteristics, including their capabilities, culture, socioeconomic background, gender, sexual orientation, and race/ethnicity.

Other methods that might be adopted by practitioners were used to establish the social relevance of the instrumental (e.g., increasing specific social skills) and ultimate (e.g., initiating conversations and forming relationships) goals of the interventions. Examples of the methods include surveying teachers, parents, peers, participants, and residential staff; observing social behavior and naturally occurring sequences; and examining the research literature that establishes relations between an outcome measure (e.g., a particular social skill) and relevant individual characteristics (e.g., likeability).

Evaluations of the interventions provide at least some evidence that the interventions can achieve the stated intervention goals. However, as previously discussed, increases in conversations, verbal responses, or other social interactions between clients and others (e.g., between students with disabilities and their able-bodied peers) in limited contexts do not necessarily demonstrate that the interactions are meaningful or that the client is socially competent. Being socially competent involves judgments or evaluations of specific social behavior within and across multiple contexts (Haring & Breen, 1992; McMahon et al., 1996).

Despite the previously mentioned problems, evaluations of the CB interventions provide suggestions for practitioners and researchers to determine whether enhanced social interactions (e.g., increases in the appropriateness, quality, and duration of social interactions; social integration into a variety of settings; social acceptance; and friendship formation) are socially meaningful to clients. Examples of these methods include observing interactions in natural settings and interviewing and surveying clients and significant others (e.g., parents, teachers, residential staff, job coaches, peers) with questionnaires requiring qualitative judgments of the relevance of the treatment gains.

Comparing outcomes with a normative sample of peers is another method for establishing the social validity of treatment results for vulnerable clients. Some researchers (e.g., McMahon et al., 1996), however, question the relevance of using the interactions of "normal" children and youths as a standard for many vulnerable clients, such as those with disabilities. For clients with multiple and/or severe disabilities, defining meaningful change must be placed in the context of their disability and capabilities. For example, improvements might be made in an autistic child's ability to initiate conversations, yet his speech does not sound natural. For some clients that might be an acceptable outcome, or their speech might eventually become more spontaneous (Stevenson et al., 2000). Identifying and measuring meaningful behaviors and goals, although important for all clients, are particularly relevant and challenging in work with vulnerable populations.

Socially relevant intervention procedures. From a social validity perspective, a serious limitation of the previously discussed interventions, and one that is important in both practice and research, was the failure to conduct individualized assessments prior to intervention. In many of the evaluations, participants frequently were referred for intervention based on someone's casual assessment that a social skills deficit was the main cause of their social isolation. Although baselines of target social skills were measured, rarely were functional assessments completed to determine other possible maintaining conditions of the low levels of social interactions. As a behavioral assessment can determine, a lack of social skills might not be the (or the only) maintaining antecedent preventing an individual from engaging in social interactions. For example, psychological problems (e.g., anxiety or depression), a lack of accommodations for a physical or cognitive impairment, poor grooming or dress, and environmental factors (e.g., home access for clients with mobility limitations and seating arrangements and meal style for residents in institutional settings) can impede social interactions even among socially skilled clients. Experiencing negative consequences, such as rejection or ridicule after attempting to initiate social interactions, would likely inhibit even socially skilled clients from future attempts to engage in social interactions with others. Practitioners and researchers will likely be more successful in assisting vulnerable clients in increasing their social resources if they conduct a thorough individual assessment before designing and implementing their interventions.

None of the studies involved participants or significant others in developing or evaluating the acceptability, feasibility, and relevance of the interventions (e.g., components of SST) before they were implemented. Practitioners and researchers, however, might learn from methods that were used in the previously described interventions to increase the social validity of their intervention materials and procedures. Examples include using models with similar characteristics as the participants, surveying and observing peers with and without disabilities to identify the high-interest conversation topics and social scenarios used in the SST, and involving elderly individuals in decision making regarding nursing home design changes. Accommodating the unique situations of clients by individualizing the materials, activities, and interventions also will likely enhance the social relevance of the interventions. For example, topics of conversation in communication books can be individualized through surveys of clients and significant others. Clients can select from predetermined situations for rehearsal only those that have personal relevance, and they can provide their own personal situations for practice and problem solving. Practitioners also can teach clients problem-solving strategies, which can assist clients in selecting responses to social situations that best solve the problem in the context of their own lives.

If their interventions are to be acceptable and feasible, practitioners also must accommodate the special characteristics and circumstances of vulnerable clients. Examples of such accommodations are incorporated into many of the interventions discussed in this chapter. For individuals with hearing impairments, the identified skills and self-management strategies can be posted on walls and floors. Peers participating in SST can be sensitized to the special communication behaviors of children with disabilities (e.g., providing instruction, examples, and having the peers simulate the children's disabilities). Puppets can be used to model social skills, and games can be incorporated into SST for clients with limited cognitive abilities. For clients with communication difficulties, mechanical or electronic devices, such as the Language Master and Touch Talker, or a specially designed communication book can be used as a communication medium. Simply reducing external distractions; keeping training tasks brief, focused, and slow paced; and teaching techniques to control psychiatric symptoms can accommodate the special needs of individuals diagnosed with schizophrenia. Finally, individuals can be recruited to assist clients in carrying out the interventions, such as writing letters for elderly clients involved in the RSVP intervention when the clients are unable to do so. All of these examples highlight the importance of practitioners and researchers assessing the need for and identifying socially relevant methods and materials that accommodate the special needs of vulnerable clients.

Evaluations of the interventions also suggest methods that practitioners and researchers might use to measure the social validity of their interventions during and after formal treatment. The methods include surveying, interviewing, and observing participants and others involved in the interventions to determine the feasibility and acceptability of the interventions. The request of school officials to continue the group intervention to enhance the social interactions of students with emotional/behavioral problems is another example of a social validity measure. In almost all cases in which the acceptability of the interventions was evaluated, the participants and significant others reported approval and satisfaction with the procedures. This suggests that practitioners need not be hesitant in offering the interventions described in this chapter to their clients and involved others. However, other social validity issues must be considered. For example, CB interventions conducted in school settings might not be feasible because of teachers' time constraints and because some teachers' philosophy of child-directed play conflicts with structured training. Issues such as time constraints and conflicts with values and philosophies certainly will limit the acceptability of interventions across settings, clients, and others involved in the intervention process. Other issues of intervention social validity that are important for practitioners and researchers to consider when using or developing CB interventions include the training required to design individual materials (e.g., for the communication book) and to carry out the interventions and the cost of specialized equipment (e.g., the Touch Talker).

Maintenance and generalization. The CB interventions discussed in this chapter demonstrate that maintaining and/or transferring treatment gains to multiple natural settings, as well as to different individuals, materials, and contexts, are frequently overlooked or inadequately measured. However, practitioners, as well as future researchers, might adopt generalization and maintenance strategies that are incorporated into the interventions. The strategies include teaching social skills in natural environments, such as work, school, and residential settings. Using multiple settings, instructors, peers, materials, and relevant examples of situations and responses and having clients practice a variety of appropriate social skills in different contexts are other strategies that appear to generalize treatment gains. However, practitioners also must assess possible negative consequences of using some of these strategies. For example, English et al. (1997) believed that peer rotation was the main reason for friendships failing to develop between the "peer buddies" and the preschoolers with developmental disabilities. The researchers speculated that rotating the peers, which was expected to increase transfer of the social skills to multiple peers, resulted in insufficient time for friendships to develop.

Assigning homework to practice the relevant skills in real-life settings and coordinating and eliciting the assistance of significant others (e.g., peers, teachers, staff, and case managers) to provide clients with opportunities to practice the skills, prompting, feedback, and reinforcement are other maintenance/generalization strategies that practitioners might use. Fading artificial prompts or monitoring devices and pairing artificial reinforcers with social reinforcers, then gradually thinning them, are additional methods.

Teaching self-management strategies to increase client awareness of performance of the identified skills (e.g., self-instruction, self-monitoring, and self-reinforcement) and teaching problem solving, instead of rote memorization, to identify appropriate responses also might increase generalization and/or maintenance of treatment gains. However, before using self-management strategies, practitioners must assess whether clients have the necessary cognitive ability, motivation, and skills for monitoring and self-reinforcing appropriate responses. Altering social environments, for example, changing classmates' perceptions of and attitudes toward students with disabilities, also is likely to enhance maintenance and/or transfer of social skills and interactions to natural settings. Finally, practitioners can hold booster sessions to refresh clients' skills and to assist them in coping with unexpected situations and obstacles, thus increasing the likelihood that the acquired skills and enhanced social interactions will be maintained or continue to increase.

Even if practitioners and researchers use the strategies incorporated into the previously discussed interventions, they likely will be challenged when assisting vulnerable clients in maintaining gains in social skills and personal interactions and in transferring the gains to multiple natural settings. For example, few methods are used to assist clients in recognizing the appropriate contexts in which to use their acquired skills, even when the skills are taught in natural settings. Another neglected area is preparing clients to cope with negative responses from others or with other adverse outcomes after using their acquired social skills and establishing relationships. The reality check incorporated into the joining-in group SST is an example of a method of preparing clients for such situations. Unfortunately, few of the interventions included such strategies, even when negative consequences were observed. For example, Breen et al. (1989) reported observing negative reactions from some co-workers after youths with autism attempted to initiate conversations with them. The researchers, however, did not report assisting the youths in coping with such consequences. If practitioners do not adequately prepare clients to cope with negative or less-than-desirable responses after they initiate or engage in interactions with others, these consequences likely will result in fewer attempts to initiate and maintain social interactions and relationships. This particularly would be the case for clients with a history of negative reactions from others because of their disability, sexual orientation, or other minority status.

If treatment gains are to be maintained and transferred to natural settings, practitioners must assess and ensure that necessary prompts and reinforcement, as well as other needed support, are in place before ending formal treatment. McMahon et al. (1996), for example, questioned whether interactions between children with mental retardation and their peers without cognitive limitations would be maintained and/or generalized to settings that include play and other materials unsuitable for children with cognitive limitations. In these circumstances, the peers might choose activities that are more interesting to them and to their peers with similar cognitive levels, which could exclude children with mental retardation. Given the limited conversation and social interaction skills of clients with some types of disabilities even after intervention (e.g., severe autism and mental retardation), whether their social initiations or relationships with peers without disabilities can be maintained and/or transferred to a variety of natural settings is unclear. For example, will peer networks and interactions with "buddies" continue without some type of support or reinforcement from adults?

For other interventions, ongoing support clearly is needed to maintain the social resources. For example, in the RSVP intervention, someone must write letters for elderly nursing home residents when they are unable to do so. These observations suggest that practitioners must evaluate the need for and ensure that required resources and support are in place before withdrawing involvement. Many times withdrawing prompts, reinforcement, and other structures (e.g., ongoing peer meetings) might be inappropriate. Such withdrawals might result in the client's loss of treatment gains and in feelings of demoralization and hopelessness.

Although many of the evaluations of the interventions described in this chapter provided evidence that the intervention gains transferred to novel individuals and settings, the individuals and settings usually were within the same organization or institution in which formal intervention took place. The majority of the interventions lack methods to coordinate treatment among various settings, such as among the school and the family and community. Providing case managers for clients diagnosed with schizophrenia is an example of coordinating efforts to maintain and transfer social skills learned in treatment settings to the family and community. Liberman and his colleagues (2002) describe the use of In Vivo Amplified Skills Training (IVAST), which incorporates case managers trained in CB techniques. The case managers serve as a liaison for clients with other treatment staff, family members, and community agencies to create opportunities for, encourage, and reinforce the clients' continued use of the acquired skills. An evaluation of the IVAST suggests that clients obtain quicker and greater improvements on measures of social functioning (including items related to relationships) compared with clients who receive only SST (Glynn et al., 2002).

Given the multiple needs of many vulnerable clients, practitioners who coordinate treatment with significant others across multiple settings likely will assist their clients in maintaining and transferring treatment gains. However, involving significant others, such as teachers and parents, in carrying out the interventions in natural settings presents other challenges. The challenges include training time, ensuring the integrity of the interventions, and determining the acceptability of the interventions as a result of significant others' socioeconomic background, gender, race/ethnicity, culture, values, and other personal circumstances.

This chapter provided multiple examples of different combinations of CB strategies that can empower the elderly; sexual minorities; and children, youths, and adults with a variety of disabilities by assisting them in enhancing their social interactions. The next chapter describes CB interventions that empower vulnerable populations by teaching skills and providing resources to increase their leisure, recreational, and related activity in residential, school, and other community settings.

ADDITIONAL READINGS AND RESOURCES

Bellack, A. S. (2004). Skills training for people with severe mental illness. *Psychiatric Rehabilitation Journal, 27,* 375–391.

Cartledge, G., & Milburn, J. F. (Eds.). (1995). *Teaching social skills to children and youth: Innovative approaches.* Boston: Allyn & Bacon.

Curl, R. M., & Hall, S. M. (1990). *Put that person to work! A manual for implementors using the coworker transition model.* Logan, UT: Utah State University.

Donohue, B., Acierno, R., Hersen, M., & Van Hasselt, V. B. (1995). Social skills training for depressed, visually impaired older adults: A treatment manual. *Behavior Modification, 19,* 379–424.

Gambrill, E. (1985). Social skills training with the elderly. In L. L'Abate & M. A. Milan (Eds.), *Handbook of social skills training and research* (pp. 326–357). New York: Wiley.

Hunt, P., Alwell, M., & Goetz, L. (1990). *Teaching conversation skills to individuals with severe disabilities with a communication book adaptation: Instructional handbook.* Conversation and Social Competence Project. San Francisco: San Francisco State University.

Kopelowicz, A. (1998). Adapting social skills training for Latinos with schizophrenia. *International Review of Psychiatry, 10,* 47–50.

Laushey, K. M., & Heflin, L. J. (2000). Enhancing social skills of kindergarten children with autism through the training of multiple peers as tutors. *Journal of Autism and Developmental Disorders, 30,* 183–193.

LeCroy, C. W. (2006). Social skills training in school settings: Some practical considerations. In R. Constable, C. R. Massat, S. McDonald, & J. P. Flynn (Eds.), *School social work: Practice, policy, and research* (6th ed., pp. 599–617). Chicago: Lyceum.

Lemanek, K. L., Williamson, D. A., Gresham, F. M., & Jensen, B. J. (1986). Social skills training with hearing-impaired children and adolescents. *Behavior Modification, 10,* 55–71.

Liberman, R. P., DeRisi, W. J., & Mueser, K. T. (1989). *Social skills training for psychiatric patients.* New York: Pergamon.

McClannahan, L. E., & Krantz, P. J. (2004). Some guidelines for selecting behavioral intervention programs for children with autism. In H. E. Briggs & T. L. Rzepnicki (Eds.), *Using evidence in social work practice: Behavioral perspectives* (pp. 92–103). Chicago: Lyceum.

Olmeda, R. E., & Kauffman, J. M. (2003). Sociocultural considerations in social skills training research with African American students with emotional or behavioral disorders. *Journal of Developmental and Physical Disabilities, 15,* 101–121.

Peeks, A. L. (1999). Conducting a social skills group with Latina adolescents. *Journal of Child and Adolescent Group Therapy, 9,* 139–153.

Pollard, N. L. (1998). Development of social interaction skills in preschool children with autism: A review of the literature. *Child and Family Behavior Therapy, 20,* 1–16.

Princeton Child Development Institute, 300 Cold Soil Rd., Princeton, NJ 08540. Private nonprofit program offering a broad spectrum of science-based services to children, youths, and adults with autism. Available at http://www.pcdi.org/

Sommer, K. S., Whitman, T. L., Keogh, D. A. (1988). Teaching severely retarded persons to sign interactively through the use of a behavioral script. *Research in Developmental Disabilities, 9,* 291–304.

Storey, K., & Provost, O. (1996). The effect of communication skills instruction on the integration of workers with severe disabilities in supported employment settings. *Education and Training in Mental Retardation and Developmental Disabilities, 31,* 123–141

UCLA Center for Research on Treatment and Rehabilitation of Psychosis, West LA VA Medical Center, 11301 Wilshire Blvd., Los Angeles, CA 90073. Ordering information for skills training modules, related assessment tools, and training materials available at http://www.mentalhealth.ucla.edu/projects/irc/index.html or through Psychiatric Rehabilitation Consultants, P.O. Box 2867, Camarillo, CA 93011. Available at http://www.psychrehab.com

Webb, B. J., Miller, S. P., Pierce, T. B., Strawser, S., & Jones, W. P. (2004). Effects of social skill instruction for high-functioning adolescents with autism spectrum disorders. *Focus on Autism and Other Developmental Disabilities, 19,* 53–62.

Wong, S. E. (1996). Psychosis. In M. A. Mattaini & B. A. Thyer (Eds.), *Finding solutions to social problems: Behavioral strategies for change* (pp. 319–344). Washington, DC: American Psychological Association.

5 Increasing Leisure, Recreational, and Related Activity

As discussed in chapter 4, individuals with physical, developmental, psychiatric, and learning disabilities and sensory impairments have a variety of limitations arising from their disability. These problems can interfere with learning the skills necessary to engage in and access available recreational, leisure, and other community activity. In addition, caregivers, residential and group home staff, and educators frequently fail to provide opportunities for those with disabilities to engage in meaningful recreational and leisure activity. The inability to accommodate the special needs of some vulnerable individuals (e.g., those with communication problems) and to teach relevant skills might contribute to these limited opportunities. The elderly who reside in nursing homes or other residential facilities frequently have low levels of involvement in meaningful recreational and leisure activity, which can contribute to boredom, social isolation, and an unrewarding life.

This chapter discusses CB interventions that empower vulnerable individuals by assisting them in learning relevant skills and in accessing leisure, recreational, and other activities in their residences, schools, and communities. Vulnerable populations include children, youths, and adults with physical disabilities, learning and developmental problems (mental retardation and autism), multiple disabilities, and severe mental illness, and the elderly. The interventions are presented first for vulnerable children and youths, then for adults. The chapter ends with a more critical summary of the interventions and draws additional applications for practitioners and researchers.

INTERVENTIONS FOR VULNERABLE CHILDREN AND YOUTHS

Advocates for students with disabilities argue that increasing their involvement in integrated physical education classes and other school activities is an important educational and social goal. These experiences not only can develop lifetime leisure and recreational pursuits but also can increase opportunities for vulnerable students to learn appropriate social behavior and to form friendships. Engaging in meaningful leisure and recreational activity in private residences, residential facilities, and other community settings also can reduce boredom; enhance psychological, social, and physical well-being; and promote community integration (Hughes et al., 2004).

CB interventions for children and youths with physical disabilities, mental retardation, autism, and multiple disabilities are described in this chapter. The interventions can be conducted in educational and vocational settings, private homes, residential facilities, and in other community settings. The six CB programs described here use a variety of strategies, many of which accommodate the special needs of children and youths with disabilities. The interventions include traditional SST, modeling, self-instruction, prompting (e.g., verbal, physical, and constant time delay), reinforcement, and booster sessions. Using a fanny pack to facilitate independently paying for restaurant food, identifying critical moments for instruction that can facilitate learning, and designing picture books to communicate the desire to engage in a particular leisure or recreational activity are examples of special accommodations.

Three of the CB intervention programs involve caregivers (e.g., parents, adult siblings, house parents, and personal assistants). One intervention involves peers with disabilities, and another recruits able-bodied peers to serve as recreational partners. All but one of the interventions were evaluated using multiple-baseline designs.

Children and Youths with Physical Disabilities

Sowers and Powers (1995) developed a behavioral intervention to assist adolescents with cerebral palsy or muscular dystrophy in achieving their personal goal of eating at a fast-food community restaurant more independently. The intervention was designed for clients who use power scooters or wheelchairs as a means of mobility and have limited communication skills and arm and hand control. Parents and personal assistants are involved in carrying out the intervention.

The general tasks targeted for learning include ordering, eating, and cleaning one's eating area in a fast-food restaurant. In developing the steps for each task, practitioners should consult the client's physical therapist to determine whether the client needs to use an adaptive strategy. If adaptations are necessary, the practitioner must identify strategies that would assist the client in performing the step with the most independence. For example, if a client has difficulty manipulating money and recognizing its value, for the step "Get money out," a strategy might be to take one $5 bill out of a conveniently positioned fanny pack (see table 1, Sowers & Powers, 1995, p. 213 for the twenty-nine identified steps and an example of a student's strategy guide). SST is then used to teach the identified steps to the client in an artificial setting (e.g., a conference room in a school) using the client's preferred food. When the client rehearses each step involved in eating in a fast-food restaurant more independently, the practitioner provides assistance only if the client is unable to successfully perform the task.

After the client masters the steps, the practitioner then uses SST to teach the client's parent or personal assistant methods to assist the client in using community fast-food restaurants more independently. The practitioner provides the caregiver with a rationale for the strategies, a strategy guide describing the specially designed methods for the client to perform each step, and six general rules for assisting and encouraging the client to participate independently. The rules include the following steps:

1. Review the steps with the client before leaving the residence.
2. Allow the client sufficient time to perform the task before assisting.
3. When assistance is given, provide only the amount necessary for the client to perform the task.
4. If an error is made, give the client the opportunity to correct it before assisting.
5. If an employee of the restaurant attempts to interact with the caregiver, direct him or her to the client.
6. After leaving the restaurant, discuss the client's feelings of pride in his or her ability to perform the tasks more independently; discuss any steps the client was unable to perform easily and provide suggestions on ways the client could perform the step more easily or independently in the future.

After the caregiver learns the tasks of eating independently in a fast-food restaurant and the general rules for encouraging independence, the client practices the tasks, while the caregiver provides any needed instruction, feedback, and assistance.

After intervention and at a six-week follow-up, the three adolescents (ages 14, 15, and 18 years) participating in the evaluation demonstrated dramatic increases in their participation and independence in eating at community fast-food restaurants. Two of the three adolescents reported being "pretty sure" they could continue to perform the steps (one indicated he was "not so sure"). All three participants reported that they were a "lot more sure" they could do other things more independently after learning to eat at the restaurants more independently. The caregivers responded to the same questions in a similar way. Two of the caregivers also reported that after intervention the youths were independently using their acquired skills in other settings.

Children and Youths with Learning/Developmental Problems

This self-instructional program can be used to increase the social leisure activity of adolescents with severe mental retardation residing in a residential facility (Keogh, Faw, Whitman, & Reid, 1984). Commercially available games (e.g., *Ants in the Pants* and *Ring Toss*) that require cooperation, turn taking, and learning game steps are used in the intervention. The practitioner begins by modeling the game steps for two or more residents while self-instructing. The residents then perform the game steps while the practitioner verbalizes the self-instructions. Following this step, the practitioner prompts the residents to use self-instruction and to perform the game steps. If a resident does not respond appropriately, the practitioner asks the other players if they could help. If the other players cannot provide the necessary assistance, instructions are given, and physical prompts and guidance are provided as necessary. To promote interactions and to enhance generalization, the practitioner prompts the residents to praise each other (e.g., "John, tell Sue she did a good job"). Edible and social reinforcers also are used when the residents appropriately and continuously play the games. If the initial intervention does not result in the resident's playing the game at a satisfactory level, other prompts can be added. For example, the practitioner can use minimal (e.g., "John, what are you supposed to do next?") and specific (e.g., "Sue, pick up a card") verbal prompts to perform a game step. Physical prompts also can be used, such as blocking inappropriate responses. If the game-playing skills do not transfer to a free play setting, the practitioner can use prompts and social reinforcers in that setting as well.

After intervention, the two male residents who participated in the evaluation increased their self-instructions, ability to play three different games requiring relatively complex skills, and verbal interactions. No changes were made in the two residents who served as controls. However, prompts and praise were necessary to maintain the skills and to transfer the game-playing skills to other settings. In addition, a booster session was required five to eighteen weeks later when a follow-up evaluation determined that game proficiency was low.

Caregivers (e.g., adult siblings, house parents, parents) can be taught a constant time delay (CTD) procedure to teach leisure skills to adolescents with moderate to severe mental retardation or autism (Wall & Gast, 1997b). Based on observations and consultations with the adolescents and their caregivers, the practitioner identifies three leisure activities for each client (e.g., playing card or table games, horseshoes, and croquet). Although the interventions are conducted in the client's residence, multiple exemplars (i.e., different types of leisure materials, recreational partners, times of day, and settings) are used to facilitate generalization of the skills. After using SST to teach the caregivers the CTD procedure described in the next paragraph (for more details, see Wall & Gast, 1997a), the practitioner assists the caregivers in using the procedure to teach the adolescents the skills involved in the first leisure activity. The caregivers then independently teach the adolescents the skills required for the other activities.

The intervention sessions begin with the caregiver providing an anticipatory cue, for example, "We had a great time playing with cards yesterday." This cue is followed by the caregiver giving an attentional cue requiring an appropriate response. For example, the caregiver asks the adolescent to show her the card game. The caregiver then makes a task request specific to the activity she is teaching. For example, for a card game, the caregiver asks the adolescent to deal the cards. The CTD procedure is used after the caregiver makes a task request or encourages the adolescent to continue the activity. The caregiver immediately follows the task request or encouragement to continue with a controlling prompt. For example, the caregiver gives direct verbal instruction or points to a correct location. During subsequent sessions, a four-second time delay is used. That is, after the caregiver gives a natural cue, a verbal task request, or encouragement, she waits four seconds. If the adolescent does not respond, only then does the caregiver use a controlling prompt. If the response is inappropriate, the caregiver interrupts the response and delivers a controlling prompt. Caregivers also provide reinforcers for appropriate responses and play. Evaluation of the intervention indicated that caregivers were successful in teaching the leisure skills to the four male adolescent participants. The game-playing skills were maintained over a two-month period.

Children and Youths with Multiple Disabilities

CTD procedures also can be used to teach purchasing skills to high school–aged students with a variety of physical and developmental disabilities (DiPipi-Hoy & Jitendra, 2004). These skills would be necessary to purchase many items related to recreational and leisure activity. Practitioners teach the CTD intervention to parents, who then use the intervention to teach their adolescents purchasing skills while shopping in community stores. Based on consultation with each parent and youth, the practitioner selects the target purchasing skills. Planning sessions also are held with the parent and youth to develop an instructional plan and to identify relevant social reinforcers (e.g., verbal praise, smiles) and prompts (e.g., "Pay the cashier").

The practitioner then teaches the parents the CTD procedures using SST techniques. The techniques include providing a rationale for using the procedures, a description of the procedures (which include task direction, verbal prompt, two-second delay, and feedback), modeling the procedures, and role playing the procedures with the parents. The parents also view a video in which a model uses the CTD procedures to teach an adolescent to withdraw cash from an ATM machine. Finally, the parents use the same procedures to teach their adolescents purchasing skills in the community. When the parent and youth arrive at the community store, the parent provides a rationale for each skill. For example, the parent might tell the adolescent that the purpose of shopping is to purchase specific items (e.g., paints and a paint brush for painting pictures). Parents precede each step in the purchasing activity with a verbal prompt, such as requesting the youth to get a specific item. The parent waits for two seconds for the youth to respond and then delivers feedback in the form of verbal praise for correct responses or verbal correction and modeling for incorrect responses. The interventions are gradually faded. The evaluation of the intervention suggested that the parents were able to successfully teach their daughters (three parent–female youth dyads participated in the evaluation) the skills needed to make purchases in the community. The skills were maintained six to eight weeks later. Social validity assessments also demonstrated that the parents and youths were highly satisfied with the intervention and its effectiveness.

This behavioral program assists severely disabled students with multiple physical, cognitive, and sensory disabilities in learning the specific skills necessary to engage in age-appropriate activities with their peers in public school and community settings (Gee, Graham, Sailor, & Goetz, 1995). Although the researchers modified the interventions to accommodate the special needs of four students, the interventions for only one student, Neil, are discussed here.

Neil was a 9-year-old student whose physical problems included a seizure disorder, quadriplegia, blindness, and a hearing impairment. Because of his multiple disabilities, Neil could only communicate through changes in affect and tone. After consultation with Neil's parents and teachers, three goals were identified. They included engaging in more integrated activities, increasing opportunities to meet able-bodied peers, and forming friendships. Consistent with these goals, the activity selected for Neil was selling ice cream with nondisabled students on the school playground. Based on a contextual analysis of students selling ice cream on the school playground (conducted by observing the activity as it was performed by other students) and clinical and educational assessments of Neil's abilities, four "critical instructional moments" to learn the specific skills needed to participate in the activity were identified. A critical moment is defined as the point at which (1) the natural setting events and social interactions within the activity provide the client with an identifiable cue to perform a specific behavior and (2) when the client performs the behavior, an easily identifiable desired impact on the social and/or physical environment results.

Because of the severity of Neil's disabilities, the skills involved small behaviors and sometimes required adaptations and/or facilitation by others. During intervention, the instructor used natural opportunities at critical moments to prompt the identified behaviors. The prompts were then faded through the gradual use of less physical assistance. For example, four critical instructional moments for one of Neil's four identified skills—holding onto items after he was assisted to grasp them—were identified. One critical moment was Neil's holding the money box while being assisted to place it on a tray. The first prompting procedure was placing the money box under Neil's arm. After he grasped the money box, the staff assisted him in holding it for a brief period. The final prompting procedure was placing the money box under Neil's palm (see table 1, Gee et al., 1995, p. 38, for the four skills, critical moments, performance criteria, and prompting procedures). Correct responses were reinforced by the natural consequence of continued participation in the activity, as well as by social reinforcers. At the end of the intervention, Neil could perform the skills needed to participate in selling ice cream on the school playground. Gee and her colleagues (1995) concluded that the results of the intervention for Neil, and also for the three other students, demonstrate the importance of intervening in natural settings. The researchers also concluded that with appropriate intervention, students with severe, multiple disabilities can participate in a variety of integrated general education and community activities.

The final intervention described in this section involves a SST program that assists students with mental retardation, speech or communication problems, and extensive educational support needs to initiate and engage in recreational activities with general education students (Hughes et al., 2004). The intervention is implemented during physical education classes after the teacher instructs all of the students to select a recreational or sport activity (e.g., volleyball, basketball, board and video games) and begin to play. First, the practitioner recruits general education students in the PE classes of the students with disabilities to be recreational partners during training sessions. The training partners are rotated randomly across the students with disabilities. Before intervention begins, the practitioner verifies with the students with disabilities that they want to engage in recreational activity and learn a described set of tasks to achieve that goal. To accommodate for the students' communication difficulties, a picture book containing two photographs is used during intervention. Using SST, the practitioner teaches the students with disabilities the following five steps (the instructional script is available from the authors):

1 Students pick up the picture book after the PE teacher instructs all of the students that "it's time to go do something."
2 Students look at and point to the first photograph depicting a youth holding an object, which prompts the students to choose an activity.
3 Students turn the page and look at and point to the second photograph showing several youths interacting with one another, which prompts them to ask a recreational partner to engage in the chosen activity.

4 Students put the picture book down and begin engaging in the activity with their partner.
5 Students self-evaluate their performance and whether they have met their recreational goals. That is, students meet with the practitioner and compare their responses to three questions—whether they chose an activity, asked a partner to participate, and initiated engagement in the activity—with their recreational goal.

All five of the African American ninth-grade students with disabilities (four females; one male) who participated in the intervention evaluation increased their initiations of recreational activities with their partners. Recreational participation in the PE classes, which was zero at baseline, became almost continuous after intervention. The students with disabilities and their recreational partners reported enjoying the interactions, and the students with disabilities reported making new friends. The students with disabilities also were able to evaluate their goal attainment accurately, and four of the five students found the picture book helpful. During the maintenance stage of the evaluation, the general education students continued to serve as recreational partners, recreational materials were placed close to the students, the instructor used the verbal cue ("It's time to do something"), and the students were handed their picture books.

INTERVENTIONS FOR VULNERABLE ADULTS

As is the case with children and youths with disabilities, increasing leisure, recreational, and related community activity for adults with disabilities is a valued personal and social goal. For adults with disabilities, the activities can enhance appropriate social and independent living skills, friendship development, physical and psychological well-being, and community integration (Wilson, Arnold, Rowland, & Burnham, 1997). Increasing the recreational and leisure activity of elderly residents in institutional facilities also can result in engagement in meaningful activity and enhanced social interactions. Before intervention, the elderly residents who participated in the programs discussed in this section spent most of their time in their rooms, where they rarely engaged in leisure/recreational activity or social interactions. In addition to enhancing social interactions and leisure/recreational activity, the CB interventions can empower vulnerable adults by assisting them in engaging in these activities more independently.

Twelve CB interventions for adults with physical disabilities, mental retardation, severe mental illness, and multiple disabilities and the elderly are discussed in this section. Several of the interventions were described in chapter 4. Because the interventions were designed to achieve goals related both to enhancing social interactions and to increasing recreational, leisure, and community activity, they also are briefly discussed in this chapter. The interventions for vulnerable adults involve a variety of CB strategies. They include enriching the environment (e.g., making a variety of leisure and recreational activities and materials available), providing instruction on the purposes and benefits of engaging in leisure/recreational activity, skills training, SST, prompting strategies (e.g., prompt hierarchies), reinforcement, and PST.

Many of the interventions accommodate the special needs of vulnerable adults. For example, communication devices (e.g., Touch Talker) are used to assist adults with physical disabilities who are unable to communicate effectively. To accommodate the special needs of clients with learning difficulties, strategies such as developing simpler versions of games and instructional materials and teaching finger counting to assist clients in paying for food at community restaurants are used. Peers, who serve as play, activity, and role-play partners, are involved in many of the interventions. Staff in residential facilities also are taught to carry out some of the interventions.

Researchers used experimental methods to evaluate several of the interventions discussed in this section (e.g., Brown & Munford, 1983; Marder et al., 1996). Other interventions were evaluated with reversal and pretest-posttest designs (Konarski, Johnson, & Whitman, 1980; McClannahan & Risley, 1975; Schleien, Kiernan, & Wehman, 1981). The remainder of the interventions were evaluated using multiple-baseline designs.

Adults with Physical Disabilities

The intervention developed by Dattilo and Camarata (1991) that teaches adults with cerebral palsy to use the Touch Talker, an augmentative communication system, was discussed in the previous chapter. Increasing clients' involvement in recreational and leisure activity, including placing food orders at a restaurant and asking others to participate in preferred recreational activities (e.g., playing cards and listening to music), is one of the goals and successful outcomes of the intervention. Practitioners working with clients who have a disability-related communication problem and desire to increase their recreational or leisure activity might find this intervention helpful.

Adults with Mental Retardation

Practitioners can increase the group home recreational and leisure activity of adults with moderate mental retardation by implementing a "leisure skills program" (Schleien et al., 1981). The program involves weekly leisure counseling sessions in which topics such as the purposes and benefits of engaging in leisure and recreational activity, the types of activities available, and the residents' interests are discussed. A variety of activities (e.g., dart game, playing cards, puzzles, billiard set, silk screening materials) are then made available, and the practitioner uses skills training to teach the residents the necessary skills for each activity. The residents also are encouraged to participate in their chosen leisure activities during their free time. A leisure skills tournament also is conducted, which begins with the residents, practitioner, and group home staff deciding on the tournament activities. A variety of reinforcers, including awards and certificates, are given to residents for demonstrating competency in the activities. Significant increases in the leisure behavior of the six residents involved in the program's evaluation were observed after intervention. However, ongoing weekly intervention was necessary to maintain the behavior.

Practitioners also can use behavioral techniques to teach adults with mental retardation to play cooperative games. For example, Nietupski and Svoboda's (1982) intervention teaches residents with severe mental retardation to play a lotto game. The game materials consist of two lotto boards, each containing four different photographs of objects the residents frequently observe in their residential facility (e.g., a bed, dresser, bus, peer, lunch tray). The call cards consist of eight photographs corresponding to those on the lotto boards. The practitioner teaches the residents to shuffle the call cards, stack them, select each call card, and match it on their own boards or pass it to their opponent until one player covers the entire lotto board. The resident then indicates that he or she is the winner. To teach the residents the lotto game skills, the practitioner uses a "systematic prompt hierarchy." This involves using the next level of intervention only if the resident needs assistance. The hierarchy is as follows.

1 Indirect verbal cue (e.g., "What do you do with the card, Jim")
2 Direct verbal cue (e.g., "Jim, give the card to Sue")
3 Modeling and rehearsal
4 Physical prompting

The practitioner also provides social and edible reinforcers for correct responses. By the end of the intervention, the six adult residents involved in the evaluation performed the lotto game without external reinforcers. Staff observed the residents initiating and playing the game two weeks later in the game room where it was taught, as well as in another room of the facility. Finally, staff observed that the residents appeared to enjoy the game.

A novel intervention developed by O'Reilly and his colleagues (O'Reilly, Lancioni, & Kierans, 2000) teaches adult group home residents with moderate mental retardation the social skills for ordering drinks in a local bar. A general task analysis of the basic social skills for ordering drinks identified the five skills that are the focus of the training. The skills include greeting the bar staff, establishing and maintaining eye contact with the bar staff during interaction, ordering a drink, accepting the drink and thanking the bar staff, and paying for the drink. The therapist implements a social skills problem-solving intervention, which teaches the clients decoding, decision, performance, and evaluation rules, to generate the appropriate social skills for ordering drinks in a bar. The questions and statements trained for the decoding, decision, performance, and evaluation skills for ordering drinks appear in table 5.1.

The intervention is designed to be implemented with pairs of clients in their group home. In carrying out the intervention, the therapist describes the social context (i.e., the bar staff asks what the client would like to drink) and then models the social rules and social skills. The therapist then role-plays the skills with one of the clients, who verbalizes the rules and social skills, as the second client observes.

After intervention, the four male and female group home residents participating in the evaluation were able to correctly perform the identified social skills in the local bar. Approximately three years later, the residents maintained their social skills of ordering a drink and also generalized the skills to two other bars. Although the therapist did not teach social skills for interacting with patrons, social interactions among all of the four residents and other bar patrons increased substantially after intervention. The residents also reported increased comfort when visiting the local bar and increased pleasure from interacting with the bar staff and other patrons.

Storey, Bates, and Hanson (1984) developed prompting strategies to teach adults with mild to severe mental retardation coffee purchasing skills in a

Table 5.1. Questions and Statements Trained for Decoding, Decision, Performance, and Evaluation Skills for Ordering Drinks

Decoding
What's happening?
The bar staff has asked me if I want a drink.

Deciding
What should I do?
I could say nothing.
I could order a drink.
I will order a drink.

Performing (see social skills provided in the text)

Evaluating
What happened when I ordered a drink?
The bar staff brought me the drink that I wanted.
Did I do the right thing?
Yes.

Note. From "Teaching Leisure Social Skills to Adults with Moderate Mental Retardation: An Analysis of Acquisition, Generalization, and Maintenance," by M. F. O'Reilly, G. E. Lancioni, and I. Kierans, 2000, *Education and Training in Mental Retardation and Developmental Disabilities, 35,* p. 254. Copyright 2000 by the Division on Mental Retardation and Developmental Disabilities. Adapted with permission.

community sit-down restaurant. The practitioner teaches the skills, which are broken down into a number of steps involving general activities (e.g., sitting down, ordering, drinking the coffee, and paying the cashier), using a prompt hierarchy of least to greatest prompts. In carrying out the intervention, the practitioner first gives the clients an opportunity to perform the step. If they cannot perform the step appropriately, the practitioner provides verbal instruction, followed by gestures, minimal physical guidance, then total physical guidance. Correct responses are followed by social reinforcers. At the end of the intervention, the six adults involved in the evaluation could appropriately order coffee as well as customers with no cognitive limitations. The adults also were able to generalize the skills to two other sit-down restaurants and one fast-food restaurant. They maintained the skills two to five months later.

Adults with Severe Mental Illness

Increasing the use of community recreational and leisure resources is among the many outcome measures of a life skills training program involving psychiatric inpatients diagnosed with chronic schizophrenia (Brown & Munford, 1983). Using group SST, group facilitators teach both nonverbal and verbal skills. Examples of nonverbal skills include eye contact, voice tone, and verbal content. Carrying on a friendly conversation and using a telephone to obtain information about community social activities are examples of verbal social skills. As homework, the patients practice the skills on the ward, and they perform tasks related to recreational/leisure activity in community settings. Examples of tasks are dining in a restaurant and obtaining information about related community resources. The program was evaluated through the random assignment of clients (N = 28 males) to the life skills training or to a traditional VA rehabilitation program. The SST group performed better on overall interpersonal skills and on self-report measures, including the use of community recreational and leisure resources.

One of the modules developed at the UCLA CRTRP contains skills training in "recreation for leisure" (Liberman & Corrigan, 1993; see chapter 4 for the SST and problem-solving intervention used to teach the skills and ordering information for the Recreation for Leisure module). The target skills include the following.

1 Identify the benefits of various recreational activities and choose activities based on their desired benefits.
2 Obtain information about the activities and determine how to use them.
3 Identify the resources needed before starting the activity.

4 Judge whether an activity is enjoyable and worth continuing.
5 Make a long-term plan for engaging in the chosen activities.

Unfortunately, research examining the effects of the different modules developed at the UCLA CRTRP failed to evaluate whether teaching a specific module, such as "recreation for leisure," results in achieving the respective goal. However, the Marder et al. study (1996) discussed in chapter 4 determined that particular groups of clients diagnosed with schizophrenia who received training in a series of modules had an advantage over clients receiving supportive group therapy. One of the advantages was increased involvement in leisure interests and activities. A later study (Liberman et al., 1998), however, found no relation between modular training and participation in leisure and recreational activity for a group of clients diagnosed with persistent schizophrenia.

Adults with Multiple Disabilities

Practitioners also can use behavioral techniques to teach adults diagnosed with mental retardation and at least one other physical or emotional disability to order and eat a meal in a fast-food restaurant. The instruction, which was developed as a component of a community survival skills program for clients with multiple disabilities, teaches four main skill areas: locating, ordering, paying, and eating and exiting (Van den Pol et al., 1981). The practitioner teaches the adults the restaurant skills in a classroom, rather than in a natural setting, by showing slides demonstrating the skills, followed by other SST strategies. Simulated materials (e.g., a counter and wall menus) are used during intervention, in addition to other techniques that accommodate the level of the clients' cognitive abilities. For example, to assist the clients in determining whether the cashier gives them accurate change, the practitioner teaches the following procedure.

> First, round up the cost of the meal to the nearest dollar and raise the corresponding number of fingers on one hand, the "cost hand."
> Second, raise the number of fingers corresponding to the number of dollars paid to the cashier on the other hand, the "amount paid hand."
> Third, match the number of fingers raised on the "cost hand" with the number of fingers raised on the "amount paid hand." The number of unmatched fingers equals the number of dollars owed.

After intervention, the three young male adults involved in the evaluation were able to successfully use their skills in a community fast-food restaurant. The skills generalized to another fast-food restaurant and were maintained up to one year later. The participants' skill levels also were judged to be comparable to the performance of a normative sample of individuals with no cognitive limitations.

Halasz-Dees and Cuvo (1986) demonstrated that behavioral methods can be used in a rehabilitation setting to enhance the leisure skills of clients with mental retardation and a variety of physical and mental health problems. This particular intervention teaches clients macrame skills and the appropriate social skills required to buy the materials needed for the activity. Using SST, the practitioner teaches the twenty-four identified tasks needed to successfully purchase the macrame material. Examples of the tasks include finding transportation to and from the store, identifying and selecting the required materials, and purchasing the materials. The clients also are taught six basic macrame knots identified from consultion of a relevant book and individuals skilled in macrame. The practitioner teaches the skills using a commercially available instructional manual adapted to meet the learning needs of the clients (e.g., the manual provides additional detail and steps) and an "error sequence correction procedure." The clients are instructed to refer to the manual for each step and are given assistance only when they do not respond, respond incorrectly, or indicate that they need assistance.

For clients needing assistance, the intervention sequence is as follows. The practitioner verbally prompts the clients by instruction while showing them (1) a finished model of the knot, (2) a series of responses shown in hand drawings for each knot, and (3) a series of steps with actual jute cord glued onto each hand-drawn picture. In the final two steps of the correction procedure, the practitioner verbalizes the procedure for each step of the knot while modeling the step and finally provides verbal instruction while physically guiding the clients through each step. The practitioner also uses social reinforcement for correct responses. After the clients learn to tie basic knots, they independently use the instructional materials to complete additional macrame projects. The five clients involved in the evaluation learned, maintained, and generalized their skills, as evidenced by their shopping independently and making a novel project.

The Elderly

Three behavioral programs that can increase the involvement of elderly residents in leisure/recreational activity within institutionalized settings are discussed here. An early intervention developed for a skilled care nursing home consists of displaying puzzles and games for one hour in a common lounge, and prompting the residents to participate (McClannahan & Risley, 1975). For example, materials are placed in the residents' hands, and they are prompted with questions or statements such as "Would you like to try this?" or "Let me show you how" or "Now you try doing it yourself." The evaluation suggests that elderly residents are most likely to participate in the leisure/recreational activity when the materials and activities are openly displayed and staff prompt them to participate.

Staff also can use other combinations of behavioral interventions to increase elderly residents' participation in an activities program (Konarski et al., 1980). The interventions involve staff personally informing each resident of the program, offering at least six different activities (e.g., games, exercising, and gardening), and, if the residents desire, assisting them into the activities area. In the activities area, the staff use verbal prompts, such as "We would like to have you join in our activities," as well as nonverbal prompts. For example, staff physically guide residents toward a desired activity and demonstrate the activity. The staff also provide other forms of encouragement and positive reinforcers, such as providing drinks and snacks at the middle and end of the activity period. The entire program and its individual components were evaluated in an intermediate care facility. The results indicated that the multiple-treatment program increased and sustained activity participation to a higher degree compared with using only individual components of the program. The participation gains were maintained ten weeks later. However, the behaviors did not generalize to another activities program within the facility and did not result in any changes in the residents' life satisfaction or their satisfaction with the facility.

More recently, Engelman et al. (1999) designed a similar behavioral intervention to increase the recreational/leisure activity of elderly residents diagnosed with dementia and living in an assisted living facility. A number of activities are made available to the residents, such as exercising, playing with a dog, drawing, painting, and reading. After the practitioner teaches certified nursing assistants (CNAs) appropriate use of prompts and social reinforcement, the CNAs make personal contact with each resident at least once every fifteen minutes during a specified period of time. If the resident is engaged in an appropriate activity, the CNA praises the resident. If the resident is not engaged, the CNA prompts the resident by giving a choice of at least two activities. After intervention, the five residents participating in the evaluation markedly increased the time they spent appropriately engaged in the activities. The number and variety of activities in which they participated also increased.

ANALYSIS AND CRITIQUE FOR PRACTICE AND RESEARCH

This chapter described a variety of CB interventions that practitioners might offer the elderly and clients with physical, developmental/learning, and multiple disabilities, and severe mental illness to increase their involvement in different types of leisure, recreational, and other community activity. The activities can be performed in educational settings (e.g., selling ice cream at lunch time and participating in PE classes), in residential facilities, in private residences, in group homes (e.g., playing cooperative games, listening to music, doing macrame), and in other community settings (e.g., ordering drinks and interacting with patrons in bars, eating in restaurants). The interventions include changing physical environments by making activities and materials available, prompting strategies, reinforcement, self-instructional training, skills training, SST, and PST. Peers with and without disabilities, caregivers (e.g., family members, personal assistants), and staff in group homes and residential facilities are frequently involved in the interventions.

Evaluations of the interventions suggest that practitioners and others, such as staff and caregivers, can use CB strategies to increase the involvement of vulnerable clients in leisure and recreational activity. The interventions also appear to facilitate school and community integration. A more critical analysis of the interventions presented in this chapter follows.

Effectiveness and Additional Applications

Although evaluations of the interventions suggest that a variety of CB strategies might assist vulnerable clients in increasing their leisure and recreational activity, they relied heavily on multiple-baseline designs and small sample sizes. The effectiveness of particular CB interventions, or combinations of interventions, for specific clients and skill development is far from determined (much of the discussion in this section of chapter 4 also is applicable here). Research on some of the interventions suggests that combining multiple CB interventions is necessary to engage some vulnerable clients in recreational and leisure activity. For example, evaluations of the interventions involving elderly residents of care facilities indicate that optimally effective programs provide and openly display recreational/leisure activities and materials and use prompting, assistance, and reinforcement.

The interventions were not inclusive of all the identified vulnerable populations or the settings in which they could be used, but practitioners might use them with other vulnerable clients and in other settings. For example, the interventions provided in the school setting for Neil, a student with multiple physical disabilities, might apply to students with other types of severe disabilities (e.g., severe mental retardation or autism) and to clients in rehabilitation and residential settings. The behavioral interventions incorporating a picture book and the Touch Talker could be applicable to any client whose disabling condition includes an inability to communicate verbally. These adaptations and interventions also might be applied to other settings, including day and foster care, residential treatment facilities, rehabilitation centers, and nursing, group, and family homes. The behavioral procedures used to teach particular skills (e.g., for game playing and eating in community restaurants) might be used to teach other recreational and leisure skills in community settings, such as playing basketball in a community recreational facility or going to a local movie theater.

As noted by O'Reilly and his colleagues (2000), teaching clients with moderate mental retardation to order their own drinks in a local bar expands the leisure activity of individuals with disabilities beyond stereotypical pursuits (e.g., engaging in arts and crafts). Learning to order drinks in a bar clearly is not applicable to all client groups, such as children, adolescents, and individuals with severe mental illness or a history of substance abuse, or socially acceptable to all agencies, clients, and significant others. Practitioners, however, might apply the problem-solving intervention to assist vulnerable clients in actively participating in other community activities, such as assisting elderly clients in engaging in senior citizen functions. This intervention also challenges practitioners and researchers to consult with vulnerable clients to increase the range of options for their engagement in recreational and leisure activity.

For some vulnerable groups, such as clients with low income, racial/ethnic minorities, and sexual minorities, engaging in and/or accessing leisure and recreational activity, or certain types of activity, will require more than skill development. For example, having few economic resources would be an antecedent condition constraining a client's ability to purchase certain types of leisure/recreational materials and to engage in some community activities. Clients with low income, as well as many racial/ethnic minorities, frequently live in low-resource communities. These communities lack many opportunities for recreational and leisure activity that are readily available in communities with more resources. Various forms of discrimination also might deter clients with a minority sexual orientation or racial/ethnic background from participating in some types of recreational or leisure activity in school, residential, and community settings. Many of these antecedent conditions cannot be changed by the CB interventions discussed in this chapter. However, practitioners might use CB interventions to teach self-advocacy, political, and job-related skills, which are discussed in subsequent chapters of this book, to change these conditions. Opportunities for conducting research on CB methods to address the unique problems of clients with low income and racial/ethnic and sexual minorities that might deter them from accessing a full range of leisure and recreational activity certainly exist.

Freedom, Control, and Social Justice

Despite some limitations, the CB interventions discussed in this chapter expand clients' freedom and control and embrace social justice in several ways. Admittedly, the interventions vary in providing opportunities for clients to establish their personal leisure/recreational goals and for choosing among relevant options. In addition, many of the interventions teach one leisure/recreational activity (e.g., macrame) or groups of activities (e.g., several games or activities/materials) chosen by the intervention designers or facility staff. However, in other interventions, the participants themselves (e.g., PE students using the picture books and clients with severe mental illness participating in the recreation for leisure module) and/or significant others (e.g., parents) are actively involved in establishing the goals and selecting the activities. Practitioners can adopt the latter methods to ensure that clients are actively involved in setting goals for participation in leisure/recreational activity, which also is important both from a social validity and empowerment perspective.

The intervention for PE students provides a good example of enhancing clients' choice and control in goal setting and in accepting the intervention. Before intervention, the practitioner verifies with the students their desire to engage in recreational activity and to learn a set of described tasks to achieve that goal. The students also are provided with multiple choices for engaging in leisure/recreational activity. Practitioners also might use a variety of prompting procedures to build on and respect the skills that clients already possess. Teaching self-evaluation, self-instruction, and problem-solving procedures also assists clients in having more control over the intervention process.

Other methods that practitioners and future developers of CB interventions might use to enhance clients' control and freedom include identifying and using adaptive strategies that facilitate their participation in leisure/recreational activities as independently as possible (e.g., the finger strategy that assists clients with mental retardation in paying for their meals at a restaurant). Almost all of the reviewed interventions enhance the clients' independence in participating in leisure/recreational activity. The clients, therefore, are not totally reliant on others, such as staff, parents, siblings, and personal assistants, to order and pay for a meal, shop, identify a recreational activity and partner, and engage in particular games and activities. Furthermore, after clients learn to perform a specific leisure/recreational activity more independently, several of the interventions suggest that clients can perform similar activities more independently as well.

Despite these opportunities for increasing client input and control, the interventions also suggest additional activity and caution if practitioners are to ensure that the interventions are empowering. Practitioners must pay particular attention to client input when interventions are conducted in schools, group homes, and institutions, settings in which individual choice and control can be easily compromised. For example, practitioners must conduct ongoing evaluations to ensure that continued intervention, such as prompting, is not coercive. Practitioners also need to evaluate whether clients, particularly those who have communication difficulties or reside in institutionalized facilities, actually are empowered by choosing and gaining natural reinforcement (e.g., pleasure and satisfaction) from engaging in the leisure/recreational activities. This is particularly applicable to situations in which ongoing intervention is necessary to maintain participation.

The goals of the CB interventions described in this chapter are consistent with a social justice perspective. Assisting vulnerable clients in learning the skills needed to engage in leisure/recreational activity is consistent with the social justice value of accessing existing social resources. Learning such skills can enhance freedom of choice, independent living, self-confidence, interpersonal relationships, and integration of vulnerable groups into school and community settings.

Social Validity

Socially relevant goals and results. The designers of the previously described interventions established the social validity of their intervention goal of increasing participation in leisure/recreational activity in a variety of ways. Emphasizing the social importance of engaging in this type of activity to individual physical, social, and psychological well-being, to socially integrating individuals with disabilities into school and community settings, and to enhancing independent living was a common method. The interventions conducted in school settings also established recreational and leisure goals consistent with students' general educational goals. As noted in the previous chapter, in order to establish socially valid goals, practitioners and researchers must take into account the capabilities of vulnerable clients and, whenever possible, recognize and build on the skills they possess. For children such as Neil, establishing limited learning goals, such as "hold on to items after assisted to grasp," is just as valid as establishing more complex goals for able-bodied children who possess a broader range of capacities (Gee et al., 1995).

The majority of the participants involved in the evaluations of the interventions learned leisure/recreational skills and increased their participation in the activities. Practitioners and researchers might infer that if clients achieve their leisure/recreational goals, or if after learning the necessary skills, they continue to engage in the activity without artificial reinforcement, the participation is meaningful. Some researchers directly assessed whether increased participation in leisure/recreational activity was socially relevant; that is, the activity was meaningful to the participants or enhanced their quality of life. Common assessment methods included obtaining feedback from participants on their confidence in performing the leisure/recreational skills; their enjoyment, satisfaction, and comfort level when engaging in the activities; and other positive outcomes from participating in the activities. The responses from most of the participants who answered such questions suggest that the intervention results were socially valid. For example, the adolescents with disabilities who enhanced their ability to independently eat at fast-food restaurants reported increased confidence in their ability to independently participate in this activity, as well as in other activities. The students with communicative difficulties who learned to use a picture book to identify and recruit recreational partners indicated, as did their recreational partners, that they enjoyed the interactions. The students also reported making new friends. The group home residents with mental retardation reported that they were more comfortable visiting the bar and were happy with their enhanced social interactions.

Only one evaluation examined whether increased participation in leisure/recreational activity in residential facilities for the elderly was meaningful to the residents. Unfortunately, neither the life satisfaction nor the satisfaction with the facility increased after elderly residents of an intermediate care facility increased their participation in leisure/recreational activity. If the residents had participated in selecting the activities, these social validity measures might have shown that the intervention gains were socially meaningful to the elderly residents. Comparing treatment results with performance of normative samples and staff reports of residents' reactions while participating in the activity (e.g., they appeared to enjoy the activity) are additional social validity measures that might be adopted by practitioners and researchers.

Socially relevant intervention procedures. In two of the interventions, professionals (e.g., physical therapists for students with a physical disability) determined the special accommodations that would be required for the intervention procedures to be feasible. No individual functional assessments were conducted to determine what other contingencies, besides a lack of skill, knowledge, or available activity and material, might be responsible for low levels of participation in leisure/recreational activity. A functional assessment might have identified other maintaining conditions, which could have suggested more relevant interventions. Maintaining antecedents could include fear of failure, social anxiety; living in dangerous neighborhoods; lack of resources, opportunity, or needed accommodations; and little interest in the available leisure/recreational options. Adverse consequences might include frustration or failure after attempting to master a skill. Depending on the results of the individualized assessment, practitioners might use interventions such as cognitive restructuring, exposure therapy, breaking the skill down into more manageable steps, and providing needed resources or a broader range of options.

The acceptability of an intervention designed to increase leisure/recreational activity might be related to issues such as cost, conflicts with values or culture, and the need for special training or resources. The previously discussed interventions provide methods to involve clients and/or significant others in individualizing the interventions and providing feedback after participating, which can increase the social relevance of current and future applications of the interventions. DiPipi-Hoy and Jitendra (2004) provide an example of involving parents and their children in identifying appropriate prompts and reinforcers. The PE students were asked whether they found the picture books helpful in increasing their PE activities. Another method practitioners and researchers might use to establish the social validity of their interventions is performing task or contextual analyses of the skills needed to perform the identified activity in natural settings (e.g., selling ice cream on the playground).

The appropriateness and feasibility of interventions also might be enhanced by practitioners and researchers making appropriate accommodations and adaptations to address clients' special needs. Examples discussed in this chapter include defining small behaviors for change and involving others to facilitate performing behaviors for students with multiple physical disabilities. Using a picture book to prompt and facilitate students with mental retardation and speech impairments to participate in PE activities and an augmentative communication system for clients with severe motor and speech deficits to enhance active participation in community activities are other examples. Using specially designed instructional books (e.g., to provide additional detail and steps) for teaching macrame skills, providing special materials (e.g., a fanny pack containing $5 bills), and teaching specific strategies (e.g., using hands and fingers to determine whether the correct change was received) for individuals with developmental and physical disabilities are yet other examples of special accommodations.

Because the majority of the interventions were conducted in schools, residential facilities, and group homes, the activities, materials, transportation, and required physical assistance were available or provided by the researcher. However, if the interventions are to be feasible in other settings (e.g., in private residences), or applied in the same settings after formal intervention, practitioners must assess whether the needed resources are or will continue to be available. For example, assessing the availability of leisure/recreational activities and materials and the money, transportation, and other assistance needed to perform the selected activity would be necessary. Such an evaluation is particularly important for vulnerable populations because of their special needs. For example, Glueckauf and Quittner (1992) observe that obstacles such as architectural barriers, unmet specialized transportation needs, and medical limitations can deter wheelchair users from engaging in a variety of home and community leisure/recreational activity.

In addition, schools frequently do not have the resources, such as staff time and transportation, to continue programs that are otherwise socially relevant. An example is Sowers and Powers's (1995) program designed to increase the ability of students with disabilities to use fast-food restaurants.

Such activities also compete with required curricula. Practitioners could partially resolve this problem by teaching parents and other caregivers to assist students in learning identified leisure/recreational skills. However, issues of school time, identifying personnel to provide the instruction, and designing specialized equipment needed for some of the interventions (e.g., picture books) must be resolved if specific interventions are to be acceptable and feasible in settings such as schools.

Maintenance and generalization. Many of the reviewed interventions are designed to be conducted in natural settings, such as in restaurants, schools, and residential facilities, which has obvious advantages for both transfer and maintenance of intervention gains. However, even when practitioners teach skills in natural settings, continued support frequently is required to maintain the client's skills and involvement after formal intervention. Examples are the physical assistance needed for Neil to continue selling ice cream on the playground and the prompts necessary for the students to continue engaging in PE activities. Continued intervention also is sometimes required to maintain and to transfer the behaviors to other settings within the same organization or facility. For example, after intervention, elderly residents failed to increase participation in another activities program in their intermediate care facility. The adolescents with severe mental retardation needed additional intervention (including prompting and reinforcement) to maintain and generalize their game-playing skills to multiple settings within their residential facility. Before formal intervention ends, practitioners must assess what supports are needed to maintain treatment gains and to generalize participation in leisure/recreational activity to other settings, individuals, and materials.

Other evaluations of the interventions discussed in this chapter suggest that in some cases acquired skills can generalize to similar settings without additional intervention, such as to multiple restaurants and bars. Some of the interventions also were conducted in artificial settings (e.g., school conference room), and the acquired skills transferred to natural settings (e.g., community fast-food restaurants). These findings suggest that practitioners can successfully use interventions in more traditional settings, particularly if they use strategies to assist vulnerable clients in generalizing and maintaining the acquired skills. The techniques include involving significant others (e.g., parents and other care providers) in carrying out the interventions; using materials similar to those in natural settings; teaching participants to socially reinforce each other; using multiple exemplars (e.g., different types of leisure materials, recreational partners, settings); teaching self-management strategies (e.g., problem solving and self-instruction); and conducting booster sessions.

Two of the interventions also resulted in generalization of the acquired skills to other types of behavior. Although the therapist only taught the group home residents with mental retardation skills for ordering and paying for their own drinks at a local community bar, their social interactions with other patrons also increased. O'Reilly and colleagues (2000) suggest that the enhanced social interactions might have occurred as a result of the residents' increased social independence, the increased opportunities for interactions created by ordering their own drinks, and response generalization. The latter explanation refers to applying the social rules that the residents had learned to order drinks to different types of social interaction. Neil and the other students with multiple, severe disabilities required a decreasing number of trials to learn the new skills for each activity. The researchers hypothesized that learning to learn might have resulted from a motivational boost stemming from the children's having caused events or acquiring some control over their environment (Gee et al., 1995). These results suggest that clients can sometimes expect additional social benefits from acquiring particular skills, and over time skills can be acquired more quickly.

Evaluations of the previously discussed interventions measured maintenance of skill acquisition and increased participation in leisure/recreational activity from a few weeks to three years. None of the interventions, however, used strategies to assist clients in maintaining the activities should negative consequences occur. For example, clients might become bored, particularly when practitioners teach only one set of skills or type of leisure/recreational activity. Negative reactions from others (e.g., from other bar patrons) also might deter subsequent participation in community activity. Researchers should develop and evaluate strategies to assist clients in coping with such possible consequences, and practitioners should engage in similar activities with their clients.

Wilson et al. (1997) also argue that collaboration between significant others, such as teachers, helping professionals, and parents, is necessary if vulnerable clients (e.g., those with disabilities) are to participate in a variety of leisure/recreational activities in different settings. The researchers also contend that if integration into community, home, and school leisure/recreational activities is to occur for vulnerable clients, relevant environments must be assessed and adapted using behavioral interventions based in research. These arguments suggest the need for practitioners to assess and adapt multiple environments and to coordinate interventions for vulnerable clients across different settings. Future research can assist in determining effective interventions, adaptations, and methods to integrate and coordinate interventions for vulnerable clients desiring to increase their leisure/recreational activity in multiple settings.

This chapter discussed examples of CB interventions that can increase the skills and participation of vulnerable populations, including the elderly, children, youths, and adults with physical, learning/developmental, and multiple disabilities, and severe mental illness, in leisure and recreational activity. The next and final chapter in part II discusses CB applications that empower vulnerable populations by assisting them in recruiting assistance to enhance social support, meet medical and emergency needs, perform routine or daily activities, and attain personal goals.

ADDITIONAL READINGS AND RESOURCES

Cather, C., Penn, D., Otto, M. W., Yovel, I., Mueser, K. T., & Goff, D. C. (2005). A pilot study of functional cognitive behavioral therapy (CfCBT) for schizophrenia. *Schizophrenia Research, 74*, 201–209.

Schlosser, R. W., Wendt, O., Angermeier, K. L., & Shetty, M. (2005). Searching for evidence in augmentative and alternative communication: Navigating a scattered literature. *Augmentative and Alternative Communication, 21*, 233–255.

Wall, M. E., Gast, D. L., & Royston, P. A. (1999). Leisure skills instruction for adolescents with severe or profound developmental disabilities. *Journal of Developmental and Physical Disabilities, 11*, 193–210.

Wilson, A., Arnold, M., Rowland, S. T., & Burnham, S. (1997). Promoting recreation and leisure activities for individuals with disabilities: A collaborative effort. *Journal of Instructional Psychology, 24*, 76–79.

Yilmaz, I., Birkan, B., Konukman, F., & Erkan, M. (2005). Using a constant time delay procedure to teach aquatic play skills to children with autism. *Education and Training in Mental Retardation and Developmental Disabilities, 40*, 171–182.

Zhang, J., Gast, D., Horvat, M., & Dattilo, J. (1995). The effectiveness of a constant time delay procedure on teaching lifetime sport skills to adolescents with severe to profound intellectual disabilities. *Education and Training in Mental Retardation and Developmental Disabilities, 30*, 51–64.

6 Recruiting Assistance to Enhance Personal Well-Being

This, the final chapter in part II, discusses CB interventions that assist vulnerable populations in recruiting assistance and in obtaining information from potential helpers and other community resources to achieve goals related to enhancing personal well-being. The goals include enhancing social and emotional support, meeting medical and emergency needs, performing routine or daily activities, and attaining individually defined goals. These goals are particularly relevant for females with low income, sexual and racial/ethnic minorities, the elderly, and individuals with disabilities. These groups commonly lack access to potential helpers and other community resources that can provide social, emotional, and other types of support and the assistance needed to meet medical, emergency, and daily needs, and to achieve personal goals. Vulnerable populations frequently experience environmental stressors, such as discrimination, segregation, and lack of economic resources, which can create high levels of stress. Individual characteristics, including physical, cognitive, and mental health limitations, all can interfere with effective communication, establishing supportive relationships, and learning help-seeking skills.

As the interventions in this chapter suggest, learning skills to recruit assistance and to obtain information from potential helpers and other community resources can assist vulnerable clients in satisfying their own needs and desires, in gaining greater control over their environment, in seeking relevant information about their medical and psychiatric treatment, and in setting and achieving their own goals. At the end of this chapter, a critical discussion of the interventions is provided, including practice and research implications.

ENHANCING SOCIAL AND EMOTIONAL SUPPORT

The CB interventions discussed now are designed to enhance the social and emotional support of pregnant adolescents or parenting adolescent mothers, women with low income, and lesbians. Several interventions discussed in chapter 4 that assist students with disabilities in decreasing loneliness and in building peer networks also are relevant here, but the evaluations of the interventions did not directly measure enhancing social and emotional support. For this reason, these interventions are not discussed again in this chapter.

Several types and combinations of CB interventions that enhance social and emotional support and related outcomes for vulnerable clients are described in this section. Interventions include group and individual SST, providing sources of information and community resources, prompting, reinforcement, homework assignments, and cognitive restructuring. Other CB interventions, such as teaching various coping strategies (e.g., self-talk, identifying and engaging in positive activities), also are used to reduce depression and stress and to enhance other measures of well-being. The interventions were evaluated using quasi-experimental, single-system, pretest–posttest, and multiple-baseline designs.

Poor, Minority Pregnant Adolescents or Parenting Adolescent Mothers

A CB program for enhancing the social support and psychological well-being of predominately poor, minority pregnant or parenting adolescents was developed during the mid-1980s by Richard Barth and his colleagues (Barth & Maxwell, 1985; Barth & Schinke, 1984; Barth, Schinke, & Maxwell, 1985). The components of the program are based on research identifying the characteristics and experiences of adolescent mothers. Studies indicate that adolescent mothers frequently experience multiple sources of stress, including poverty, social isolation, biological changes, and family conflict. Adolescent mothers also commonly lack the cognitive and behavioral skills for building, accessing, and maintaining the social support networks that can mitigate the adverse influence of the stressors on their parenting and mental health.

In addition to research findings, information gathered from students in parenting programs and responses to questionnaires identified stressful situations and coping skills relevant to the adolescents. A second sample of parenting adolescents then evaluated the stressful situations based on their frequency, difficulty, and future likelihood of occurring. Problem situations were related to child care, conflicts at home and with partners, and engaging in important activities, such as attending school and finding employment. These problem situations guided the choice of the specific examples used in the SST and the homework assignments, as well as the coping and social skills targeted by the program. The skills fall into four main categories: coping with unwanted advice or criticism, refusing unwanted requests, handling significant others' offensive behavior, and decreasing personal distress.

During the group intervention, facilitators use SST to teach the adolescents specific coping and social skills. These skills include nonverbal behavior, help seeking, negotiation and comprising, problem solving, identifying and using positive cognitions, coping with depression, and dealing with criticism and stress while remaining calm. Examples of strategies for coping with depression are identifying and engaging in positive activities and identifying and drawing on members of the adolescents' social support networks. For successfully handling criticism and stress, adolescents are taught to identify and use self-talk during stressful exchanges and to reinforce or acknowledge when they remain calm. Examples of self-talk are "Hang in there, you're staying calm" and "That was all right. I said my mind and I didn't give up or get too upset" (Barth & Schinke, 1984, pp. 528–529). Group facilitators also provide the group members with a handout prompting them to identify members of their social support networks who might be able to provide various types of support (see Barth & Schinke, 1984, p. 529, for the handout). To assist the adolescents in meeting their various needs, group leaders encourage them to identify, discuss, and access a wide range of available resources beyond immediate family, such as extended kin, peers, and neighbors, and to evaluate the personal costs of using the resources. Group members also identify potential social supports to assist with specific problems, such as obtaining transportation. Quizzes and homework assignments are given to encourage the adolescents to use the skills in their homes and communities.

The adolescents (N = 79) involved in the program's evaluation were attending alternative high schools and volunteered to join the treatment or comparison group. After intervention, the adolescents participating in the group intervention had stronger social support networks compared with the comparison group. The treatment gain was maintained at the four-month follow-up, as indicated by three of the four social support measures, including the "Asking for Aid Scale." The adolescents also reported satisfaction with the program and its benefits.

Women with Low Income

Women with low income also are at risk of experiencing low levels of social support. Despite their greater need, these women have fewer social contacts and receive lower levels of material, emotional, and social support compared with women with more economic resources. This lack of support, in turn, can contribute to negative outcomes, such as psychological distress and impaired parenting practices (Belle, 1982; Klebanov, Brooks-Gunn, & Duncan, 1994). More than thirty years ago, Miller and Miller (1970) developed a reinforcement intervention to increase the attendance of women with low income at self-help groups. The developers of the intervention realized the difficulties many women with low income have in attending self-help and related groups even when the groups can provide benefits, such as social support. They therefore used positive reinforcement to increase the attendance of these women at self-help group meetings.

Practitioners assisting women with low-income in enhancing their social, emotional, and even material support might find this intervention applicable for two reasons. First, the self-help meetings can provide support for their members. For example, in one of the group's activities, the group leader invites the women to identify personal problems, after which group members discuss and offer solutions for the problems. Second, the reinforcers that the consulting practitioner provides for attendance are related to material and community resources. For example, reinforcers include concrete goods (e.g., kitchen appliances and utensils, furniture, clothing, toys), which can be solicited from higher-income neighborhoods, services (e.g., assistance in negotiating a welfare benefit grievance, locating housing, negotiating housing improvements with a landlord, resolving legal problems), and information (e.g., on obtaining benefits from social service agencies). Attendance at the meetings (N = 52) increased dramatically from an average of three participants before intervention to an average of fifteen after reinforcement. Attendance at the self-help meetings also was associated with participation in other self-help activities.

A multicomponent behavioral intervention also can be implemented in self-help or mutual-aid groups to enhance the social support of low-income women (Paine, Suarez-Balcazar, Fawcett, & Borck-Jameson, 1992). This intervention was designed to assist a mutual-aid group, which was led by a low-income agency's nonprofessional staff person, in achieving the group's goals by enhancing the skills of the group leader. The goals include providing and receiving support and encouraging and assisting one another in finding solutions to common life problems. Examples of problems include coping with an alcoholic, abusive spouse, living on a limited income, and finding suitable day care and employment.

The intervention is conducted using a self-help group leader's handbook that develops leadership skills for the types of support measured by the Self-Help Behavioral Assessment Instrument. The instrument was developed through a relevant literature review, an analysis of audiotapes of the mutual-aid group meetings, and consultation with experts in the area of self-help and social support. The types of support identified include sharing personal problems, providing empathetic responses, and discussing possible solutions to problems. Leadership skills, such as coping with difficult situations (e.g., members who frequently come late) and opening and closing group meetings, also are targeted in the handbook. The handbook, which was developed in collaboration with the mutual-aid group leaders, is not meant to be prescriptive. Instead, the handbook encourages group leaders and members to choose the elements that they find helpful (for information on acquiring the Self-Help Behavioral Assessment Instrument and *The Self-Help Group Leaders Handbook*, see Research and Training Center on Independent Living in "Additional Readings and Resources" at the end of this chapter).

During the training sessions, the practitioner uses SST to teach the group leader the content of the handbook, which focuses on the identified support behaviors and leadership skills. In a typical session, the group leader reads the relevant chapter, answers exercises and study guide questions, and practices the skills through role play, which is followed by the practitioner providing performance feedback. The leadership skills are then practiced in a mock mutual-aid group. Comparing pretraining and posttraining observations demonstrated increases in the group members' disclosures of personal concerns and a variety of support behaviors (e.g., providing alternatives, general information, and statements of support) during the mutual-aid meetings after intervention. Ratings of two experts on the assistance and support group members provided to one another during the self-help meetings also increased after intervention. Other social validity measures indicated that the group leader was highly satisfied with the importance, usefulness, and ease of the intervention. However, the intervention appeared to have no effect on member satisfaction with the group meetings.

One of the goals of the survival skills workshop developed by Thurston and her colleagues (Thurston, 1990; Thurston, Dasta, & Greenwood, 1984) for low-income, urban, and primarily minority women is to enhance the participants' social support. The workshop is conducted by peer trainers using SST and prepared materials. Skill areas, which were identified as necessary for advancing educational and employment goals, were chosen through a survey of urban women and professionals working with low-income women and through analysis of requests for assistance from a local community action agency. Examples of the identified skill areas, which are the focus of the workshop, include assertiveness, child management, self-advocacy, coping with crises, employment, and obtaining community resources. The interventions, such as role playing and group discussion, maximize opportunities for the women to interact, engage in supportive social interactions, and form relationships that will continue after workshop completion. The women also are given materials, such as informational handouts, resource lists, and worksheets, to increase their awareness and use of various community and personal supports. Transfer of the skills to the women's natural environments is accomplished through the assignment of weekly homework related to the workshop content and the women's own goals. An example of a goal is identifying and engaging in an assertive response to a specific difficult situation (for additional information on the survival skills workshop, see Survival Skills Education & Development in "Additional Readings and Resources" at the end of this chapter).

The workshop was evaluated using pretraining and posttraining interviews and scores on a survival skills knowledge test and by group members providing evidence of completing weekly homework assignments. The results of fourteen workshops involving more than 200 women demonstrated an increase in the women's survival skill knowledge test scores after intervention. Almost 50% of the women provided evidence supporting their performance of the identified behaviors. The women also reported applying the workshop information to handle current problems, an enhanced capacity for meeting their future goals, and an increase in their social interactions. The women's ratings of their satisfaction with the program and the workshop's materials, relevance, and impact on their ability to handle current problems and attain future goals were high (ranging from 4.4 to 4.6 on a five-point scale).

Lesbians

Safren and Rogers (2001) reported a case study using CB interventions to assist Anne, a 24-year-old white woman experiencing difficulties with attention and concentration, which resulted in several job losses during the previous three years. Anne's problems appeared to stem from her inability to cope with the realization that she was a lesbian. As part of Anne's treatment, the therapist used CB methods to assist her in the coming-out process, in reducing her anxiety, and in increasing her social support.

During the beginning stages of therapy, Anne articulated her concerns, negative judgments, and mixed beliefs and feelings about lesbians. Anne feared lesbians, yet she wanted to identify with them. To assist Anne in resolving her ambivalent beliefs and emotions, the therapist used cognitive restructuring. After the therapist asked Anne to write down her automatic thoughts about lesbians in general and what it would mean for her to be a lesbian, Anne was able to identify several negative beliefs she held about lesbians (e.g., they are angry, man-hating, unhappy) and negative beliefs about herself as a lesbian (e.g., she couldn't have children, she would be estranged from her family, she always would be lonely). Anne also was frightened to admit that she was "one of them." The therapist assisted Anne in finding evidence for alternative statements and beliefs, and together they developed a homework assignment in which Anne would test her automatic thought that "lesbians are angry." Anne agreed to go to a local lesbian bookstore, where she interacted with lesbians and read literature depicting images of lesbians inconsistent with Anne's automatic thoughts. In between sessions, Anne also recorded her thoughts about lesbians and her sexual orientation in order to identify her negative beliefs about herself and other lesbians. Anne then learned to examine the evidence for these beliefs and to identify more functional alternative beliefs.

After Anne made progress in changing her automatic thoughts and beliefs about life as a lesbian, the therapist used cognitive restructuring to assist

Anne in identifying and changing the thoughts that prevented her from frequenting places where she could meet other lesbians. After building a small group of close friends and acquaintances, Anne became increasingly anxious over her desire to come out to her family. After exploring with Anne the reason for the timing of her decision and the pros and cons of coming out, the therapist had Anne make a list of the people to whom she wanted to share her sexual identity and needed the therapist's assistance to do so. The therapist then rehearsed with Anne her disclosure. They began with the persons causing Anne the least amount of anxiety (e.g., her sister) and progressed to her mother, the person causing her the most anxiety. When treatment ended, Anne was experiencing less anxiety and depression about her sexual orientation and other aspects of her life. Anne also was much more comfortable with her lesbian identity, had a social support system in the lesbian community, and was able to come out to the persons important to her.

MEETING MEDICAL AND EMERGENCY NEEDS

The CB methods discussed now are designed for adult clients with a chronic health condition, mental retardation, and severe mental illness, and the elderly. The interventions are based on an important assumption. That is, in order for individuals with disabilities and the elderly to be fully and successfully integrated into the community, they must possess the necessary skills to recruit assistance for handling emergencies and for obtaining information about their medical and/or psychiatric treatment. The interventions that enhance vulnerable clients' ability to meet their medical and emergency needs include individual and group SST, problem solving, prompting strategies, reinforcement, and homework assignments. Two of the interventions were evaluated using experimental designs (Brown & Munford, 1983; Dow, Verdi, & Sacco, 1991). With the exception of the first group intervention (which was not evaluated), the remaining interventions were evaluated using single-system, multiple-baseline, and pretest-posttest designs.

Adults with Chronic Disease

This CB group intervention is designed for adults with type 1 diabetes, a condition usually diagnosed during childhood in which the body cannot produce the insulin necessary for it to convert sugar, starches, and other food into energy (Petrides et al., 1995). The intervention assists adults with type 1 diabetes in coping more effectively in social situations involving their chronic health condition. The practitioner begins by assisting the clients in determining the amount of health information that is appropriate to share, depending on the person involved (e.g., intimate friend, colleague, work supervisor, stranger) and the social context (e.g., residence, work, store).

The clients then learn to identify persons who can assist them, to identify appropriate information and explanations to provide to potential helpers, and to ask for specific assistance in a variety of contexts. For example, group members identify potential helpers when they require a glucagon injection for severe hypoglycemia (low blood sugar) or food for an insulin reaction at their place of employment. Based on the particular individual and context, the clients discuss and develop strategies, modify them, and practice the skills in role plays. Unfortunately, the effectiveness of the intervention was not evaluated. The intervention is described here because practitioners might find it applicable to clients with many different types of chronic health problems or disabilities.

Adults with Mental Retardation

Risley and Cuvo (1980) designed this behavioral intervention, which involves prompting and reinforcement strategies, to teach adults with mental retardation to make emergency telephone calls to the fire station, police, and doctor. In developing the intervention, the researchers used a variety of techniques to identify and then modify the specific steps required to reach four subgoals related to seeking emergency assistance by phone. The techniques included observing a skilled individual with mental retardation perform the behaviors, obtaining relevant information and feedback from a telephone company business consultant and local fire and police departments, and observing a training film on using the telephone. The four subgoals are as follows.

1 Make a decision on whom to call.
2 Find the telephone number of the emergency person in a directory.
3 Dial the number.
4 Provide the necessary information.

The intervention uses a specially designed telephone directory accommodating the clients' special learning needs. The directory contains a page for each emergency service provider, which displays a picture of the relevant person (e.g., fireman, policeman, or doctor), a printed occupation, and a telephone number. Pictures of emergency situations for each type of emergency, such as a kitchen stove on fire for a fire emergency, also are used during training. During the intervention, the practitioner presents the clients with one of the pictures, asks the clients whom they would call on the telephone if the event in the picture occurred, and prompts the clients to use the telephone and telephone directory. If the client does not respond or responds incorrectly, the practitioner uses a verbal prompt, for example, "Lift the telephone off the hook and listen for the dial tone." If the task is not successfully performed, the practitioner uses verbal instruction plus modeling, for example, "Let me show you. See how I picked up the receiver and listened for the dial tone? Now you try it." If necessary, the practitioner uses physical guidance, and praise is given for correct responses. To provide feedback and additional reinforcement, the practitioner also constructs a poster board "thermometer" depicting the identified steps of emergency calling. After each step is performed correctly, the clients move a ribbon up the thermometer and "win the game" when the ribbon reaches the top. The multiple-baseline design across the three clients participating in the evaluation demonstrated that they all learned to successfully make emergency calls in the three types of situations. The skills were maintained one to two weeks later.

Adults with Severe Mental Illness

The SST program discussed in the previous chapter (Brown & Munford, 1983), which teaches inpatients with chronic schizophrenia a variety of social skills, also teaches the patients relevant skills to access information about their medication needs. For example, the patients are taught to set up an appointment with a busy doctor to discuss the side effects of their medication. The patients practice the skills on the ward, as well as in the community. Self-reports and role plays indicated that the SST group performed better than individuals in a traditional rehabilitation program in making appointments and discussing medication issues with their physicians.

Two of the training modules developed at the UCLA CRTRP—Medication Self-Management and Symptom Self-Management—assist clients diagnosed with severe mental illness in successfully coping with problems related to medication issues (see chapter 4 for a discussion of the basic components of the training modules and for ordering information). Examples of skills practitioners teach clients in the Medication Self-Management module include obtaining information about their psychiatric medications, identifying side effects and methods to alleviate them, and negotiating medication issues with health-care providers. Examples of skills taught in the Symptom Self-Management module include identifying and managing warning signs of relapse, for example, developing an emergency plan and monitoring relapse signs with assistance from others.

Based on the Medication Self-Management module, Dow et al. (1991) evaluated a group Medication Communication Skills Program (MCSP) for psychiatric inpatients with a variety of diagnoses (primarily schizophrenia, major depression, and bipolar disorder). In implementing the MCSP program, group facilitators use SST to teach the patients a variety of nonverbal (e.g., eye contact and voice volume) and verbal (e.g., making specific requests and asking medication-related questions) communication skills. Group facilitators also teach group members additional skills for identifying and using resources to improve patient-physician communication. The skills include making phone calls, arranging transportation to the physician's office, and recording side effects. To enhance generalization of the skills, the patients role-play the skills with staff members from another unit and ask their unit physician medication-related questions. For example, the patients ask their physician to describe common side effects and options to alleviate them. Group members also learn the problem-solving component of the modular training, and group facilitators initiate a discussion on methods to cope with problematic patient-physician situations. The situations include a physician refusing to address medication side effects, a physician missing a scheduled appointment, and a patient running out of medication and having no available funds. Finally, group facilitators elicit and discuss problematic situations that patients experience with their own physicians.

Psychiatric inpatients ($N = 48$) were randomly assigned to the MCSP group or to a medication education group. Psychiatrists found that the MCSP group engaged in longer conversations and asked more specific medication-related questions, as compared with the comparison group. Ratings of the MCSP group on assertiveness in seeking treatment-related information and acquiring information about a newly prescribed medication, exhibiting appropriate social skills and eye contact, and compliance with their medication regime also were higher.

The Elderly

Ruben (1987) based this group SST on research indicating that elderly persons frequently have inaccurate or incomplete knowledge of their prescribed medications, because they fail to adequately question their physicians and pharmacists. Failure to obtain this information contributes to medication errors and dissatisfaction with physicians. Although the intervention was designed for elderly women residing in the community and receiving antidepressant medication, it could be applied to elderly individuals receiving any type of medication. The intervention involves a practitioner using group SST to teach group members relevant questions to ask their pharmacists and physicians. A simple recording form listing specific questions and statements is used during the training (see Ruben, 1987, pp. 9–10). An example question follows.

> I have a few questions to ask you about one of my medicines. The name of my medicine is _____. What is the medicine for? It says on the label _____. What does this mean? What side-effect does the medicine have?

The group members practice using the form during a telephone conversation with another group member, and during three telephone calls to local area pharmacists, and then generalize the skills by calling local physicians. As indicated by the preintervention and postintervention measures, the group members ($N = 20$) increased their ability to obtain information on their medications from local pharmacists and physicians after intervention.

The case study of a 65-year-old widowed female with a psychiatric diagnosis of major depression and a visual impairment, discussed in chapter 4, also used SST to teach the client to recruit assistance from others (Donohue, Acierno, Van Hasselt, & Hersen, 1995). An example of a scenario used for role playing in the area of asking someone for transportation to a doctor's appointment follows from Donohue, Acierno, Hersen, and Van Hasselt (1995).

> You have an important appointment with your eye doctor. You were supposed to get a ride with a relative, but the relative is sick and can't take you. Just then, your phone rings, and it's a friend. You want to ask this person to take you to the doctor. The person says to you: "Hello, _____, how are you?" (pp. 389–390)

The SST resulted in the client increasing her requests for such assistance.

PERFORMING ROUTINE OR DAILY ACTIVITIES

Individuals with some types of disabilities commonly are unable to perform routine or daily activities without assistance from others. CB interventions that empower vulnerable clients by teaching them skills to obtain the necessary assistance from others when it is needed are discussed here. The interventions teach children and youths with mental retardation, learning disabilities, and/or multiple types of disabilities to recruit others to assist them in completing class assignments and engaging in routine activities within school settings. Behavioral interventions that teach adults with physical disabilities and the elderly to recruit help to perform routine activities also are discussed.

The CB strategies presented here are combined in a variety of ways to form unique intervention packages. The strategies include SST (including assertiveness training), identifying and changing cognitions related to anger control and self-efficacy, relaxation techniques, think-aloud strategies, prompting, reinforcement, homework assignments, and general case instruction. With one exception (Glueckauf & Quittner, 1992), all of the interventions were evaluated using single-system, multiple-baseline, or multiple-probe designs.

Adults with Physical Disabilities and Visual Impairments

This group assertiveness skills program is designed to teach adult wheelchair users with a variety of physical disabilities, including spinal cord injuries, multiple sclerosis, and cerebral palsy, to achieve goals related to asserting their needs (Glueckauf & Quittner, 1992). Among the multiple goals of the program are to (1) appropriately use assertion skills in situations such as obtaining information about wheelchair accessibility and requesting assistance from a stranger (evaluated by role plays); (2) decrease social anxiety caused by a variety of wheelchair-related activities, such as asking for assistance to mount a curb (measured by a social discomfort scale); and (3) increase the inclination to perform wheelchair-related activities (evaluated by self-report). Therapists use SST techniques to teach the relevant assertive skills. The techniques include discussions and role plays of structured vignettes and audio-visual and therapist modeling. Other interventions involve discussing the previous and the next week's homework assignments (i.e., practicing the skills in natural settings and relevant readings), identifying and changing cognitions related to anger control and self-efficacy, teaching relaxation techniques, and implementing individual assertiveness goals. Although no significant differences between pretest and posttest scores were found in the wait-list control group, the assertion training group significantly increased performance on the three outcome measures (N = 34 whites). With the exception of the role-play test, the treatment group maintained the gains six months later.

Practitioners also can teach assertive skills to adults with visual impairments to increase their help-seeking behavior (Everhart, Luzader, & Tullos, 1980). In this intervention, the group facilitator incorporates SST into an interactive group format. The group members set group objectives, such as requesting assistance outside of the rehabilitation center, telling a bus or cab driver where they want to go, and asking for assistance to find items in a store. Group members also identify three personal goals. In subsequent sessions, the successes and failures of attempting to accomplish the personal goals are shared, and some experiences are role played. All group members (N = 8) participating in the group intervention at a rehabilitation center for the blind passed an evaluation of their performance on role-play situations based on the group goals. Staff at the center also reported positive changes in all but one group member, and five of the clients reported that the group was helpful. However, no baselines of the behaviors were taken to assess whether the group members increased their help-seeking behaviors.

An intervention developed by Dattilo and Camarata (1991), which uses behavioral techniques to teach the use of an augmentative communication system (Touch Talker) to increase the conversational skills of young adults with severe motor and speech problems, was discussed in chapter 4. One of the results of the evaluation is applicable to this chapter as well. That is, the frequency with which the clients signaled their care providers for assistance increased after intervention.

Individuals with Learning, Cognitive, and Developmental Disabilities

Mental retardation. This intervention teaches elementary school students with mild to moderate mental retardation the skills for recruiting their teachers' assistance and feedback on class assignments when attending a general education classroom (Craft, Alber, & Heward, 1998). The behavioral program consists of three components. First, the practitioner uses SST to teach the students to recruit teacher assistance. A think-aloud technique is used to model the recruiting skills, for example, "OK, I'm done with half of my work. Now I'll look to see if the teacher is busy. She's free. I'll raise my hand." After discussing circumstances appropriate for seeking teacher assistance (e.g., when the students do not understand the assignment and the teacher is available), the practitioner teaches the students appropriate recruiting behaviors. The behaviors include the students raising their hands two or three times per class period or walking to the teacher's desk. If other students are at the desk, the students are taught to wait in line until the teacher recognizes them. At that time, the students make a statement (e.g., "I don't understand this question," "I'm finished") or ask a question (e.g., "Can you help me, please?").

Second, the practitioner prompts the students to recruit before entering the general education classroom each morning. The practitioner also draws three small boxes at the top of the students' classroom assignments (e.g., a spelling worksheet) and instructs them to check one of the boxes each time they recruit and to stop recruiting when all three boxes are checked. Finally, at the end of the school day, the practitioner reviews the students' progress. The practitioner prompts the students if they do not recruit and provides inexpensive reinforcers (e.g., a sticker, pencil) if they do recruit. Prompts and artificial reinforcers are gradually phased out, and a social reinforcer (teacher praise) is used as appropriate.

The evaluation (a multiple-baseline design across four students) demonstrated that after intervention all of the students increased their recruiting behavior, as well as the percentages of completed and correct worksheet items. After intervention, the general education teacher provided feedback more frequently and reported that the students appropriately asked for assistance. All four students reported accomplishing more work when they recruited and feeling good and happy when they received praise from their classroom teacher. Maintenance of the skills and outcomes were measured for only five class periods.

Learning disabilities. Teachers in regular classrooms frequently have insufficient time to provide all of the assistance required by students with special needs. As this intervention demonstrates, teaching students to recruit peer assistance can supplement teacher assistance (Wolford, Heward, &

Alber, 2001). This behavioral intervention teaches junior high school students with LD to recruit peers with no disabilities to assist them in completing class assignments during cooperative learning group (CLG) activities in a general education classroom. A special education teacher, who is trained to carry out the intervention, discusses with the students appropriate times to ask for help. Examples of the times are when the student begins the assignment and does not understand the directions, has completed approximately one-half of the assignment, and completes the assignment. The teacher then uses SST to teach each student the following help-seeking behaviors.

1. The student gets the peer's attention by lightly tapping him or her on the arm or back, and saying, "Excuse me" and/or saying the peer's first name.
2. If the peer does not respond within five seconds, the student attempts to get the peer's attention by repeating the behaviors.
3. The student asks the peer questions that are likely to generate positive attention or a relevant response, for example, "Did I answer this question right?" "Can you give me some help with this question?" or "Can you tell me how I am doing so far?"
4. After the peer responds, the student thanks the peer.

The teacher also provides students with a cue card listing the recruiting steps and encourages them, if necessary, to refer to the card during the CLG. At the end of the school day, the teacher reviews the recruiting behaviors and reinforces the students with inexpensive items for appropriately recruiting. These activities are gradually discontinued.

The multiple-baseline design across four students (each CLG consisted of one student with LD and three peers with no disabilities) demonstrated that the students increased their recruiting responses, instructional feedback and praise from peers, and the number and accuracy of their completed language arts assignments after intervention. The recruiting behaviors also transferred to another classroom. During the maintenance phase, the rate of recruiting responses decreased but remained far above baselines and within the desired range. Qualitative information gathered from students, peers, and teachers generally indicated satisfaction with the students' help-seeking behaviors and the effectiveness of the intervention in teaching the students with LD to appropriately seek assistance from peers.

Individuals with Multiple Disabilities

General case instruction (i.e., using multiple examples of help-seeking situations, prompts, and reinforcers) also can teach help-seeking behaviors to individuals with mental retardation and multiple physical impairments (Chadsey-Rusch et al., 1993). This intervention is designed for clients who encounter daily situations in which they need assistance and have the ability to either sign or ask for assistance but rarely initiate requests for help without being prompted by someone else. The intervention is implemented in situations in natural settings where the clients need assistance to engage in a variety of tasks. Examples of tasks include accessing food, operating drinking fountains, opening doors, and walking in school (e.g., in the cafeteria, classroom, and hallway) and in community settings (e.g., vocational training and work sites and shopping malls).

During the general case instruction, the practitioner sets up five opportunities a day for each client to request help. An example is giving a client an unopened bag of chips in a school cafeteria. The practitioner waits for the client to ask for or sign "help" or to attempt to help himself or herself. If the client requests assistance, the practitioner assists him or her. If the client does not request the required assistance, the practitioner gives a verbal or sign prompt to the client to request help. After the client responds with a help request, the practitioner reinforces the response with assistance. The spontaneous help-request behaviors of two of the three female adolescent students participating in the evaluation increased after intervention (a multiple-probe design across participants was used). For the two students who improved, their gains in help-seeking behavior generalized to novel situations, and the skills were maintained for five to eight weeks.

The Elderly

A case study discussed in chapter 4 and in the previous section of this chapter also demonstrates the use of SST to increase the help-seeking behavior of a 65-year-old widowed female client with major depression and a visual impairment (Donohue, Acierno, Van Hasselt, & Hersen, 1995). An example of a role-play scenario for requesting assistance follows from Donohue, Acierno, Hersen, and Van Hasselt (1995).

> You are walking to your apartment from the parking lot. You have just finished talking with a friend for a long time, and you have forgotten how to get home. In addition, you are having a tough time walking because of some uneven pavement in the parking lot. Just then you hear someone walk by and you want to ask this person to take your arm and guide you to your apartment. The person says to you, "You look like you're lost." (p. 408)

ATTAINING INDIVIDUALLY DEFINED GOALS

Three similar SST programs were developed by Fabricio Balcazar and his colleagues to teach vulnerable youths skills to recruit assistance from potential helpers to attain their personal goals. Although some of the interventions discussed in the previous two chapters provide for clients defining their own goals, the programs discussed here are unique. In addition to establishing their own goals, the youths learn specific skills to recruit potential helpers to achieve the goals, and goal attainment is evaluated. Students with physical disabilities, African American students, and institutionalized youths with emotional or behavioral disorders, or LD participated in the evaluations of the interventions. The first of the three interventions is described in more detail, followed by briefer descriptions of the remaining two interventions (see Balcazar, Garrate-Serafini, & Keys, 1999, in "Additional Readings and Resources" at the end of this chapter to obtain information on the interventions).

Adults with Physical Disabilities and Sensory Impairments

This SST program teaches adults with seeing, hearing, and mobility impairments to recruit assistance to achieve their personal goals (Balcazar, Fawcett, & Seekins, 1991). The interventions were based on a situational analysis that identified the contexts in which help-recruiting behaviors for individuals with disabilities were most likely to occur. The analysis used information obtained from interviewing experts on and individuals with physical disabilities and reviewing relevant literature. Examples of the identified situations include asking for assistance to clarify goals, to obtain referrals, to remove obstacles that might impede goal attainment, and to secure information about available opportunities, and asking for advice. Role-play scenes were prepared based on these identified situations. The researchers identified the help-recruiting skills targeted for intervention by reviewing relevant literature, by interviewing individuals with physical disabilities, and by asking individuals experienced in working with individuals with disabilities to evaluate a videotape depicting simulated help-recruiting situations. Table 6.1 presents the twenty-five help-recruiting skills targeted for intervention.

Practitioners teach the identified skills to clients individually using a prepared training manual. The practitioner begins by reviewing the lesson content, which includes definitions of the responses used during conversations with potential helpers and examples of these conversations. Clients then complete written exercises requiring them to list relevant responses. The clients practice the skills using role-play exercises, while the practitioner provides performance feedback and social reinforcers as appropriate. The clients also establish personal goals related to health, education, and social relationships and meet with relevant individuals in the community or in educational settings (e.g., professors and graduate students in a university) to request help to achieve their goals. Examples of short-term goals include

Table 6.1. List of Help-Recruiting Skills

Opening Statements
1. Greet and introduce yourself.
2. Make a comment to initiate an informal conversation.
3. Mention the person who referred you (if applicable).
4. State your general goal.
5. State your situation.
6. State your strengths and abilities.

Making a request
7. Describe what you have done.
8. State your personal resources and experiences.
9. State the specific request.
10. State the potential benefits of the assistance.
11. Request confirmation of your goal.

Handling refusals to your request
12. Ask the helper what he/she would do in your situation.

If the helper has a suggestion:
13. State whether the suggestion is compatible with your goal.
14. State the feasibility of the suggestion.
15. State whether you will follow the suggestion.

If you decide to follow a suggestion, or the helper agrees to assist you:
16. Ask when, where, or how the assistance will take place.

If you decide not to follow a suggestion:
17. Ask for additional advice.

If no additional advice is provided:
18. Make a different request.
19. Ask for a referral.
20. Ask how the referred person might help.
21. Ask for permission to use the helper's name when talking to the referral.

Closing statements
22. State your appreciation for the helper's time and assistance.
23. Summarize your understanding of the agreements.
24. State your enjoyment of the meeting.
25. Make a final closing statement.

Note. From "Teaching People with Disabilities to Recruit Help to Attain Personal Goals," by F. E. Balcazar, S. B. Fawcett, and T. Seekins, 1991, *Rehabilitation Psychology, 36,* p. 34. Copyright 1991 by the Division of Rehabilitation Psychology of the American Psychological Association. Reprinted with permission.

locating note takers for a class, finding summer employment, and obtaining needed equipment to practice wheelchair racing.

Preintervention and postintervention ratings of the role-play exercises by helping professionals experienced in working with individuals with disabilities indicated that performances of the recruiting skills were significantly higher after intervention for all four college students participating in the evaluation. Ratings of the quality of the students' videotaped meetings with potential helpers (professors and graduate students in the universities the students were attending) were higher after intervention. Of the twenty goals proposed by the students, 75% of the goals were attained; 47% of the attained goals were attained with better than expected results. The size of the participants' social support networks, including individuals who provided material aid, advice, positive feedback, physical assistance, and social support, significantly increased from baseline to four months after intervention. The participants' ratings of their satisfaction with the intervention (mean of 6.5 on a seven-point scale) indicated that they were highly satisfied.

African American Youths

Other vulnerable populations also can have difficulties in accessing adequate social resources. For minority racial/ethnic populations, discrimination, disproportionate economic disadvantage, and residential and educational segregation all can limit access to social support networks that could assist them in achieving personal goals. Based on this research, Balcazar, Majors et al. (1991) developed a SST program to teach African American high school seniors attending inner-city schools to recruit help to attain their educational and personal goals. Techniques similar to those described in the previous intervention were used to identify typical situations that African American students can experience in requesting assistance from others, as well as to identify effective skills involved in the help-seeking process.

As does the previous behavioral program, this program divides a typical meeting with a potential helper into four main phases, including thirty identified skills for opening the meeting, making a request, handling rejections and suggestions, and closing the meeting. Practitioners instruct the students to write observable goal statements by starting the goal with the word "to." This word is then followed by an action verb clearly specifying one main result when the goal is accomplished. Examples of goals include "to find a summer job," "to apply for scholarships to attend college," and "to learn to use a word processor." A training manual with procedures similar to those described in the previous intervention is used to teach the students the identified skills for requesting assistance to attain their established goals. An African American consultant reviewed the manual's training examples and language to ensure that they were appropriate for the youths' age and culture. During the group sessions, the practitioner and students role-play the help-seeking situations identified for each lesson. An example of a situation follows.

> You have been thinking about what classes you will be taking during your first semester in college. You would like to get an idea from someone with

experience. Tell me who you might ask for help and approach me as if I am that person. (Balcazar, Majors, et al., 1991, p. 448)

Preintervention and postintervention ratings of the role-play performance of the three students involved in the evaluation demonstrated significant increases in their help-seeking behaviors after training. Evaluation of in vivo help-seeking behaviors, in which each student met with a different minority professional before and after intervention (e.g., two students aspiring to be accountants requested assistance from an accountant and bank vice president), also demonstrated significant improvements in the identified skills. Student reports of their goal attainment also were positive. Of the twelve goals proposed by the students, ten of the goals were attained at or above expected levels of success three months after intervention. None of the established goals resulted in an unfavorable outcome, but two goals were achieved with less than expected success. All three students entered college the fall semester following the completion of the project.

Youths with Behavioral/Emotional Disorders and Learning Disabilities

Balcazar and his colleagues (Balcazar, Keys, & Garate-Serafini, 1995) developed a similar SST program to teach youths with emotional/behavioral disorders, mild mental retardation, or LD to set "transitional" goals and to recruit potential helpers to assist in attaining their goals. The youths who participated in the evaluation were separated from their families by court order, attended a residential school for students with severe behavioral/emotional problems, and were expected to transition into the community in the near future. The main phases of the help-recruiting process (opening the meeting, making a request, the person agrees to help or handling rejections, and closing the meeting), the help-seeking skills, and the role-play scenarios were identified using a similar process as described in the first help-seeking intervention.

Practitioners conduct SST in groups with the use of a training manual containing content divided into two phases (samples of lesson plans are provided in the article). In the first phase, practitioners teach the youths to identify personal strengths; to set personal transitional goals in the areas of education, employment, social life, and independent living; and to develop a plan of action while identifying potential helpers. In the second phase, practitioners teach help-recruiting skills using instructional content similar to that described in the first help-recruiting intervention. During the SST, situations involving problem areas such as inquiring about and applying for jobs and colleges, seeking information on financial aid and scholarships, locating health care, and increasing community involvement and social relationships are role played. In addition to practicing prepared role-play situations, the youths suggest and role-play situations based on their personal experiences with vocational, educational, and independent living problems.

Pretraining and posttraining role-play assessments and evaluations of the male youths' (two African Americans; four whites) actual help-seeking interviews demonstrated increases and improvements in their help-seeking skills. Of the seventeen goals set by the youths, 65% were achieved, and 23% were still in progress at the end of the evaluation. The size of the participants' social networks, including individuals who provided assistance in at least one of seven areas, also increased. The youths' ratings indicated satisfaction with the training and content of the materials (5.2 and 4.5, respectively, on a seven-point scale). One year after intervention, five of the six students were employed or were in vocational training with jobs funded by rehabilitation services.

ANALYSIS AND CRITIQUE FOR PRACTICE AND RESEARCH

This final chapter in part II discussed CB strategies that empower vulnerable populations, including women with low incomes, racial/ethnic minorities, lesbians, elderly individuals, and children, youths, and adults with disabilities, by teaching them to recruit assistance and obtain information to achieve four main goals. The goals include (1) enhancing social and emotional support, such as receiving empathy and advice, information, and assistance to resolve common life problems; (2) meeting emergency and medical needs, such as learning skills to receive emergency assistance, obtaining information on medications, negotiating medication needs and problems, and keeping appointments with medical providers; (3) performing routine and daily activities, such as completing school assignments, mounting curbs, operating drinking fountains, and having personal needs addressed by care providers; and (4) attaining individually defined goals, such as locating note takers for a college class, applying for scholarships to attend college, and obtaining employment.

Results of the evaluations of these interventions suggest that a range and different combinations of CB strategies can be used individually or in groups to achieve the identified goals. The interventions include SST, PST, prompting strategies, reinforcement, providing sources of information and community support cognitive restructuring, homework assignments, relaxation techniques, think-aloud strategies, and general case instruction. The following sections discuss these interventions more critically and suggest implications for practice and future research.

Effectiveness and Additional Applications

As was the case in the previous two chapters, evaluations of these CB interventions have a number of limitations. The interventions primarily were conducted with volunteers, frequently used single-system and multiple-baseline designs instead of random assignment, combined CB interventions in different ways, and involved a small number of participants with specific characteristics. Therefore, determinations of which CB interventions, or combinations of interventions, are effective for achieving particular goals for specific clients are far from conclusive and require further research. Despite the limitations of current research and cautions regarding the applicability of the evaluation results to other individuals or groups (e.g., Paine et al., 1992, found that the leadership training that was effective in increasing supportive interactions in a low-income woman's mutual-aid group was not effective for a group of individuals with multiple sclerosis), many of the interventions might be applicable to other vulnerable populations desiring to achieve similar goals.

The CB interventions that assist individuals in enhancing emotional and social support were conducted with low-income racial/ethnic minority females, but similar interventions also might apply to other vulnerable groups. The groups could include racial/ethnic minority males, sexual minorities, the elderly, and clients with physical, learning, or sensory impairments. Practitioners could implement the group SST that teaches adults with diabetes to recruit assistance for medical or other emergencies in a variety of settings (e.g., hospitals, rehabilitation centers, nursing and group homes, mental health clinics). The SST also might be used to assist clients experiencing other chronic health problems or disabilities in requesting needed assistance. The interventions designed to teach clients with severe mental illness to obtain information about their medications and psychiatric condition, to discuss and negotiate their medications, and to obtain resources to keep medical appointments also appear to be relevant to youths and adults with other types of disabilities and chronic medical problems.

In addition to teaching students with physical and developmental disabilities to recruit others to assist them in performing school work and other routine tasks, practitioners might use similar behavioral methods in other settings and with other vulnerable clients. For example, practitioners could use SST to teach students from low-income and some racial/ethnic minority backgrounds, who tend to perform less well academically compared with higher-income and white students, to recruit assistance in completing homework assignments and in acquiring related resources in the school, residential, and other community settings. The behavioral interventions designed to teach African American youths and students with disabilities to establish personal goals and to recruit others to assist them in achieving their goals might be applicable when individual assessment for any vulnerable client reveals that an inadequate social network, or a lack of social skills for accessing an existing social network, is impeding goal attainment. Practitioners also could use similar interventions for other racial/ethnic and sexual minorities, low-income clients, and females.

Similar SST programs also might be relevant for some recent immigrant groups. In the United States, individuals are expected to be assertive in identifying and recruiting others to help achieve their personal goals. However, individuals from other ethnic groups (e.g., Asians and Latinos) might expect that others will automatically provide support, because their culture emphasizes interdependence. Finally, practitioners might find that the SST program developed for vulnerable youths transitioning from a residential setting to independent living is applicable to clients making other kinds of transitions. Examples include child welfare clients (who are disproportionately poor and African American) transitioning from a group or foster care home to independent living and patients being discharged from rehabilitation centers, long-term care facilities, and psychiatric hospitals into the community.

Freedom, Control, and Social Justice

The previously discussed CB interventions demonstrate several methods that practitioners and future researchers might use to enhance individual freedom, control, and input into the intervention process. For example, in the case study of Anne, cognitive restructuring was used to assist her in the coming-out process. By examining, challenging, and changing the thoughts that were causing her difficulties, Anne was able to control the intervention process, and ultimately her own thoughts and behavior. By offering interventions, such as the content of the leadership training for the low-income mutual-aid group, as suggestions, practitioners and researchers can recognize the need for group leaders and members to use their own strengths and to maintain their autonomy. Similar to the studies discussed in the previous two chapters, the interventions examined in this chapter use a variety of prompting strategies that recognize and build on client strengths. Practitioners also can provide opportunities for client input into the intervention process by asking clients to identify their own goals, high-risk situations, social supports, and unique self-talk. Additional examples of individualizing the CB procedures are discussed in the next two sections.

CB interventions that teach clients to monitor their own psychiatric symptoms, to make emergency plans, and to seek assistance for personal problems, emergencies, school work, and performing routine activities in the home, school, and community, enhance clients' freedom and control. After acquiring such skills, vulnerable clients do not have to wait for someone to notice and assist them. The clients themselves are in control of when, whom, and how to ask for the needed assistance. Clients who learn to ask relevant questions about their medications can make informed decisions about their medical and psychiatric treatment. Vulnerable youths who learn skills to recruit assistance and obtain information from community sources can exert greater control over their environment, satisfy their own needs and desires, and achieve their personal goals.

The interventions assist vulnerable groups in obtaining resources, assistance, and information to achieve their own goals; to enhance their social support, academic work, and performance of daily routines; and to meet their medical and emergency needs. These outcomes are consistent with a social justice perspective. Finally, if achieving these goals results in successful integration of vulnerable groups into the community, this also is consistent with the value of social justice.

Social Validity

Socially relevant goals and results. The interventions discussed in this chapter demonstrate several methods that practitioners and researchers can use to establish the social validity of their instrumental and ultimate treatment goals. An example is identifying supporting research, such as establishing the importance of social support to the well-being of adolescent mothers and of learning relevant skills to recruit assistance to handle emergencies and obtain needed resources and information. Acquiring the latter skills also can enhance successful integration of vulnerable groups into schools and communities. Surveying individuals with similar characteristics as the clients (e.g., low-income women) and professionals with relevant experience (e.g., those working with individuals with disabilities) also can identify socially relevant skills. Analyzing interactions in the context in which the behaviors are to be performed is another method to identify skills for which socially valid intervention goals are established. An example is reviewing audiotapes of mutual-aid group meetings to determine supportive behaviors. Creating opportunities for clients to establish and work toward their personal goals also should enhance the acceptability, desirability, and importance of the intervention goals. An example of an intervention goal that might be less socially valid is increasing attendance at self-help group meetings without establishing a goal related to gaining some benefit from the meetings.

With few exceptions (e.g., Petrides et al., 1995), the evaluations of the interventions provide evidence that the interventions can assist clients in accessing or increasing social resources that most people likely would consider socially relevant. The social resources include acquiring assistance from others to complete class work assignments, perform other daily/routine activities, resolve personal problems, learn knowledge related to medications and medical treatment, achieve personal goals, and increase social support networks. In other studies where measuring the client's actual use of the skills to obtain social resources would be difficult (e.g., accessing police, fire, or medical services to assist with emergencies), evidence was provided that participants learned the relevant social skills. However, whether increases or improvements in other outcomes (e.g., size of social support networks, likelihood scales, survival skills tests, skills exhibited in role plays) were actually meaningful or relevant to the participants' lives is not always clear.

Practitioners and researchers might adopt additional methods from the previously described interventions to establish the social validity of their intervention results. Examples include surveying and interviewing clients and relevant others (e.g., teachers, peers) to determine their satisfaction with the intervention gains. Experts and others involved in the interventions can assess the quality of the acquired skills and ultimate outcomes (e.g., help-seeking skills and supportive behaviors in natural settings). Determining increases in the percentage of completed and correct class assignments for students with disabilities who increase their help-seeking behavior is another example of a socially relevant measure. Finally, clients can evaluate the success of their goal achievement. With the exception of an evaluation of whether striving to attain personal goals resulted in unfavorable outcomes for African American youths, none of the evaluations of the interventions reported assessing negative outcomes as a result of the interventions.

Socially relevant intervention procedures. As was the case with the interventions discussed in the previous two chapters, functional assessments were not completed before implementation of any of the interventions described in this chapter. If antecedent conditions such as physical or other barriers (e.g., access to transportation, a telephone, the necessary economic resources), depression or anxiety, or negative perceptions of anticipated outcomes exist, even socially skilled clients would be less likely to access community supports, potential helpers, and other resources. This suggests the need for practitioners and researchers to conduct functional assessments to ensure that their interventions are socially relevant, that is, that the interventions address the maintaining conditions of identified behaviors, such as recruiting skills.

Various rationales were provided for the selection of intervention materials, such as role-play situations and the responses that participants learned and practiced. For example, the interventions developed by Balcazar and Barth and their colleagues used detailed and extensive contextual analyses (based on Goldfried & D'Zurilla, 1969) to ensure that the content of the interventions was sensitive to the participants' characteristics and situations. Practitioners and researchers might use other techniques, such as incorporating relevant literature and surveying or interviewing clients themselves, individuals with similar characteristics as the clients (e.g., physical disabilities, racial minority status, gender, age, income), and relevant professionals and experts to develop and modify intervention materials to ensure their social appropriateness. The intervention described by Petrides et al. (1995) uses strategies that are particularly sensitive to the social context in which individuals with type 1 diabetes might share information and use help-recruiting behaviors to seek emergency medical assistance. Assessing the satisfaction of clients and involved others with the intervention procedures and materials is another method that practitioners and researchers can use to determine whether their interventions are socially valid.

The previously discussed interventions also suggest a variety of methods that practitioners and researchers might use to individualize treatment, which also should enhance the acceptability and applicability of their interventions. Examples include teaching clients to identify their own high-risk situations, unique self-talk to assist them in handling high-stress situations, and positive activities to combat depression. Clients identify members of their own social support networks to assist them in a variety of ways, complete homework assignments relevant to their unique problems, practice skills necessary to achieve their individual goals, and choose among a variety of reinforcers.

In addition to the special accommodations discussed in the previous two chapters (e.g., Touch Talker), the interventions presented in this chapter suggest additional accommodations and adaptations that practitioners and researchers might use to enhance the acceptability and feasibility of their interventions. Using specially constructed emergency telephone directories adapted to the cognitive abilities of clients with mental retardation is an example. Teaching and prompting students with learning and developmental problems to keep track of recruiting their teacher's assistance by marking boxes on their class assignments and providing cue cards to assist students with LD in remembering the steps of recruiting peer assistance are yet other examples. The absence of reports of special accommodations or adaptations for participants in some interventions, such as teaching relaxation techniques to wheelchair users with physical disabilities, is surprising.

Maintenance and generalization. Evaluations of the interventions previously discussed frequently neglected to determine whether gains in social skills or ultimate outcomes were maintained after formal intervention ended. If maintenance of intervention gains was measured, it usually was measured for a short period (e.g., a few weeks). As discussed in the two subsequent chapter summaries, practitioners and researchers must realize that for many reasons the acquired skills, or the use of the skills, will not always be maintained or transfer to other settings, individuals, and contexts. The reasons include adverse experiences with others (e.g., medical providers or members of social support networks), worsening of physical or psychiatric conditions, and changes in social support networks. For example, individuals who had provided some type of support or information might no longer be available, or a student might be assigned a new classroom teacher or learning group. Reinforcing attendance of women with low income in self-help groups might not result in long-term attendance if the women do not receive emotional support and/or assistance from group members or other impediments, such as lack of transportation or child care, are not addressed.

The research evaluating the interventions frequently, but not always, examined whether the intervention gains transferred to environments outside of the intervention setting. As already noted, determining whether skills used infrequently, such as seeking police, fire, and medical emergency services, generalize to actual emergencies is very difficult. Even when researchers evaluated the transfer of intervention gains to natural settings, they frequently neglected to assess whether the gains transferred to multiple settings, individuals, and contexts. For example, the acquired skills of students with mental retardation to recruit their teacher's assistance and feedback on class assignments were evaluated on only one type of assignment, in one class, and with one teacher. The college students with disabilities recruited assistance for attaining their individual goals only from college personnel. If the client's goal is to transfer the acquired skills to other materials, settings, situations, and/or individuals, then the acquired skills must be assessed under those circumstances. And, when necessary, practitioners and researchers must use the same or develop additional strategies to enhance generalization of the skills.

To assist clients in maintaining and transferring their intervention gains, practitioners and researchers might adopt the techniques used in the interventions discussed in this chapter. For example, clients can complete homework assignments in a variety of natural settings and practice the identified skills, such as medication-related information-seeking and negotiation skills, with multiple individuals, including relevant individuals in natural settings (e.g., physicians and pharmacists). Clients can practice problem-solving exercises to identify and develop methods to cope with problematic situations, such as between themselves and their physician. Multiple situations can be set up across multiple natural settings for clients to practice help-seeking skills, and clients can be taught strategies to cope with rejection when recruiting assistance from potential helpers. Phasing out prompts and artificial reinforcers also might enhance maintenance and generalization of the skills. However, none the interventions (as was the case with most of the interventions discussed in the two previous chapters) involved significant others to coordinate intervention between the treatment and other settings (e.g., between the school and home). This analysis suggests the need for practitioners to assess and, when necessary, resolve barriers that interfere with the transfer and maintenance of intervention gains before closing a case. Researchers also need to continue to evaluate effective methods to enhance maintenance and transfer of intervention gains to multiple materials, settings, individuals, and situations.

The three chapters of part II discussed CB interventions that practitioners can use to assist vulnerable clients in accessing and increasing a variety of social resources. Although research has provided some evidence for the effectiveness of all but a few of the interventions, many of the interventions and evaluations have limitations that continue to present challenges for practitioners and researchers. The limitations are related to the research design, applicability of the findings to similar or other vulnerable clients, and establishment of socially valid intervention methods, goals, and results. The challenges include identifying and providing special accommodations and adaptations for the special needs of vulnerable clients, individualizing assessment and treatment, and maintaining and transferring the treatment gains to other relevant materials, settings, contexts, and individuals. Despite these challenges, part II provides a rich source of interventions and information for practitioners to use to assist vulnerable clients in accessing and increasing their social resources and for researchers interested in developing and evaluating CB interventions to achieve related outcomes.

Part III contains three chapters discussing CB interventions that empower vulnerable populations by assisting them in acquiring, maintaining, and increasing their economic resources. The specific goals are securing employment by learning job-seeking skills; maintaining and advancing in employment by increasing on-the-job productivity, work quality, and relevant social skills; and acquiring economic-related resources from public benefits programs and private sources.

ADDITIONAL READINGS AND RESOURCES

Alber, S. R. (2000). Teaching students to recruit positive attention: A review and recommendations. *Journal of Behavioral Education, 10,* 177–204.

Balcazar, F. E., Garrate-Serafini, T., & Keys, C. B. (1999). *A road-map for success: Setting goals and recruiting mentors.* Department of Disability and Human Development. Chicago: University of Illinois at Chicago.

Cipani, E. (1990). "Excuse me: I'll have . . .": Teaching appropriate attention-getting behavior to young children with severe handicaps. *Mental Retardation, 28,* 29–33.

Donohue, B., Acierno, R., Hersen, M., & Van Hasselt, V. B. (1995). Social skills training for depressed, visually impaired older adults: A treatment manual. *Behavior Modification, 19,* 379–424.

Research and Training Center on Independent Living, University of Kansas, Dole Center Room 4089, 1000 Sunnyside Ave., Lawrence, KS 66045-7555.

Survival Skills Education & Development. 436 Spring Garden Street, Greensboro, NC 27401. Available at http://www.ssed.org

Thurston, L. (1994). *Survival skills for women: Facilitator manual & materials.* Manhattan, KS: Survival Skills Education and Development.

PART

THREE

Acquiring and Increasing Economic Resources

7 Obtaining Employment

Social work historically has been concerned about the inequitable distribution of economic resources and the adverse effects of economic deprivation on the well-being of individuals and families (Brieland, 1995). The profession's concerns about poverty and unemployment are reflected within the core value of social justice in the NASW (1999) Code of Ethics. Social workers are challenged to advocate social policies that enhance the economic well-being of all individuals and to assist individuals in accessing needed resources. Poverty is an economic condition that places individuals at risk for multiple adverse outcomes and disproportionately affects vulnerable groups. Chapter 7, and the next two chapters in part III, describe CB interventions that empower vulnerable populations by assisting them in attaining three goals related to increasing their economic well-being: securing employment, maintaining and advancing in employment, and acquiring economic and related resources from social support networks, government programs, and community sources.

This chapter focuses on CB strategies that assist vulnerable clients in obtaining employment by learning job-seeking skills, which include locating job leads, preparing application materials, interviewing, and recruiting mentors and potential helpers. First, an overview of the economic resources of vulnerable populations is presented and the reasons for and consequences of poverty and low earnings among vulnerable groups are discussed. This is followed by a discussion of CB interventions that assist low-income and older individuals, racial/ethnic minorities, recent immigrants, and individuals with mental retardation, severe mental illness, and physical disabilities in securing employment. The final section addresses practice and research implications of the interventions, including effectiveness and additional applications, and issues related to freedom, control, and social justice, and social validity.

ECONOMIC RESOURCES OF VULNERABLE POPULATIONS

In the United States, approximately 37 million people (12.6% of the population) have an income below the level that the federal government defines as needed to provide basic necessities, such as food, housing, and clothing (U.S. Census Bureau, 2006). Poverty places adults and children at risk of numerous negative outcomes, including health and mental health problems, criminal activity, impaired cognitive development, low educational achievement and attainment, teenage pregnancy, marital conflict, and homelessness (e.g., Duncan & Brooks-Gunn, 1997; Eamon, 2001, 2005; Luthar, 1999). Job loss, even if it does not result in poverty, can increase the risk of mental health problems, low self-esteem, and low life satisfaction (Caplan, Vinokur, Price, & van Ryn, 1989).

Because poverty places individuals at risk of a variety of adverse outcomes, individuals living in poverty are considered to be a vulnerable group. Other groups traditionally considered to be at risk also are disproportionately poor (U.S. Census Bureau, 2006). While this country's poverty rate is approximately 8% for non-Hispanic whites, approximately 22% of Hispanics and 25% of blacks live in poverty. Poverty rates for children and adolescents (approximately 18%) follow a similar pattern: 10.0% of non-Hispanic white, 28.3% of Hispanic, and 34.5% of black children are poor. A disproportionate percentage of individuals who are foreign born also live in poverty (16.5% vs. 12.1% of native born). The last statistic is particularly important because the number of foreign-born people in the United States has recently more than doubled (Tumlin & Zimmermann, 2003). Single women are more than twice as likely to be poor (28.7%) than are single men, and five times as likely to be poor compared to married couples.

Women of racial/ethnic minority backgrounds are particularly vulnerable to poverty, as are some racial/ethnic minority elderly persons. The poverty rate for individuals at least 65 years of age is relatively low (approximately 10%), but the rate is almost double for elderly Hispanics and African Americans. Many older adults, such as displaced homemakers and adults with insufficient income, either must enter or continue to participate in the workforce or must face a life of poverty (Braddy & Gray, 1987; Mor-Barak & Tynan, 1993). Census 2000 highlights the economic disadvantage of yet other vulnerable groups. For example, approximately 19% of individuals with physical or mental disabilities live in poverty, a rate double that of able-bodied individuals (U.S. Census Bureau, 2003). Openly gay and bisexual men also experience an income disadvantage (30–32%) relative to their heterosexual peers. Although lesbian and bisexual women have lower wages than comparable males, they actually have higher wages compared to their female heterosexual peers (Blandford, 2003).

Not surprising, poverty rates are tied to employment and earnings. Less than 3% of full-time workers are poor, compared with approximately 13% of part-time workers, and 22% of the unemployed (U.S. Census Bureau, 2006). Unemployment rates and earnings follow a pattern similar to poverty rates, with nonwhites, women, noncitizens, and individuals with disabilities being disproportionately disadvantaged (U.S. Census Bureau, 2003, 2006; U.S. Department of Labor, 2006). Since 1996, when Congress passed the Personal Responsibility and Work Opportunity Reconciliation Act (PRWORA), locating and sustaining employment has been particularly important for low-income mothers. PRWORA ended the entitlement of low-income families with children to cash benefits, imposed a five-year limit to Temporary Assistance to Needy Families (TANF), required states to initiate strong work programs, and strengthened sanctions for recipients failing to comply (Kim, 2000). Unfortunately, even when disadvantaged populations, such as former TANF recipients, secure employment, they frequently work in low-paying jobs with few benefits (Long, 2001; Zedlewski, 2002).

In addition to a lower minimum wage and lower levels of social program benefits, compared with other Western industrialized countries with much lower poverty rates (Rainwater & Smeeding, 2003), other factors are responsible for the unemployment and low earnings that can result in poverty among vulnerable groups in the United States. These include hiring and wage discrimination, social stigma, and attitudes of professionals, family members, consumers, and employers. Economic incentives of social insurance programs and lack of access to vocational services, supportive employment, and work accommodations can be additional barriers to securing adequate employment. Cognitive, physical, medical, and psychiatric problems, as well as inadequate education, job skills, and job-seeking skills, can interfere with achievement of vocational goals for many vulnerable groups. Residence in areas with high unemployment rates, lack of transportation, and inadequate child care also constrain secural and maintenance of employment (Blandford, 2003; Drake, McHugo, Becker, Anthony, & Clark, 1996; Montague, 1988; Sauter & Nevid, 1991). For recent immigrants, additional barriers to employment include lack of English proficiency, limited work histories, and cultural customs or values (Jung & Jason, 1998; Tumlin & Zimmermann, 2003).

Older workers (defined as individuals age 50 years and older by the U.S. Department of Labor) also have particular difficulties in securing and maintaining employment. Older adults are especially vulnerable to economic and labor market changes, including company reorganizations, plant closings, and layoffs. Older workers are more likely to have lower educational levels, to possess outdated job skills, and to face negative stereotypes regarding their productivity and work contributions. Older workers also frequently become discouraged and prematurely terminate their job search (Braddy & Gray, 1987; Mor-Barak & Tynan, 1993; Rife & Belcher, 1994).

Having responsibility for and increased control over one's economic well-being can be empowering. And, for most individuals, employment offers additional social and psychological benefits. Work is an important part of fulfilling adult role expectations, and employment provides structure and opportunities for daily activity and social interactions. Employment can enhance self-esteem, a sense of identity, social status, and problem-solving and social skills and can facilitate integration into the community (Corrigan, Reedy, Thadani, & Ganet, 1995; Tice, 1994; Tsang, 2003; Twamley, Jeste, & Lehman, 2003). Many older adults living long and healthy lives choose employment as one way to continue a meaningful involvement in society (Mor-Barak & Tynan, 1993). Reviews of research on vulnerable groups indicate that most of them desire to be employed (e.g., Bond, 2004; Braddy & Gray, 1987; Lovett & Harris, 1987).

SECURING EMPLOYMENT BY LEARNING JOB-SEEKING SKILLS

CB strategies that empower vulnerable populations, including individuals with disabilities and low income, older persons, women, recent immigrants, and minority racial/ethnic groups, by assisting them in obtaining employment by teaching them job-seeking skills are discussed now. Job-seeking skills are related to finding job openings, navigating the application process, interviewing, and recruiting assistance from mentors and potential helpers. The Job Club, a behavioral approach that teaches multiple job-seeking skills, also is described.

A number of other CB interventions designed to increase the job-seeking skills of vulnerable groups are not included in this section. For example, SST can be used to assist high school seniors with LD (Mathews & Fawcett, 1984), adults with work-related disabilities (Mathews, 1984), women with mild to moderate mental retardation (Hall, Sheldon-Wildgen, & Sherman, 1980), African American and Latina adolescent mothers (Schinke, Gilchrist, Smith, & Wong, 1978), and low-income youths and adults (Barbee & Keil, 1973; Heimberg, Cunningham, Stanley, & Blankenberg, 1982) in learning to effectively complete employment applications and interview for jobs. CB interventions also can assist low-income racial/ethnic minority adolescent mothers (Staab & Lodish, 1985), unemployed low-income women with a history of psychiatric problems (Arnold & Parrott, 1978), and individuals with a variety of physical, cognitive, and psychiatric disabilities (Farley, 1987; Farley & Akridge, 1987) in learning job-seeking skills and methods to manage anxiety, other negative emotions, and self-defeating thoughts and behaviors that interfere with the job search process.

Although evaluations of these CB interventions indicate that most of the participants enhanced their job-seeking skills and/or learned to manage negative emotions, behaviors, or cognitions, they failed to determine whether the participants secured employment after intervention. Consistent with the definition of empowerment discussed in chapter 3, this section focuses on CB interventions for which some evidence is provided that the enhanced job-seeking skills resulted in participants actually obtaining employment.

Interviewing Skills

As the designers of the CB interventions discussed here have argued, the interview process is extremely important to obtaining employment. Once a job applicant secures an interview, an employer's assessment of the applicant's interview behavior is the next critical step in the hiring process. Many vulnerable individuals are unfamiliar with the job interview process and lack the social skills necessary to present themselves in a positive way, which frequently results in their inability to secure employment.

The interventions discussed now use SST procedures to enhance the job interviewing skills of individuals with mental retardation and severe mental illness. An SST program also targets skill development for former Asian refugees. The SST programs identify a variety of job interviewing skills and are conducted individually, in groups, or by peers. The SST program developed for Asian refugees is unique, because it identifies skills, knowledge, values, and cultural issues that are important for recent immigrants to learn in order to effectively interview for a job. All of the interventions were evaluated using multiple-baseline designs.

Adults and youths with mental retardation. This group SST program was designed to improve the job interviewing skills of clients with mild mental retardation (Kelly, Wildman, & Berler, 1980). The behavioral intervention focuses on three main skill areas, which research has identified as important predictors of favorable evaluations of job candidates by personnel managers. The identified skill areas are as follows.

1. Appropriately disclosing positive information about the interviewee's interests, experience, training, and work skills
2. Conveying interest in the position
3. Asking the interviewer relevant questions

As part of the SST, the group members view three modeling tapes in which the skills are demonstrated. Afterwards, the group facilitator discusses the importance of the skills and provides further examples, and group members identify and rehearse their own appropriate responses. During this process, group members and the group facilitator provide appropriate feedback. Evaluation of the group SST (N = 4 adolescent males residing in a brief residential treatment program) demonstrated that the training improved job interview performance during role plays and during job interviews at a fast-food restaurant. Global evaluations of the interviews, including the adolescent's interest, experience and training, competence, and ability, and the likelihood of their hiring the adolescent, made by experienced personnel interviewers also improved after training. Six months later, two of the four adolescents were employed.

Schloss and colleagues (Schloss, Santoro, Wood, & Bedner, 1988) developed an employment interview training for clients with mild mental retardation that can be implemented either by peers or by practitioners. The interview questions used in the intervention were obtained from employers in relevant job areas (e.g., service and light industry). Appropriate answers for the questions then were developed in consultation with the clients and employers. Based on the client's difficulty in appropriately answering them, the practitioner selects twenty interview questions from a pool of eighty questions covering three general areas (personal, work, and education). Interview question index cards are then prepared for each client, which contain a type-written question on the front of each card and appropriate answers on the back. The back of each card also contains a column of ten boxes each labeled "+" and a second column of ten boxes each labeled "−". A poster that illustrates the steps to be used in the peer- and practitioner-directed instruction also is prepared. Finally, an "order card" assists the clients, who serve as peer trainers for each other, in remembering the tutoring activities. Using similarly prepared question cards, the practitioner teaches the clients the peer-training procedures through modeling, a system of least prompts (allowing for independent performance, followed by a verbal then a modeling prompt), rehearsal, feedback, and praise.

To implement the peer-directed procedure, one of the clients (the "tutor") places a token on the first square of the order card and reads the question printed on the first card in the interview question card deck. If the client's response matches the response on the back of the card, the tutor follows the prompts on the poster, which indicate that he or she should acknowledge the correct answer (e.g., "That is right"), mark the first "+" box on the interview question card, and go onto the next question. If the response does not match the response on the back of the card, the poster provides instruction to give feedback on the correct answer, repeat the question, and mark the first "−" box on the interview question card. The tutor then moves the order token to the second square and repeats the question. If on the second try, the client's response is correct, the tutor acknowledges the response. If this response is also incorrect, the tutor moves the token to the third square and reads the interview question again. A correct response is acknowledged. If the response is incorrect, the tutor asks the question again and turns the card to face the other client. The tutor follows the reading of the correct answer with verbal acknowledgment. When three "+" marks are checked in a row for the first attempt, the card is removed from the deck. Practitioner-directed instruction is similar to the peer-directed instruction. An evaluation of simulated interviews indicated that both methods resulted in substantial increases in the client's (N = 2 females) appropriate responses to the three types of questions. At a six-month follow-up, the skill level of only one of the clients was maintained, but after training both clients were hired in competitive employment settings.

Adults with severe mental illness. Kelly and his colleagues developed and evaluated two SST programs that teach job interview skills to formerly hospitalized psychiatric patients. The first program teaches the skills individually to the clients (Furman, Geller, Simon, & Kelly, 1979), and the second uses a group format (Kelly, Laughlin, Claiborne, & Patterson, 1979). When implementing the individual program, the practitioner selects target skills for each client based on an initial assessment using a standard interview training script. Although the skills vary by client, common skills include providing positive information on education and/or work experience, using appropriate gestures, expressing interest or enthusiasm in the position, and asking the interviewer appropriate questions. The individual training program involves four main components.

1. The practitioner reviews a videotape of a previously conducted interview and provides the client with feedback on his or her performance.
2. The practitioner coaches the client on ways to improve performance on the identified skill; the client practices the skill and is prompted to incorporate the skill into the next interview.
3. A role-play job interview is conducted and videotaped.
4. The videotape is reviewed, and the practitioner provides feedback and reinforcement as appropriate.

The identified skills for the group SST are similar to the common skills taught in the individual SST. Consistent with SST, the group facilitator uses videotaped modeling, group discussion, behavioral rehearsal, feedback, and reinforcement. The evaluation demonstrated an increase in the job interview skills for all of the clients ($N = 3$ in the individual program; $N = 6$ in the group program). Assessments by actual personnel managers also indicated improvement in all of the skills for eight of the nine clients after involvement in one of the programs. Two of the clients, who were unsuccessful in obtaining employment for two years prior to the individual SST, secured paid employment after intervention. The jobs were maintained at a three-month follow-up. Despite a year-long history of being unsuccessful in finding employment, five of the clients in the group SST obtained paid employment in competitive or vocational settings after intervention.

Recent immigrants. Jung and Jason (1998) developed a unique four-day job interview SST program for former Asian refugees. The individual training targets fourteen behaviors identified from a skills checklist (developed by Mathews, Wang, & Fawcett, 1984) and twenty-six additional behaviors representing four areas of Western values and social customs determined to be important for successful job interviews. The skills taught in the SST are categorized into four main areas: appropriate social greetings (e.g., making eye contact), assertiveness in expressing job qualifications and clarifying job information, communicating an ability to work independently and to be socially compatible, and expressing determination and perseverance. During the first training session, the practitioner provides the client with information on cultural differences (e.g., deference vs. assertiveness) and similarities (e.g., succeeding through hard work) between Asian and Western values. The practitioner discusses the ways in which the values are perceived in the two cultures and encourages the client to express the shared values during the interview. The practitioner also uses SST (the practitioner serves as a model) to teach the client to engage in appropriate social greetings. During the next three training sessions, SST is used to teach the skills in the three remaining skill categories.

After intervention, the participants (two females; one male) demonstrated an increased understanding of Western social customs and the interview process, an enhanced performance in simulated interviews, and an increase in their self-confidence. A one-month follow-up determined that the participants had increased their employment searches, and one had a job offer. Significant others also reported an increase in the participants' motivation to seek employment, an improvement in their social skills, and an increase in their self-confidence about seeking employment as a result of the SST.

Recruiting Skills

As discussed in the introduction to chapter 6, minority racial/ethnic groups and individuals with disabilities are at risk of discrimination, economic disadvantage, and residential and educational segregation. Such conditions limit access to social networks that might assist these individuals in achieving personal goals, such as securing employment. Using SST to teach skills to recruit mentors and potential helpers can increase employment opportunities.

As described in the previous chapter, three SST programs developed by Balcazar and his colleagues assisted African American high school students (Balcazar, Majors, et al., 1991), college students with physical disabilities (Balcazar et al., 1991), and adjudicated youths with emotional/behavioral disorders, LD, and mild mental retardation (Balcazar et al., 1995) in learning help-recruiting behaviors to attain their personal goals. Because some of the participants set and attained goals related to obtaining jobs, these help-recruiting interventions are relevant to this chapter as well. A goal set by two of the three African American students was "to find a summer job"; after intervention, both students secured summer employment. A personal goal set by one of the four college students with physical disabilities also was finding a summer job. After intervention, the student obtained two summer jobs. Job-related goals, such as inquiring about job openings, applying for job positions, and securing job interviews, were among the transitional goals set by the adjudicated youths with emotional/behavioral disorders and learning problems. At a follow-up one year after intervention, three of the six youths were employed in competitive jobs, and two of the youths were receiving vocational training and had jobs funded by rehabilitation services.

The Job Club Method

The Job Club method is a standardized group approach to job seeking that follows lesson plans directed toward attaining specific objectives. As a result of the 1996 welfare reform, which imposes time limits for cash benefits and emphasizes work, developing and using effective job-finding methods to assist current and former welfare recipients in finding employment are extremely important. The Job Club program has been incorporated into many Welfare-to-Work programs to assist TANF recipients in locating jobs (Brooks, Nackerud, & Risler, 2001), as well as to assist other low-income individuals, older workers, and individuals with physical and psychiatric disabilities in locating employment.

Azrin and Besalel (1980) describe the Job Club as an example of applying the principles of behavioral psychology to the processes of vocational counseling and to obtaining employment. The goal of the Job Club method is to "obtain a job of the highest feasible quality within the shortest feasible time period for all participating job seekers" (p. 1). The program is a comprehensive approach because it assists job seekers in every area believed to influence securing a job (Azrin, Flores, & Kaplan, 1975). The areas include expanding vocational choices; overcoming discouragement in job seeking; accessing support and information from family, peers, and other members of social support networks; obtaining transportation, professional advice, and job leads; and learning to prepare resumes, obtain and perform appropriately in job interviews, and schedule time for job-seeking activities.

The Job Club method also is empowering. It focuses on the job seeker's strengths and is an effective method for teaching self-help skills that can increase the economic resources of vulnerable populations through employment. The Job Club program provides assistance to job seekers until they obtain employment, regardless of the length of time. If workers lose or quit their jobs, they can immediately re-enroll in the program. The following four paragraphs, which are summarized from the *Job-Club Counselor's Manual* (Azrin & Besalel, 1980), provide a brief description of the expectations and responsibilities of the job seekers, followed by a description of the job counselors' responsibilities, counseling style, and methods.

Job Club members are expected to attend group meetings, to perform the designated activities, and to treat job seeking as a full-time job. They are expected to obtain job leads and interviews and to schedule time for these activities. Because social network members are considered primary sources of job leads, job seekers are expected to contact friends, relatives, and acquaintances and to follow up on leads. The Job Club manual provides forms, examples, and practice scripts for job seekers to use when performing these activities and to assist in scheduling and keeping records.

The main responsibilities of Job Club counselors are to provide job seekers with the necessary facilities and supplies, support, instruction, and opportunities to practice the relevant skills needed to carry out their responsibilities. The counselors' style is directive; it emphasizes progress and final outcomes, but it also is supportive and encouraging. Counselors teach job seekers to enlist various types of support from their family, including emotional support, encouragement, job leads, job search suggestions, transportation assistance, and allowances for the long hours spent in the job search. Counselors also encourage group members to provide support to one another, and they assign each group member a "buddy" who provides encouragement, advice, and practical assistance in job-seeking activities. The buddy assists with activities such as writing letters, monitoring phone calls, reading want ads, transportation, and practicing for interviews.

Job Club counselors are committed to assisting every Job Club member in obtaining employment. They provide each job seeker with frequent individual attention and perceive all job seekers as employable, regardless of their employment and educational background, disability, or past experiences. Counselors constantly emphasize and praise the job seekers' positive characteristics, appropriate performance, and progress, while withdrawing attention from the job seekers' deficits and any perceptions that they may lack employment opportunities. Counselors collect and provide job leads, give instruction, and facilitate practicing job-seeking skills. The skills include writing resumes, filling out job applications, finding job leads, making telephone calls, arranging transportation, placing job-wanted ads in local newspapers, and appropriately answering interview questions.

Job Club counselors teach job seekers to emphasize their personal, social, and work skills in their applications, resumes, initial job contacts, and interviews. They also teach job seekers methods to de-emphasize, discuss, and reframe in a positive way any apparent disability or other perceived deficit, such as a prison record. Counselors teach the job seekers methods to obtain interviews for unpublicized jobs. Methods include accessing their social network, making telephone contacts, using the yellow pages section of telephone books, turning unsuccessful job inquiries into job leads, and approaching former employers. Job seekers learn to consider many types of positions, and, if necessary, to obtain a job in another location.

Evaluations of the Job Club method for job seekers who are diagnosed with a severe mental illness or another disability, unemployed, on public assistance, and older are discussed next. The rigor of the evaluations ranges from simply reporting the percentage of participants who secured employment after participating in the Job Club to randomly assigning the participants to a Job Club group or to a control or some other type of employment services group. The first section on applying the Job Club method to clients with a psychiatric diagnosis also discusses special accommodations and adaptations that meet the special needs of this vulnerable group.

Adults with severe mental illness. In the first of the three Job Club programs described here for clients with severe mental illness, a number of revisions were made to meet the special needs of hospitalized psychiatric patients (Jacobs, Kardashian, Kreinbring, Ponder, & Simpson, 1984). Full-day, instead of half-day, client participation is required to provide structure and support. Other accommodations include daily goal setting, establishing communication between the Job Club staff and the clients' ward treatment staff, providing transportation, using monetary reinforcement for program attendance, assisting with problems involving daily-living skills, and providing job maintenance services for clients who find jobs. The latter involve teaching problem-solving strategies to assist with problems related to social interactions and managing stress and psychiatric symptoms. After intervention, 56% of the psychiatric patients (N = 97) found employment during the first eight months, and 10% entered full-time job training programs. A six-month follow-up of the clients entering jobs or training indicated that after 30, 60, 90, and 180 days, 80%, 75%, 80%, and 67.5%, respectively, were still employed or continued in their job-training program. No comparison or control groups were used in the evaluation.

Jacobs and his colleagues (Jacobs, Collier, & Wissusik, 1992) later developed a Job-Finding Club module (available from the first author), which built on previous work modifying the Job Club method for individuals with psychiatric disabilities. The module, which includes a technical manual, a trainer's manual, a client workbook, and a skills video, is designed to assist clients with psychiatric diagnoses who have adequate personal, social, and job skills in finding competitive community employment. The seven skill focus areas include readiness for work, job interests, finding job leads, contacting potential employers, completing job applications, job interviewing, and finalizing the job offer. Evaluations of this module with persons diagnosed with a variety of psychiatric disabilities reported job placement rates ranging between 35% and 60%. These rates contrasted with much lower rates (5–15%) for patients leaving most inpatient psychiatric facilities. However, employment rates for individuals with the most persistent and serious mental illness, such as schizophrenia, were one-half to one-third lower compared with employment rates for individuals with other diagnoses (e.g., depressive disorders).

Corrigan et al. (1995) also evaluated the Job-Finding Club module with mental health outpatient clients diagnosed with a severe mental illness. Of the forty-four clients, 70.5% dropped out before completion, and 34% reported obtaining competitive jobs or positions in on-the-job training programs six months later. However, no significant differences were found in obtaining employment between those who remained in or dropped out of the program.

The Job Club method also was adapted to the special needs of state hospital clients with various psychiatric diagnoses (primarily schizophrenia, other psychotic disorders, and affective disorders) referred from inpatient facilities, halfway houses, and outpatient clinics (Brey, Zadny, Gonzalez-Huss, & Ament, 1989). The accommodations include the following.

1. Clients are not assigned "buddies." Because of the Job Club members' varying capabilities and temperaments, assigning a buddy can create stress.
2. Sessions are limited to two hours per day, which frees time for clients to attend their mental health treatment activities. However, clients are encouraged to spend as much time as possible on job-search activities.
3. Record-keeping activities are completed only during the sessions and limited to the contacted employers.
4. Minimal requests are made to family and friends for assistance and support because most clients are estranged from these sources of social support.
5. Job-wanted ads are not placed in local newspapers.
6. Economic type assistance is given as needed (e.g., providing appropriate clothing, living stipends, and bus passes).
7. A phone number and post office box are provided to place on job applications for clients with no residence outside of the hospital.
8. Clients sign a contract at the beginning of the program that establishes mutual responsibilities. The clients' responsibilities include informing the Job Club staff if they find the activities too stressful or they experience suicidal ideation and refraining from substance abuse.

After intervention, 78% of the clients (N = 122) found jobs in competitive employment.

Unemployed and clients receiving public assistance. Azrin et al. (1975) conducted one of the first evaluations of the Job Club method. The evaluation was conducted in a small college town with no public transportation and a long history of above-average unemployment. The researchers recruited participants from a variety of sources and included anyone who was employed less than full time, was not receiving unemployment compensation, and desired full-time employment. After matching participants on an index of employability, they were randomly assigned to a control or Job Club group. The average job seekers in the Job Club group started working in fourteen days (median time), versus fifty-three days for those in the control group. Within two months, 90% of the Job Club participants had obtained full-time employment, compared with 55% of the control group. The average starting salary was approximately one-third higher for the Job Club participants.

Azrin and Phillip (1979) conducted a subsequent study on the Job Club method (N = 154), in which 86% of the clients were receiving financial assistance from some public agency and exhibited some type of problem that limited employment opportunities. The problems included a physical, emotional, or intellectual disability and chronic unemployment. The clients were randomly assigned to the Job Club or to a two-day lecture, discussion, and role-play program. At the six-month follow-up, 95% of Job Club clients had obtained jobs, while only 28% of the comparison group had found employment. The jobs of Job Club clients were obtained sooner (average of ten vs. thirty days) and were maintained over the study period. Although the median salaries of Job Club participants were 22% higher than those of the comparison group, salaries were close to a minimum wage.

Azrin and his colleagues (Azrin, Philip, Thienes-Hontos, & Besalel, 1980) also evaluated the Job Club method with clients receiving public assistance and residing in five different cities (N = 979). At each site, the clients were randomly assigned to the Job Club program or to an existing job-counseling program. The unemployment rate in the cities ranged from 4.6% in Wichita to 15% in Harlem. Of the clients actually participating in the programs (22% of the Job Club group and 31% of the comparison group dropped out), 80% of Job Club clients, compared with 48% of clients in the alternative program, were employed at the six-month follow-up. At the twelve-month follow-up, the percentages were 87% and 59%, respectively. The Job Club program was more effective in each of the cities (86% of Job Club clients in Harlem obtained jobs), regardless of the client's gender, education, race/ethnicity, disability status, and age, and whether they were required to participate. The jobs obtained by Job Club participants also were more likely to be long term, unsubsidized, and acquired through their own efforts. The Job Club clients' jobs were comparable to the control clients' jobs in terms of mean salary, full-time status, and type. Job Club members secured employment in a median of six sessions (mean of eleven), and 90% obtained jobs within twenty-three sessions. A six-month follow-up also found that more Job Club clients reported being satisfied with their jobs (84%) compared with clients participating in the other program (78%).

Two more recent studies evaluating the Job Club program for public assistance recipients reported similar results. Stidham and Remley (1992) determined that 70.8% of Job Club participants (N = 116) secured employment, compared with the overall agency placement rate of 29% during the same fiscal year. An evaluation of four two-week Job Clubs for TANF recipients in Georgia determined that 62.5% of the participants found work. However, the study lacked a control or comparison group (Brooks et al., 2001). When the researchers examined differences in perceived barriers to employment between TANF recipients who did and did not find employment, they found that unsuccessful job seekers were more than twice as likely (54% vs. 24%) to perceive transportation as their biggest barrier to employment. A larger percentage (69%) of unsuccessful job seekers, however, reported owning a car compared with successful job seekers (56%). The researchers suggested that for some participants, perceptions might be more important than reality in influencing job-seeking behavior. Job Clubs might be more successful if strategies were used to evaluate clients' perceptions of employment barriers.

Older workers. This first of four evaluations of the Job Club method for older workers described here randomly assigned clients (N = 46) receiving employment services for older workers to normally available services or to the Job Club program (Gray, 1983). At a twelve-week follow-up, 74% of Job Club participants had secured employment versus 22% of participants in the comparison group. The type of employment was comparable for both groups, but Job Club participants earned more money and worked more hours. However, salaries and job status tended to be low in both groups.

In a subsequent study, thirty-five older job seekers were randomly assigned to a Job Club group or to a group provided with the job seeker's manual used in the Job Club program (Braddy & Gray, 1987). Participants in the latter group also were encouraged to use the job information and referral assistance offered by the senior employment service and other community agencies. After twelve weeks, 89% of Job Club participants were employed, compared with only 25% of participants in the alternative group. Characteristics of the jobs were comparable.

Gray and Braddy (1988) conducted a similar evaluation of a Job Club program with clients (N = 48) who were involved with an employment service for older workers in an area with an unemployment rate of 10%. The older adults were randomly assigned to an abbreviated version of the Job Club program or to a normal services group. At a twelve-week follow-up, 83% of Job Club participants were employed, compared with only 26% of the control group. The study also identified increases in job-seeking knowledge and in the participants' social networks as the mechanisms accounting for Job Club's effectiveness. To further examine the importance of social support provided within the Job Club, the researchers randomly assigned thirty-five older unemployed workers in areas with low unemployment rates (3–5%) to the Job Club program or to a group using only the Job Club search handbook and normal services. Almost all of the Job Club participants (94.7%) obtained employment, compared with 38% of the control group.

The analysis only partially supported the hypothesis that social support accounted for the better outcomes of Job Club participants.

Finally, Rife and Belcher (1994) evaluated the Job Club method for older unemployed workers (N = 52) who applied for employment services with a community agency. The unemployed workers were randomly assigned to a Job Club program or to a state government job service and community referral program. After twelve weeks, 65.4% of Job Club participants were employed, while only 26.9% of the control group found employment. Measures of continuous employment, income, and number of hours worked all were significantly higher for Job Club participants. However, wages tended to be low for both groups, and the work was usually part time.

ANALYSIS AND CRITIQUE FOR PRACTICE AND RESEARCH

This chapter focused primarily on behavioral interventions that empower vulnerable populations by assisting them in securing employment by teaching them job-seeking skills. The skills include finding job leads, preparing application materials, interviewing, and increasing and accessing social support. Vulnerable populations include older individuals, racial/ethnic minorities, recent immigrants, and individuals with mental retardation, severe mental illness, physical disabilities, and low income. CB strategies primarily involve SST, including modeling, prompting, rehearsal, feedback, and reinforcement. Requisite resources also are provided (e.g., work area and supplies, job leads, postage, and transportation) and problem-solving strategies are taught to assist clients in maintaining employment. The interventions can be conducted individually or in groups, and in one intervention, peers train each other. Conducting interventions in groups, such as in Job Clubs, has the added advantage of providing a variety of support to members, including encouragement, job contacts, and transportation. A more critical evaluation of the interventions and the research that evaluated them follows.

Effectiveness and Additional Applications

Evaluations of the CB interventions demonstrated that many of the participants obtained employment after intervention. Multiple-baseline designs were used to demonstrate effectiveness of the SST programs discussed in "Interviewing Skills" and "Recruiting Skills" to achieve the instrumental goal of enhancing job-seeking skills. Researchers then reported the number of participants achieving the ultimate goal of obtaining employment. Without random assignment, determining whether the SST programs increased the participants' job-seeking skills is difficult to establish, let alone whether the interventions resulted in participants actually securing employment.

Many, but not all, of the evaluations of the Job Club method used experimental designs. The latter studies demonstrated that Job Club participants were more likely to secure employment compared with control or other intervention groups. In some studies, differences in the employment rates between the Job Club and comparison groups were dramatic.

Practitioners, however, must use caution when referring particular clients to or including them in Job Clubs. Evaluations suggest that the program has better results for some clients (e.g., individuals with a work history), more mixed results for other clients (e.g., public assistance recipients), and relatively poor results for clients with severe mental illness. Brooks et al. (2001) also reported that more than 50% of the public assistance clients assigned to the Job Club program did not attend the first session, even when attendance was mandatory. In addition, some clients are not eligible for Job Club participation, because of severe cognitive or physical disabilities, mental illness that is not managed (e.g., psychosis or disruptive behavior), serious alcohol or drug problems, and certain types of medical problems. Azrin et al. (1980) also pointed out other barriers, such as high unemployment rates and lack of transportation and child care, that, if not addressed, can reduce the effectiveness of Job Clubs.

Despite these cautions, evaluations of these SST and Job Club programs suggest that practitioners might use these methods with many vulnerable clients to increase their job-seeking skills and to assist them in finding employment. The Job Club method also has been adapted to the special needs of other vulnerable populations, such as clients with hearing and seeing impairments (Amrine & Bullis, 1985; Dickson, 1979; Dickson & McDonnel, 1982) and students with disabilities transitioning from high school (Lindstrom, Benz, & Johnson, 1996). Because these programs were described but not evaluated, they were not discussed in this chapter; the effectiveness of these Job Club programs must be established by future research. Job Clubs also might be successful for persons living with HIV and AIDS. Because of more effective medications, these individuals are increasingly resuming normal activity, including returning to the workplace (Arns, Martin, & Chernoff, 2004). Practitioners and researchers also might adapt the interventions developed by Jung and Jason (1998), which increased the knowledge of Western values and customs and enhanced job-seeking skills for Asian immigrants, for other immigrant groups.

Practitioners might use the previously discussed interventions in mental health, health and rehabilitation, school, and community-based gerontology settings, as well as in community action and public social service agencies. Although occupational social workers can practice in these types of settings, the majority of social work practice and research in this area involve employed clients served in employee assistance programs (Iversen, 1998). Iversen argues that the social work profession also should focus practice knowledge, skills, and research on enhancing the employment skills of the unemployed and working poor. Iversen's review of the literature on Welfare-to-Work programs suggests that the most successful programs provide multiple services individually tailored to meet client needs. Depending on individual assessment, the interventions discussed in this chapter might be one or the sole component of comprehensive services that assist the unemployed and working poor in securing employment at a livable wage.

Freedom, Control, and Social Justice

Assisting vulnerable populations in improving their economic status and in achieving economic independence through employment is consistent with enhancing individual freedom and control and with a social justice perspective. Compared with many other employment programs, the Job Club method appears to be more effective in helping some vulnerable clients to secure employment, secure it more quickly, and in some cases obtain jobs with more hours and higher pay. Azrin and his colleagues (1980) addressed another important question from a social justice perspective: Is one client's secural of a job achieved at the expense of other clients? The researchers argued that since approximately 55% of the jobs secured by Job Club participants had not been publicly advertised, many of the jobs were created or made available sooner by Job Club members' job-search activities. A job secured by one participant, therefore, does not necessarily take a job away from another.

Although the majority of the participants involved in the previously described CB programs indicated that securing employment was a personal goal, this likely will not be the case for all individuals. Some clients participating in Job Clubs, particularly those on public assistance, may prefer to remain unemployed. Instead, they participate to avoid negative consequences, such as discontinuation of welfare benefits. Even after the job-seeking skills are learned and clients choose to be employed, problems such as living in areas with high unemployment rates, low educational levels, and limited work history may leave many clients with few job choices. In addition, securing employment does not necessarily translate into a better quality life or result in an increase in economic well-being, compared with remaining on income support programs when possible. These issues are discussed more fully in the next section.

Several methods are used in these job-seeking interventions that increase clients' input into and control over the intervention process. The methods include graduated prompting strategies and clients identifying and rehearsing their own interview responses, serving as peer tutors and supports for one another, and seeking their own mentors or other social supports to assist them in finding employment. Clients also control the use of their job-seeking skills, such as choosing for which jobs to apply.

Social Validity

Socially relevant goals and results. The social relevance of the instrumental goals of enhancing specific job-seeking skills, such as those related to job interviews, was established in a variety of ways. For example, relevant skills were identified through reviews of the employment literature, interviews of employers in relevant job areas, and a validated skills checklist. Although the ultimate goal, securing employment, may not be a desirable goal from the perspective of all individuals, most members of society, including vulnerable populations, generally value being employed. Employment also is related to adult well-being.

Evaluations of the programs discussed in this chapter, particularly the Job Club method, suggest that these interventions can increase employment for many vulnerable clients. By that measure, at least, the results of the interventions are socially valid. As noted in the previous section, some of the evaluations of the Job Club method also reported that Job Club participants secure jobs more quickly, obtain higher salaries, and work more hours compared with participants in other employment programs. Azrin and his colleagues' (1980) evaluation also found that 84% of Job Club public assistance participants were satisfied with their jobs, compared with 78% of clients participating in another employment program. These outcome measures all indicate that the results of the Job Club method are socially valid. The evaluations also suggest that agencies and practitioners should have little hesitancy in offering the intervention to many vulnerable client groups.

Many evaluations, however, failed to report the worker's salary or whether the employment was full-time. When salaries were reported, they tended to be low. None of the studies evaluated whether employment resulted in benefits, such as health insurance, in a higher income than public assistance recipients had previously received, or in an improved quality of life. The evaluations also failed to examine whether securing employment resulted in unpredicted or negative effects on the participants or their families. Negative outcomes might include a decrease in income and/or benefits, poor-quality child care, a lower quality of life, high stress levels, or exacerbation of psychiatric or physical symptoms. Practitioners and researchers might use more comprehensive socially valid measures of clients' secural of employment, which would include a livable wage, benefits, desired working hours, and an enhanced quality of life for the workers and their families.

These last measures are particularly important given recent welfare reforms and the results of research evaluating government work programs, many of which have incorporated Job Clubs. Many work program participants make approximately the same income as control groups after combining income from earnings and government benefits, such as food stamps and public assistance (Michalopoulos, Schwartz, & Adams-Ciardullo, 2000). Although the majority of recipients who leave welfare are working, most have unstable jobs with low pay and limited benefits (Zedlewski, 2002). Job search programs are insufficient to assist many clients in making a successful transition from public assistance to acquiring and maintaining employment that results in financial independence. For many current and former public assistance recipients, other strategies, such as the Earned Income Tax Credit (EITC), state tax credits, and postsecondary education, must be used to achieve employment and financial goals (Long, 2001).

Socially relevant intervention procedures. None of the CB interventions discussed in this chapter preceded intervention with an individualized functional assessment, which could have assisted in designing more relevant interventions. Such an assessment might have identified other maintaining conditions, besides a lack of skill, that were responsible for the participants' failure to obtain employment. The need for practitioners and researchers to assess and address other maintaining conditions of job-seeking behaviors is suggested by Brooks et al.'s (2001) study. The inability of some Job Club members to secure employment appeared to be the result of their perception that they had transportation problems, when, in fact, many had available cars. For other individuals, lack of transportation, particularly in rural areas, might be a maintaining antecedent for failure to use the job-seeking skills and/or to secure employment. Other research suggests that factors such as anxiety, dysfunctional beliefs (e.g., related to performance), low educational levels, disability, number of children, and limited English proficiency are maintaining antecedents of failure to use job-seeking skills and/or to obtain employment (Farley, 1987; Kim, 2000). An individualized assessment can assist practitioners in determining appropriate interventions.

Socially valid intervention materials, such as role-play situations and job-interviewing responses, were developed in many of the programs through consultation with the participants, potential employers, and personnel managers. The SST program developed by Jung and Jason (1998) is particularly sensitive to culturally defined social skills and incorporates content on cultural similarities and differences between the social norms in this country and the home countries of the Asian American participants. The final section of chapter 6 provides a discussion of the social relevance of the interventions conducted by Balcazar and colleagues that assist vulnerable clients to recruit potential helpers to attain personal goals.

To enhance the social relevance of interventions, researchers and practitioners also can adopt methods used to individualize the standardized behavioral procedures discussed in this chapter. For example, clients can focus only on job-interviewing skills and questions with which they have problems, and they identify and rehearse their own interview responses. Other interventions use videotape practice interviews, and practitioners provide individual feedback. Despite the structured, standardized approach to teaching job-seeking skills, the Job Club method individualizes the interventions and uses many strategies consistent with empowerment and a systems approach to treatment. For example, the practitioners speak with each Job Club member individually and frequently, reinforce their strengths, and focus on positive behaviors, while downplaying or ignoring weaknesses and negative behaviors. Agencies also provide resources (e.g., work space, telephones, job leads, and assistance in locating transportation), and practitioners teach and encourage Job Club members to access resources from multiple sources (e.g., family, other members of their social support networks, former employers, group members).

Most of the special accommodations incorporated into the interventions described in this chapter are made in Job Clubs designed for clients with severe mental illness. The accommodations were described in detail earlier in this chapter. The intervention developed by Schloss and colleagues (1988) also incorporates special accommodations to teach adults with mild mental retardation interview skills. These include specially designed interview question cards and an order card to facilitate peer instruction. With the exception of the studies conducted by Balcazar and his colleagues, evaluations of the programs failed to report whether the interventions were acceptable to participants and others affected by or involved in the interventions. The Job Club method, however, has been used with many types of clients and in a variety of settings, suggesting that the program is feasible and acceptable to many clients, agency personnel, and social policy makers (e.g., in terms of costs, values, resources required, and ease of administration). In addition, one evaluation of the Job Club method for unemployed low-income clients reported that 22% of Job Club participants dropped out, compared with 31% of participants in an alternative program (Azrin et al., 1980). However, dropout rates among some Job Club groups, such as those for individuals with severe mental illness, are exceptionally high. This indicates that the Job Club method is not acceptable to all clients and that practitioners and researchers must assess and, if possible, address maintaining conditions that deter participation.

Maintenance and generalization. For clients whose goal is to obtain employment, job-seeking skills must transfer to natural settings and be maintained long enough for them to secure a job. In Job Clubs, members are assisted in filling out actual job applications and in developing personal resumes, but the length of time these behaviors are maintained and whether they transfer to other job applications and to revisions of resumes is unknown. With the Job Club method, maintaining job-seeking skills generally is not a serious issue, as job seekers, at least theoretically, can remain in the Job Club until they locate employment. Former Job Club members also can return if they need additional assistance. In one Job Club evaluation, approximately 50% of the psychiatric clients who lost the jobs they had secured from participating in a Job Club took advantage of this open door policy (Jacobs et al., 1984). Some clients, however, chose not to return because of the stigma of the psychiatric hospital where the Job Club was located. This latter finding suggests that employment programs must be offered in locations associated with successful employment.

Several of the evaluations of the SST programs discussed in the first two intervention sections of this chapter measured transfer of interview skills to natural settings by assessing participants' interviews with potential employers in actual employment settings. However, rarely did the studies investigate whether participants maintained their performance or whether their skills transferred to different types of settings or interviewers. The one study that did evaluate maintenance of the job-interviewing skills determined that the skills of one of the two participants declined by the six-month follow-up. This finding suggests the need for practitioners to offer booster sessions for clients who do not immediately secure employment. Only one SST evaluation reported whether participants maintained their employment, and the follow-up was only three months.

Assessing maintenance of employment is important, particularly for vulnerable populations. Vulnerable groups are likely to face the same types of problems after employment that were barriers to securing employment in the first place. The problems include symptoms of severe mental illness, limitations caused by physical and cognitive disabilities, inappropriate social interactions, lack of transportation or child care, and local economic conditions. Maintaining continuous employment also is important for reasons such as qualifying for benefits (e.g., health insurance and unemployment compensation), advancement, and increased salary, and because of the absence of a guaranteed safety net for low-income families with children. From an empowerment perspective, losing employment involuntarily or resigning because of unresolved problems when a worker desires to remain employed surely is not empowering.

Although the Job Clubs' evaluations reported percentages of workers who were employed at different times following Job Club participation (e.g., 30–180 days), the studies suffer from methodological problems. First, the longer the follow-up period, the fewer former Job Club members could be located. Second, the researchers rarely determined whether unemployment was involuntary and, if unemployment was involuntary, the reason for the job loss. Jacobs et al.'s (1984) follow-up data on the effectiveness of the Job Club method for psychiatric patients determined that one-third of the members who secured employment were unable to maintain their jobs. Work-related stress, psychiatric symptoms, and layoffs because of downturns in the economy all were significantly related to job loss. As these findings and research discussed in the next chapter indicate, job loss rates of many vulnerable populations are high. Many vulnerable workers require initial and ongoing supportive interventions to enhance productivity, work quality, and job-related social skills if they are to maintain or advance in employment. CB interventions to address these outcomes are discussed in chapter 8.

ADDITIONAL READINGS AND RESOURCES

Agran, M., & Moore, S. C. (1994). *How to teach self-instruction of job skills.* Washington, DC: American Association on Mental Retardation.

Azrin, N. J., & Besalel, V. A. (1980). *Job-Club counselor's manual: A behavioral approach to vocational counseling.* Baltimore: University Park Press.

Elksnin, L. K., & Elksnin, N. (1991). The school counselor as job search facilitator: Increasing employment of handicapped students through Job Clubs. *School Counselor, 38,* 215–220.

Goldman, B. (1989). Job search strategies for women on welfare. In S. Harlan & R. Steinberg (Eds.), *Job training for women* (pp. 389–413). Philadelphia: Temple University Press.

Mathews, R. M., & Fawcett, S. B. (1985). Assisting in the job search: A behavioral assessment and training strategy. *Journal of Rehabilitation, 51,* 31–35.

Mathews, R. M., Whang, P. L., & Fawcett, S. B. (1984). *Learning job-finding skills.* Lawrence, KS: Research and Training Center on Independent Living, University of Kansas. Available at http://www.rtcil.org/produ cts/index.shtml

Rusch, F. R., Hughes, C., & Wilson, P. G. (1985). Utilizing cognitive strategies in the acquisition of employment skills. In W. O'Donohue & L. Krasner (Eds.), *Handbook of psychological skills training: Clinical techniques and applications* (pp. 363–382). Boston: Allyn & Bacon.

Wong, S. E. (1996). Psychosis. In M. A. Mattaini & B. A. Thyer (Eds.), *Finding solutions to social problems: Behavioral strategies for change* (pp. 319–344). Washington, DC: American Psychological Association.

8 Maintaining and Advancing in Employment

Obtaining employment provides no assurance of equality or protection against discharge for vulnerable employees. Vulnerable workers employed in sheltered workshops or in integrated, competitive work settings frequently receive low wages, fail to advance, and maintain employment only for a short period of time. These negative outcomes commonly are the result of inadequate accommodations and support, low productivity and work quality, inappropriate social behavior, a need for constant supervision, difficulties coping with psychiatric symptoms, and a variety of other psychosocial stressors (Corrigan et al., 1995; Elksnin, Elksnin, & Sabornie, 1994; Grossi & Heward, 1998). The CB interventions discussed in this chapter are designed to assist vulnerable workers in resolving or managing many of these problems. Workers who successfully resolve these problems are more likely to maintain their jobs, increase their wages, and secure more fulfilling and higher-paying jobs. For workers employed in sheltered workshops, the interventions can assist them in obtaining positions in integrated, competitive work settings. These successes can empower vulnerable workers.

This chapter begins with a brief discussion of the components and goals of supported employment, followed by a description of CB interventions that assist vulnerable workers in increasing their work productivity and quality. A description of CB strategies that enhance job-related social skills, which can result in vulnerable workers maintaining or advancing in employment, follows. The final section provides an analysis and critique for practice and future research, including issues of effectiveness and additional applications, freedom, control, and social justice, and social validity.

SUPPORTED EMPLOYMENT

Traditionally, vocational rehabilitation programs have used three main approaches to assist vulnerable workers (primarily individuals with mental retardation, severe mental illness, and physical disabilities) in finding and sustaining employment (Twamley et al., 2003). The first approach is sheltered workshop employment, where workers usually perform factory-type jobs in group settings segregated from workers with no disabilities. Perhaps because clients in sheltered workshops are rarely taught the skills necessary for competitive employment, less than 5% of them obtain community employment. The second approach is the psychosocial rehabilitation work program. This program involves prevocational training (i.e., teaching job and job-search skills) and transitional or trial employment, such as working part time at less than a minimum wage or working as a volunteer before securing a competitive job. This approach has been criticized because it fails to provide supportive services long enough to assist clients in succeeding in competitive employment. Despite criticisms of the sheltered workshop and psychosocial rehabilitation work approaches, they are the most commonly available vocational services for workers with disabilities.

The third approach to assist vulnerable workers is supported employment, designed for workers who cannot work independently in competitive jobs without intensive ongoing support services (Twamley et al., 2003). The objectives of supported employment differ from those of sheltered workshops and psychosocial rehabilitation. Supported employment programs focus on quickly locating and placing clients into integrated, competitive work settings that pay at least a minimum wage. Supported employment specialists provide workers with on-the-job training, make modifications to adapt jobs to their special needs, plan strategies for maintaining the acquired job skills, and provide continuous open-ended follow-up intervention to assist workers in maintaining employment. Intervention includes assisting with transportation and coordinating services with the clients' co-workers, supervisors, other service providers, and significant others.

Clients working in supported employment earn more than their peers in sheltered workshops, and they have opportunities for interacting with co-workers without disabilities and other community members. Research suggests that supported employment programs are effective for increasing the competitive employment of workers with a variety of disabilities (Kregel, Wehman, & Banks, 1989; Rusch & Hughes, 1989; Twamley et al., 2003). CB methods have played an important role in supported employment programs through job-task analysis and training, modifying the antecedent conditions in work settings, teaching workers independence strategies, and enhancing workers' communication and social skills (McDonnell, Nofs, Hardman, & Chambless, 1989; Wacker, Fromm-Steege, Berg, & Flynn, 1989).

All of the CB interventions described in this chapter were developed for workers with some type of disability. To assist other vulnerable workers, such as the economically disadvantaged, in obtaining and maintaining employment, the federal government has funded various employment activities through Job Opportunities and Basic Skills (JOBS) and Job Training Partnership Act (JTPA) programs, and more recently through Welfare-to-Work programs. Job training, case management, and supported work activity (e.g., on-the-job training and other postemployment services) have been provided in the majority of these programs (Greenberg, Meyer, Michalopoulos, & Wiseman, 2003; Perez-Johnson, Hershey, & Bellotti, 2000). These practices suggest that policy makers recognize that on-the-job training is an efficient and preferred method of teaching many job tasks, and many low-income and former public assistance recipients require ongoing support if they are to maintain employment.

Although numerous evaluations of government work programs have been conducted, the contribution of CB methods to assist clients in learning job and related social skills in these programs is extremely difficult to assess. The difficulty stems from the programs' being administered through hundreds of different local agencies and sites. This has resulted in variations in program components and the manner in which they have been administered. Formal evaluations of specific CB methods incorporated into the multicomponent programs also are rare (Bloom & Michalopoulos, 2001; Greenberg et al., 2003). Because of these problems, the interventions discussed here are limited to well-defined CB interventions that meet three criteria. First, the interventions were designed to enhance workers' job skills and related social skills in employment settings. Second, the interventions were evaluated to determine their effectiveness. Third, the evaluation provided some evidence that by improving their job skills and related social skills, the workers were able to maintain or advance in their jobs.

INCREASING WORK PRODUCTIVITY AND QUALITY

CB interventions designed to increase the work productivity and quality of workers with physical disabilities, mental retardation, and severe mental illness who are currently employed in sheltered workshops or competitive employment settings are discussed now. The interventions include various combinations of CB methods, such as prompting strategies (e.g., use of graduated, picture, photograph, verbal, and recorded prompts), reinforcement (e.g., praise, recognition, money), modeling, and other SST techniques. Many of the interventions incorporate a variety of self-management strategies, including self-reinforcement, self-monitoring, and performance feedback (e.g., graphs, stacked tokens, timers, recruiting praise, and a self-operated auditory prompting system), self-instruction, problem solving, and setting production goals. All but two of the discussed interventions (Bell, Lysaker, & Bryson, 2003; McNally, Kompik, & Sherman, 1984) were evaluated using multiple-baseline or single-system designs.

Additional CB interventions not included in this section have been used to teach vulnerable workers basic job skills. Evaluations of these interventions, however, did not determine whether learning the skills resulted in participants securing, enhancing, or maintaining employment. For this reason, these interventions are not described in detail in this or the previous chapters. Instead, the studies are cited in the following relevant sections. Practitioners interested in additional methods that might enhance or maintain employment of vulnerable workers by teaching or improving job skills are referred to those sources.

Workers with Physical Disabilities

This older case study involved Eric, an 18-year-old male with cerebral palsy and a severe speech impairment (Wehman, Hill, & Koehler, 1979). The case study describes placing an individual with disabilities into competitive employment with support from a job coach and advocate through Project Employability. The goal of this project was to demonstrate the employment potential of individuals with severe disabilities and no formal job training.

Eric was hired to operate a freight and passenger elevator at a large hospital. His job duties involved routine tasks such as operating the elevator and using clear language at the appropriate time (e.g., "Going up"). Eric also learned how to handle the elevator in emergency situations. During on-the-job training, the job coach provided verbal prompts, followed by more intrusive prompts when necessary. As Eric learned the job tasks, the coach gradually placed herself at the rear of the elevator and began riding the vehicle on a gradually decreasing schedule. The job coach also advocated for Eric regarding his disability with other staff who regularly rode the elevator, which helped staff develop an understanding of Eric's abilities and limitations. After intervention, Eric established a friendly relationship with many hospital staff, and the staff advocated for Eric in the presence of strangers on the elevator. Eric went from part-time to full-time employment.

Grossi (1998) describes two case studies of using a self-operated auditory prompting system to increase the work performance of two supported employees with severe physical disabilities. Both workers desired to keep their jobs; but to do so, they needed to improve their work performance. Gina suffered from osteoporosis and severe epilepsy with recurrent seizures, which required her to use a wheelchair to prevent injury during seizures. Gina worked for a large retail store, and her duties included arranging the merchandise, restocking, and light dusting. Several behaviors were jeopardizing Gina's continued employment. They included problems staying on task, working too slowly, and interacting inappropriately with others (e.g., interrupting co-workers and customers). Rob, who had severe epilepsy and cerebral palsy, was one of six men working on a janitorial mobile crew responsible for cleaning several buildings. His job duty was cleaning sink areas, tables, and conference rooms. Rob frequently became distracted, had verbal outbursts when he didn't get his way, telephoned his mother frequently during working hours, and inappropriately roamed the building.

Although a job coach provided on-the-job supervision and support, both Gina and Rob required an unacceptable amount of staff time to redirect and prompt their return to work.

To prompt the two employees to stay on their job tasks, a self-operated auditory prompting system was designed and was used by the workers. After the employees selected their own music tapes, the job coach embedded the tapes with auditory prompts on a variable schedule (averaging about thirty seconds). The auditory prompts reminded Gina and Rob to evaluate whether they were working and to continue their job activity. Examples of the prompts are "Gina are you working? (pause) Keep working!" and "Are you working? (pause) Keep those hands moving." While completing their job duties, the employees wore headphones and carried their tape players in a way that did not interfere with their work (e.g., in a pouch).

For both workers, the reversal design demonstrated that the intervention improved their work performance (e.g., increased time on job tasks and accuracy of performing the job tasks). The workers and their supervisors were satisfied with the intervention and found it helpful. After intervention Gina used the auditory prompting system for one year, at which time she was reassigned to work in two different departments within the same company. She continued to use the system when needed. Rob was referred for an individual job placement based on his improved performance and was given a raise.

Workers with Mental Retardation

Sheltered workshops. The four CB interventions discussed here were developed to increase the job performance of sheltered workshop employees. This first behavioral intervention improves the work productivity of adults with mild to severe mental retardation by reducing worker distractions and using prompts and reinforcement (Martin, Pallotta-Cornick, Johnstone, & Goyos, 1980). To reduce worker distraction, partitions are constructed to divide the production table into four sections, with two workers to a section. In front of each worker, the practitioner posts pictures and mounts items depicting the relation between the product the workers are completing (e.g., airline coffee packs) and the money they can earn. Workers are then instructed to work hard, look at their picture prompts, and make lots of the product to earn money to buy goodies after work.

The practitioner also implements a reinforcement and feedback system to increase the workers' productivity. First, instead of receiving their earnings weekly, the workers are given the money daily based on the number of production items completed. Second, supervisors are trained to provide the workers with ongoing feedback on their productivity. In order to do this, a specially constructed receiving tray is attached to the partition in front of each worker. The tray is divided into a number of sections, the size of which is determined by the average hourly rate of production during baseline. During each work session, supervisors collect products from the completed sections of the receiver trays and calculate the number of coins (e.g., nickels, quarters, etc., depending on the production rate) the workers earned. Feedback is then provided for each worker by way of a a frequency bar graph. The workers observe as the supervisors construct a bar graph by putting one "x" for each earned coin into the spaces of the graph paper. The workers are encouraged to try and get their line of x's higher than the previous session. Supervisors also use praise as reinforcement.

The production rate of all workers (N = 16) participating in the evaluation increased after intervention, with the range varying from a few percentage points to 150% of baseline production. The supervisors and workers, who were given multiple choices to work at the production table or under the previous workshop conditions, preferred the production table. The evaluation also suggests that the intervention must be continued to maintain the workers' increased productivity.

In this CB intervention, self-monitoring is added to performance feedback and reinforcement to increase the productivity of sheltered workshop employees with mental retardation ranging from borderline to severe (McNally et al., 1984). In implementing the self-monitoring procedure, the supervisor provides the workers with a number of pink tokens (one fewer than the mean number of production units completed daily during baseline) stacked on top of several blue tokens. The supervisor then instructs the workers to remove a token from the top of the stack and place it into their container each time they complete a unit of production (e.g., screwing a cap on a bottle). Workers also are told that their goal is to reach the first blue token, which indicates achievement of their baseline performance. When the workers reach their first blue token, they are instructed to tell the floor supervisor. The supervisor then turns on a light, which remains lit for the remainder of the workday, publicizing the workers' attainment of their goals. Production goals are reset every several days based on the mean production rate of the previous day. Goal achievement also is reinforced by the thirty minutes of leisure activity workers are given at the end of the day. In addition, at the end of each work day, the supervisor removes the blue tokens from the workers' containers and attaches them to a bar graph displayed on the wall. The three workers earning the most blue tokens during a work week are taken out to lunch. The A-B-A reversal design demonstrated that the intervention was associated with large increases in the productivity rates of the thirteen workers involved in the evaluation. Although only one worker's productivity consistently approached the industrial rate, 95% of the time the workers met or exceeded their daily goals.

Hughes and Petersen (1989) added self-instructional training to prompting, performance feedback, and reinforcement strategies to increase the on-task behavior and work performance of workshop employees with mild to moderate mental retardation. The intervention begins with the trainer providing a rationale for improving work performance, for example, "If you work better, your supervisor will praise you more and won't criticize you and tell you what to do so often; you also might be able to get a competitive job." The trainer shows the workers dollar bills while discussing the relation between production and earning more money on payday. The trainer also asks the workers what they like to buy with their money. The workers then are shown brightly colored bar graphs of their on-task behavior during baseline and are told that the graphs indicate poor work performance. The trainer suggests that working better could improve the graphs, which are updated and shown to the workers at the end of each workday to provide performance feedback.

The trainer uses self-instructional training to teach the workers to self-instruct while performing their job task. However, the training ends with the workers completing the job task while whispering the self-instructions, instead of saying the instructions silently to themselves. Although the workers are encouraged to develop individual adaptions of the self-instructions, the following are examples of statements for the job task of stuffing envelopes.

1 "What does _____ want me to do?" (task performance question)
2 "First I pick up the envelope. Then I put in the yellow letter, the green letter. Now I put down the envelope." (statement to guide performance)
3 "Now check back. Good, I did a good job. Next one." (self-reinforcement and prompting statement)
4 "Check back. Oops. Better fix it." (error-correcting statement)

In addition, the workers are shown a photograph of themselves working in the workshop. The workers then are told that after using self-instruction to complete each task, they should look at the picture, self-reinforce, and tell themselves to continue working by saying, "Next one." During the work sessions, the trainer provides a variety of reinforcers contingent on the workers' attention and correct performance. After formal training, the intervention is withdrawn, with the exception of the photograph, which prompts the workers to stay on task. The on-task behavior of all four workers involved in the evaluation increased substantially following the training and transferred from the training to the work setting. The on-task behaviors were maintained at a three-week follow-up. The intervention had mixed effects on the workers' task completion.

In this final CB intervention, which was developed to increase the productivity of sheltered workshop employees with mild to moderate mental retardation, the workers learn a "recruitment-of-praise package," in addition to a self-monitoring procedure (Hildebrand, Martin, Furer, & Hazen, 1990). Before teaching the workers to self-monitor their productivity, the trainer constructs self-monitoring sheets containing a chain of vertically drawn boxes. The self-monitoring sheets then are placed in front of each worker's receiver box, in which the worker places the finished product. The trainer uses skills training to teach the workers to draw a diagonal line through the next box in line on their self-monitoring sheets after completing each product.

After the workers master the self-monitoring procedure, the trainer teaches them to solicit praise for reaching their production goals. For each worker, the trainer draws a pink line under the box representing the completion of the worker's short-term production goal. After workers meet their short-term production goal (by marking the relevant box as indicated by the pink line), the trainer uses SST to teach them to solicit praise by raising their hands or by flipping the white side of a small card to the pink side. In response, the trainer provides a social reinforcer, and the workers select and use a stamp to mark their monitoring sheets (e.g., a happy face). The trainer then sets a new production goal by drawing a pink line under the appropriate box on the worker's self-monitoring sheet. If the self-monitoring is inaccurate or the solicitation for praise inappropriate, corrective feedback is given and the short-term goal repeated.

After intervention, two of the three workers involved in the evaluation demonstrated increased production rates, and rates remained high at the one-month followup. The two workers with increased productivity worked at 91% and 93% of the normative rate. The intervention, however, appeared to decrease productivity for the third worker. Production accuracy, which was high at baseline, increased slightly during the recruitment intervention. All three workers preferred the recruitment package, and staff continued to use the intervention for the two workers who had increased their productivity.

Competitive employment. The goal of the first of seven CB applications designed to increase the work performance of employees with mental retardation working in competitive employment settings is to reduce the amount of time required to perform job tasks (Crouch, Karlan, & Rusch, 1984). During intervention, the workers are given a wristwatch, and before a task (e.g., managing the dishwashing machine, stocking serving lines, sweeping, mopping) is started, co-workers are instructed to prompt the workers to begin and complete an assigned task at a specific time. A few minutes before the workers are to begin a designated task, the co-workers instruct them to state when they will begin and complete the task. The workers also are asked to describe how the start and completion times look on their wristwatches or the wall clocks. For example, for 9:15, the big hand will be on 3 and the little hand will be on 9. At the midpoint of the allotted time for the respective task, the co-workers prompt the workers to say when they will finish the task. The co-workers also socially reinforce the workers after they perform the activities and make the statements. After intervention, all three employees involved in the evaluation improved their work performance and, with few exceptions, met the supervisor's time criteria for each job task.

Rusch and his colleagues (Rusch, Morgan, Martin, Riva, & Agran, 1985) also used self-instructional training to increase the performance of job tasks of employees with mild to moderate mental retardation. The training is similar to that developed by Hughes and Petersen (1989) previously discussed in this chapter. The only difference between this self-instructional training and the previously described training is that the workers are taught to covertly self-instruct while performing the job tasks. After intervention, both workers involved in the evaluation increased their job performance on at least one of three tasks related to their jobs as kitchen helpers in university dormitories. Their time spent working also increased, and the workers met or exceeded the production standards of nonprobationary co-workers without disabilities. The skills were maintained at a two-week follow-up.

Christian and Poling (1997) designed a CB intervention combining three self-management procedures—self-timing, self-instruction, and self-recording—with prompting and reinforcement to improve the productivity of competitive employees with mild mental retardation. In the first phase of the intervention, the practitioner teaches the self-management strategies while the workers complete a task (e.g., setting tables, rolling silverware into napkins) that they can perform at an acceptable rate. The practitioner models appropriate use of a timer set to signal the expiration of the designated time for a specific task, self-instruction, and data recording. Acceptable times for particular tasks are written in a notebook, which the employees use to record whether they complete a task within the designated time. The practitioner verbally prompts the employees to perform the behaviors and reinforces them for accurate recording and for completing the task within the acceptable time. In the second phase of the training, the practitioner chooses an acceptable time for a task performed too slowly (based on the workers' speed in performing the task during baseline), and the employees perform the task using the self-timing, self-instruction, and self-recording procedures. Reinforcers are gradually faded. After intervention, the productivity of the two participants increased; they were at or above 75% of the rate of able-bodied co-workers. The increased productivity was maintained for up to two months. The intervention procedures were acceptable to the workers, co-workers, and supervisors. Both of the workers kept the jobs that they were at risk of losing, and one worker's performance earned her a salary increase.

This CB program developed by Browder and Minarovic's (2000) involves teaching sight words, in addition to self-management strategies, to assist employees with moderate mental retardation in increasing self-initiated job tasks. From a list of job tasks that the employees are expected to self-initiate, the trainer identifies key sight words. For example, for a bagger at a grocery store, for "Replace bags at checkout" the key sight words are "fill bags" (see table 1, p. 80 of the article, for a list of job tasks and sight words for jobs related to working as a bagger and custodian in a grocery store, a cook's assistant in a cafeteria, and a seamstress in a clothing factory). After identifying the sight words, the trainer teaches the employees the words using a progressive time-delay procedure. To do this, the words are placed on flash cards, which are presented to the employee. In the beginning of the instruction, if the employee fails to respond correctly, the trainer immediately models the correct response. Later, the trainer gradually increases the amount of time after showing the card before modeling the response. The trainer praises the employee's correct responses.

During the second phase of the intervention, the trainer models the following "Now-Did-Next" self-instruction strategy to teach the employees to self-initiate tasks.

1. The trainer points to the words "fill bags" on a checklist and says, "NOW I'm going to fill the bags," then role-plays stocking bags.
2. The trainer states, "I DID fill the bags, so I check off bags like this," then the trainer checks the words "fill bags."
3. The trainer states, "NEXT, I am going to sweep," while pointing to the word "sweep."

After the trainer introduces each step, the employee practices the self-instruction sequence. The procedure is repeated until all words are checked off the checklist. If the intervention is conducted in another setting and does not transfer to the work site, the trainer encourages the use of the self-monitoring strategies by using a hierarchy of verbal prompts as follows.

1. Nonspecific prompt about the list: "What do you need to remember?"
2. Specific prompt about the list: "Use your list."
3. Nonspecific prompt about self-management: "How do you use the list?"
4. Specific prompt about self-management: "Use your "Now-Did-Next."

After intervention, all the employees involved in the evaluation (N = 3) demonstrated mastery of their sight words for job assignments, used the sight word checklist, and independently initiated their work assignments. The employers' satisfaction with the employees' work also increased. The use of the sight word list was acceptable to the supervisors, and informal observations and reports from significant others indicated that the interventions were highly acceptable to the three employees.

Grossi and Heward (1998) designed a more comprehensive self-management training program, which includes goal setting, self-monitoring, and self-evaluation, to increase the work productivity of employees with mild mental retardation. In this program, skills training is used to teach the self-management procedures that assist workers in proficiently learning job tasks (e.g., scrubbing pots, sweeping and mopping floors) that are identified through a task analysis. The practitioner assists the employees in setting their own work goals by showing them a simple line graph depicting their baseline production measures in comparison to the competitive standard (an area on the graph that is shaded). The employees then are taught to self-monitor their work performance by using a stopwatch or countdown timer to measure and then record the number of work units completed or the amount of time required to complete each task. The employees then record their performance in a notebook by circling the appropriate number that matches the number on their counter or stopwatch. Finally, the practitioner teaches the employees to self-evaluate by comparing their performance against their previously set goal or the competitive standard. Depending on their performance, the workers make adjustments in their performance goal. The employees also are taught to verbalize whether they are in the competitive range—for example, "Good, I'm in the area" of the shaded area.

The employees (N = 4) involved in the study learned to set goals, monitor their work productivity, and evaluate their performance against the competitive standard. After intervention, each employee's work productivity improved for each task while work quality was maintained. Three of the four employees positively evaluated the intervention, but the fourth found it to be too stressful. The supervisors also were satisfied with the program and reported that self-monitoring improved the workers' productivity and work quality and increased their independence. After intervention, all four of the workers, who were in a community-based work training program receiving a training wage, obtained a competitive job with the support of a job coach.

This behavioral intervention involving a self-monitoring procedure and social and self-reinforcement was designed to assist employees with moderate mental retardation in staying on their job tasks (Kaplan, Hemmes, Motz, & Rodriguez, 1996). The intervention begins with the practitioner taking photographs of the workers performing their assigned tasks (e.g., sweeping and mopping floors, clearing tables, wiping tables and trays), which are placed into a small wallet the workers carry in their pockets. The workers then are taught to recognize when they are on or off task. To do this, by the workers and their supervisors rate whether they are on or off task at various times during the workday, after which the supervisors provide the workers with feedback regarding the accuracy of the workers' ratings. The employees then are given a timer with a compartment filled with nickels set to buzz every thirty seconds. When the timer sounds, the workers evaluate whether they were on task immediately before the signal. If they were on task, the workers take a nickel from the timer, place it in their pockets, reset the timer, and return to work. If the workers were off task, they refer to the relevant photograph in their wallet to determine which task they should be performing. At the end of the day, the workers keep the nickels they earned. Based on their performance, the supervisors also provide feedback or social reinforcement. If the workers' self-evaluations of their on-task behavior differ by no more than one on-task observation, they receive an additional fifty cents. After formal intervention, the workers continue to use their timing devices and are provided with a choice of reinforcers to self-administer.

The evaluation involving seven workers determined that including self-reinforcement (using nickels instead of steel washers, which also was evaluated) was more effective in increasing six of the seven men's on-task behavior and productivity, compared to using only the self-monitoring procedure and social reinforcement. The employees also preferred the intervention including self-reinforcement. The workers and their supervisors reported improvements in the employees' work performance and on-task behavior after intervention. The improvements were maintained several weeks after formal intervention was discontinued.

As described in the case study of Mr. Jones, picture prompting also can be used to assist workers with severe mental retardation in working more independently (Wilson, Schepis, & Mason-Main, 1987). Mr. Jones, a 36-year-old man with severe mental retardation who had been institutionalized for more than twenty years, was working in a family-owned restaurant. Mr. Jones's job required him to perform food service tasks, such as packaging silverware and dishwashing. During the first phase of the picture prompt training, his job coach taught Mr. Jones to use a previously constructed booklet, which consisted of photographs depicting Mr. Jones performing each step of his assigned job tasks. In the restaurant, the job coach introduced each page of the picture booklet, which represented a sequence of tasks for performing each job. The coach verbally explained what the picture represented, pointed out relevant information in the photograph, and modeled the task. After the task was performed and the relevant information in the work environment matched the picture, the job coach marked an "x" in the box provided on the page and then turned the page. Mr. Jones then practiced the behaviors. Sometimes part of the relevant task depicted in the photograph had already been completed, which confused Mr. Jones. For example, when the picture prompted Mr. Jones to fill the sink with soapy water, the sink was already filled. To teach his client to adapt his behavior to these types of situations, the coach arranged the work environment so that occasionally the task depicted in the photograph was completed before Mr. Jones was shown the picture prompt. When this occurred, the coach introduced the photograph stating, "It looks like someone has already done _____." The coach then followed the previously described training procedures.

In the second phase of the intervention, Mr. Jones used his picture prompt booklet to assist him in completing the assigned job tasks while the job coach observed. If Mr. Jones performed the task appropriately, he was intermittently praised. If he made an error or failed to initiate the appropriate response, the coach used the previously described strategies. After Mr. Jones became more proficient at completing the tasks more independently, the coach gradually faded his assistance, and the restaurant assumed supervisory responsibility. The picture prompts also were faded, and in approximately two months Mr. Jones was performing his work tasks without assistance. Twenty months later, Mr. Jones remained employed by the restaurant, and the owners rated him one of their best employees.

Other studies have evaluated a variety of CB interventions designed to enhance the job skills and performance of individuals with mental retardation. Because these evaluations did not determine whether research participants secured, enhanced, or maintained employment after intervention, they are only briefly mentioned here. Prompting strategies were used to teach adolescents and adults with moderate to severe mental retardation janitorial skills (Cuvo, Leaf, & Borakove, 1978; Simmons & Flexer, 1992). Skills training assisted a young man with severe mental retardation in learning the job skills of a bus person in a community restaurant (Certo, Mezzullo, & Hunter, 1985) and taught co-workers to teach food preparation skills to women with mild mental retardation (Likins, Salzerg, Stowitschek, Kraft, & Curl, 1989). Graphic feedback was used to increase the speed of a woman with moderate mental retardation who stripped trays in the dishroom of a hospital (Davis, Bates, & Cuvo, 1983). A variety of self-management techniques, including self-instruction, self-reinforcement, and establishing production goals, assisted adults with mild to severe mental retardation in performing a variety of job tasks (Agran, Fodor-Davis, & Moore, 1986; Salend, Ellis, & Reynold, 1989) and in increasing their productivity (Moore, Agran, & Fodor-Davis, 1989). Self-management techniques also assisted high school students with mental retardation in performing job tasks independently (Sowers, Verdi, Bourbeau, & Sheehan, 1985).

Workers with Severe Mental Illness

The only CB intervention discussed in detail in this section was developed in a transitional employment setting for clients diagnosed with schizophrenia or schizoaffective disorder (Bell et al., 2003). The intervention is a component of a job support program, which involves employees and supervisors providing the clients on-the-job training. A job coach is assigned at the client's request. The support program provides other supportive services, including ongoing contact with supervisors, arranging special accommodations, and assisting with crises. The CB intervention is conducted for sixteen weeks in groups of six. Group facilitators use the Work Behavior Inventory to conduct biweekly assessments of the clients' work performance through observation and supervisor interviews. The inventory, which is specifically designed for clients with severe mental illness, consists of five subscales, including work habits, work quality, and various job-related social skills.

During the group sessions, group facilitators provide workers with feedback on their scores for each work behavior scale and on particular items that might have lowered or raised their scores. The workers also are given graphs depicting their ratings on each subscale. Group members then discuss the ratings and engage in problem solving to identify strategies to improve specific areas in which they are having difficulty. Following this activity, the workers set specific work performance goals for the next two weeks. The group members then write the goals on their time sheets used for recording daily work hours. At subsequent group meetings, the workers discuss progress in meeting their goals. If a goal is attained, a new goal is set. The male workers participating in the study (N = 63) were randomly assigned to the CB intervention or to a usual support services group. The workers participating in the CB intervention improved their overall work performance to a greater extent and worked 36% more hours and 22% more weeks than the comparison group.

Although no evidence was provided that the behavioral techniques resulted in the research participants securing, maintaining, or advancing in employment, the following two studies suggest that the interventions can enhance the job skills of individuals with severe mental illness. Sauter and Nevid's (1991) evaluation indicates that skills training can increase the productivity rates of piecework jobs completed by hospitalized patients diagnosed with chronic schizophrenia. A later study suggests that errorless learning (the task is performed until it is automatic and done without error) is more effective than standard skills training in increasing the productivity and accuracy in assembly tasks among clients diagnosed with schizophrenia or schizoaffective disorder (Kern, Liberman, Kopelowicz, Mintz, & Green, 2002).

ENHANCING EMPLOYMENT-RELATED SOCIAL SKILLS

CB interventions designed to teach job-related social skills, such as following instructions, appropriate dress and grooming, responding to criticism, and engaging in a variety of other social interactions that are necessary to maintain or advance in employment, are discussed now. Vulnerable workers include those with mental retardation and severe mental illness. The interventions include SST, self-instruction, punishment, and problem solving. With three exceptions (Bell et al., 2003; Tsang, 2001; Wallace, Tauber, & Wilde, 1999), the interventions were evaluated using single-system and multiple-baseline designs.

Because evaluations of certain other CB methods designed to assist vulnerable clients in learning job-related social skills did not determine whether learning such skills resulted in any employment-related outcomes, they are only briefly mentioned in the sections that follow. Evaluations of the interventions generally demonstrated that the programs were effective in enhancing the participants' job-related social skills. These interventions might be relevant to practitioners or agencies providing services to vulnerable clients desiring to learn job-related social skills to acquire, maintain, or advance in employment.

Workers with Developmental and Physical Disabilities

This case study demonstrates the use of several behavioral interventions to teach appropriate social behaviors to Phil, a young man with moderate mental retardation working in a supported competitive employment setting (Wheeler, Bates, Marshall, & Miller, 1988). Phil worked as an animal caretaker in a university lab, where his basic job duties involved caring for and feeding of animals and maintaining equipment and facilities. Following extended supportive work training, interviews with supervisors and co-workers and formal observations identified seven inappropriate social behaviors that placed Phil's continued employment at risk. The behaviors were failing to shave, to respond to greetings, to follow instructions, and to initiate social interactions, and belching, discussing excessive drinking, and pouting. The job coach used SST to teach Phil to respond to greetings and to initiate social interactions. The remaining five behaviors were listed on a piece of laminated poster board in the form of a checklist and placed in Phil's work locker. The job coach used the following procedures to teach Phil to use the checklist.

1. When Phil arrived at work, the job coach accompanied Phil to his locker.
2. The job coach verbally stated each behavior on the list and provided examples. An example for following instructions was telling Phil that after a supervisor gave him instructions, he should begin carrying them out within five seconds.
3. The job coach instructed Phil to self-record at noon by placing a plus

sign next to any behavior that he exhibited appropriately, and a minus next to any behavior he performed inappropriately.
4 The job coach informed Phil that he would provide feedback to him throughout the day and that Phil should do his best.
5 At noon, the job coach accompanied Phil to his locker and prompted Phil to perform the self-recording.
6 The job coach prompted Phil to re-evaluate his performance and, if Phil did not accurately self-record, to do so accurately.
7 The job coach gradually withdrew prompts, feedback, and his presence.

Phil's seven social behaviors improved after intervention. Co-workers' evaluations of Phil's job performance also indicated significant improvement, and Phil's three subsequent employment evaluations fell within the average to above-average range. Phil also was given additional and more complex job responsibilities and attained civil service status. Phil's improved behaviors were maintained over a thirty-eight-week period, during which time Phil required only minimal support from his job coach.

In this second case study, behavioral interventions assisted Jim, a 26-year-old employee with moderate mental retardation, in maintaining his employment (Rusch & Menchetti, 1981). Jim was employed as a full-time kitchen worker, but his employment was threatened because he refused to do specific assigned tasks (e.g., cleaning the grill) and to provide assistance throughout the day when requested by his co-workers (e.g., assisting cooks to lift a heavy item). Jim also was currently in an apartment training program, where he was learning to live semi-independently. Residential training staff agreed to participate in the intervention, because if Jim lost his employment, he would return to an intermediate care facility. Intervention consisted of traditional SST techniques. Prior to Jim's work shift, the trainer provided instruction on and Jim practiced the following behaviors.

1 When asked by a co-worker or supervisor to do a job, immediately stop what you are doing.
2 Respond with "ok" or "yes" in a friendly voice to acknowledge that you heard the request.
3 Perform the job correctly.
4 When the job is completed, return to your original job.

The trainer also told Jim that if he refused a request, the shift supervisor would send him home, which was the standard consequence for workers' failure to comply with work requests. The residential staff and Jim agreed on a set of procedures if Jime were to be sent home. Jim would immediately go to his apartment, call his residential placement coordinator, and remain in the apartment until the coordinator arrived. The coordinator then would discuss with Jim the reason for his being sent home and would prompt Jim to describe an appropriate response. After intervention, Jim exhibited a dramatic increase in the percentage of compliant behaviors. Jim was sent home only once for refusing a work request. In a follow-up evaluation eighteen months later, Jim's supervisor reported that Jim met all requirements for the position, and he was an asset to the work setting.

Other evaluations suggest that CB interventions can enhance the job-related social skills of clients with a variety of disabilities. The interventions include problem solving to increase appropriate responses to job-related criticism for young adults with moderate mental retardation (Collet-Klingenberg & Chadsey-Rusch, 1991). Problem solving also can enhance a variety of job-related social skills, such as appropriately responding to criticism, negotiating when disagreements occur, and offering assistance to complete a task, for workers with brain injuries (O'Reilly, Lancioni, & O'Kane, 2000) and adolescents with mild to moderate mental retardation (Park & Gaylord-Ross, 1989). SST techniques can teach adults with moderate to severe mental retardation to appropriately accept job-related criticism (Eckert, 2000), request assistance from their supervisors (Morgan & Salzberg, 1992), and initiate job behaviors (McCuller, Salzberg, & Kraft, 1987). In addition, SST can teach job-related social skills to high school students with LD and emotional/behavioral disorders (Montague, 1988; Whang, Fawcett, & Mathews, 1984). The social skills include offering and accepting compliments, accepting instruction and criticism from a supervisor, providing constructive feedback, and explaining a problem to a supervisor.

Another study involving high school students with mild mental retardation compared the effects of four types of instruction—teacher modeling, videotaped modeling, problem solving, and behavioral rehearsal—on increasing social skills related to interacting more appropriately with supervisors and co-workers (Foss, Autry, & Irvin, 1989). Several evaluations suggest that self-instructional training can increase job-related social behaviors for workers with learning and physical disabilities. Examples include informing a supervisor when work materials run out and when assistance is required to complete a job for employees with moderate to severe mental retardation and autism (Agran, Salzberg, & Stowitschek, 1987); increasing initiative in seeking assistance for work-related problems interfering with completion of job tasks for workers with severe mental retardation (Hughes & Rusch, 1989); and increasing requests for production supplies when they are needed for a high school student with a combination of severe mental retardation and cerebral palsy (Rusch, McKee, Chadsey-Rusch, & Renzaglia, 1988).

Workers with Severe Mental Illness

Research suggests that supported employment services, such as the Integrated Placement and Support (IPS) program, are more effective than traditional vocational rehabilitation programs in helping clients with severe mental illness to secure employment (Drake et al., 1996). Clients who participate in IPS programs, however, are no more likely to retain employment compared with clients receiving traditional vocational rehabilitation services. Problems related to social functioning, which are frequently neglected in employment support programs for severely mentally ill clients, appear to be a main reason for job termination. Integrating SST into supported employment programs might enhance the ability of employees with severe mental illness to handle interpersonal interactions, such as dealing with customers, accepting criticism from supervisors, and coping with stigmatizing attitudes of co-workers (Tsang, 2003; Wallace et al., 1999).

To overcome the limitations of employment support programs, Wallace and his colleagues at the UCLA CRTRP developed a comprehensive and structured treatment program, the Workplace Fundamentals module. The workplace module, which is designed to be integrated into supported employment services, is one of the social and independent living skills modules developed by the UCLA Center. Information gathered from relevant research, the clinical literature, and interviews with professional staff, employers, and workers with severe mental illness was used to develop and validate the module content.

The module assists clients with severe mental illness in retaining their jobs by teaching them a variety of strategies in multiple skill areas. The skill areas include identifying ways in which work changes clients' lives, learning expectations for job performance, and identifying personal strengths and preferences, then identifying mismatches with current employment. Clients also learn to apply general problem solving to cope with stressors and substance use as it affects employment, to manage symptoms and medications at the employment site, to recruit social support, and to interact and socialize appropriately with co-workers and supervisors. Practitioners teach the workplace skills using the same CB strategies used in other modules designed to teach a variety of social and community living skills to clients with severe mental illness (see chapter 4 for a discussion of the basic components of the training modules and for ordering information).

Wallace and his colleagues (1999) conducted a pilot study of the Workplace Fundamentals module with ten clients (five in an employed group; five in an unemployed group) receiving services from a contract vocational agency. The module training resulted in both groups substantially improving their knowledge of the material and their performance of the skills after intervention and at a six-month follow-up (a one-way repeated-measures analysis of variance was used to analyze each group). Clients in the employed group sustained their employment during the nine months of the study, which for four of the five clients was the longest they had ever been employed. Three of the five unemployed clients secured and maintained employment.

A similar work-related SST program was evaluated by Tsang (2001) with unemployed clients diagnosed with schizophrenia (N = 97) in Hong Kong. The nine residential community facilities in which the clients resided were randomly assigned to one of three groups: an SST group with follow-up support, an SST group without follow-up support, and a control group receiving a standard intervention. Clients in the two SST groups, compared with the control group, had higher self-perceived competence in work-related situations and exhibited better work-related social skills. The SST group with follow-up support had an employment rate of 46.7%, and maintained their jobs at the three-month follow-up. Only 23.1% of the clients without follow-up support and 2.4% of the control group found employment. Clients in the training group with follow-up support were generally satisfied with their jobs and developed harmonious relationships with their supervisors and co-workers. The results suggest that integrating SST into vocational rehabilitation programs might enhance employment rates and employment tenure for individuals with severe mental illness.

The CB goal setting and feedback intervention for supported work employees diagnosed with schizophrenia or schizoaffective disorder discussed in the previous section (Bell et al., 2003) is also relevant here. Three of the subscales of the Work Behavior Inventory, including social skills (e.g., interest in others, appropriately expressing feelings), personal presentation (e.g., hygiene, mannerisms, dress), and cooperativeness (e.g., appropriately accepting constructive criticism, listening attentively to instruction, and following instruction without resistance), assessed job-related social skills. The evaluation indicated significantly greater improvements in the skills for the CB intervention group, as compared with a control group. Clients in the intervention group also worked for more hours and for a longer period of time.

This final case study used SST to assist a 28-year-old African American man with a long history of psychiatric problems, including depression, sleep terrors, schizoid personality disorder, and intermittent explosive disorder, in maintaining competitive employment (Mueser, Foy, & Carter, 1986). The client worked for an office machine service company, which frequently required him to repair machines at different office sites and to interact with customers. At the time treatment was sought, the client's supervisor had received four customer complaints regarding his inability to control his temper and his rudeness while on repair assignments. Based on interviews with the client and supervisor, the therapist constructed thirteen situations to assess the client's social skills. The situations involved interactions with customers, security guards, co-workers, and the supervisor. As a result of the assessment, the therapist and client selected the following behaviors for training: combinations of voice volume, affect, and eye contact; responsiveness (e.g., acknowledging the customer's feelings); eliciting suggestions (e.g., in solving problems, such as gaining access to an office); requesting clarification when someone criticized the client's work; and appropriately self-asserting when the client perceived that the supervisor's criticisms were unjustified.

The client practiced the skills in role plays with a variety of individuals playing various roles, such as a customer, security guard, and supervisor. During behavioral rehearsal, the therapist used verbal instruction, modeling, and praise and made positive requests for behavioral change. The client also practiced the skills in his job settings. After intervention, the client's five behaviors substantially improved over baselines and were maintained three months later. Three work performance ratings by the supervisor—overall job performance, response to criticism, and quality of interactions with customers—also substantially improved after treatment and were maintained up to three months later. Finally, after treatment and up to eight months later, the supervisor received no complaints from the client's customers.

ANALYSIS AND CRITIQUE FOR PRACTICE AND RESEARCH

This chapter presented a number of CB strategies that can empower workers with mental retardation, physical disabilities, and severe mental illness by increasing their job productivity, work quality, on-task behavior, and related social skills. These work improvements can result in these workers maintaining or advancing in employment, as indicated by increases in salary, promotion, and placement from a sheltered workshop into a competitive work setting. The interventions designed to increase job and job-related social skills include traditional skills and SST, prompting, feedback, reinforcement, punishment, and a variety of self-management strategies.

The evaluations of the interventions suggest that practitioners working in mental health, vocational, and employment settings (e.g., employee assistance programs) can use CB interventions to assist vulnerable clients in improving social skills interfering with job tenure or advancement. Interventions that enhance behaviors related to job productivity and quality also can be taught in employment, vocational, and rehabilitation settings. An analysis of the interventions presented in this chapter follows.

Effectiveness and Additional Applications

Evaluations of the CB interventions, with few exceptions, involved a small number of participants and used single-system or multiple-baseline designs.

The limitations of these types of research designs were discussed at the end of chapter 4. Despite these limitations, evaluations of the interventions reviewed in this chapter, along with other summaries (e.g., Agran & Moore, 1994; Lagomarcino, Hughes, & Rusch, 1989; Martin & Hrydowy, 1989), suggest that CB interventions can be effective in enhancing job performance and related social behaviors. Relations between enhancing job and job-related social behaviors of vulnerable workers and maintaining and advancing in employment are more difficult to establish. The content of this chapter, however, provides some evidence that the interventions can enhance job and job-related social behaviors, which can assist even workers with severe disabilities in improving their employment situation.

Evaluations of the interventions revealed that not all workers improved their job performance and related social skills, and there was wide variation in improvements when they were found. One evaluation determined that a worker's productivity actually decreased. These findings suggest the need for practitioners and researchers to conduct ongoing assessments and to determine factors related to variation in effectiveness of their interventions. Another important issue related to effectiveness, which has been addressed in previous chapters, is the lack of knowledge regarding which CB interventions, or combinations of interventions, are effective for a particular skill or client. This suggests the need for further research in these areas.

The interventions discussed in detail in this chapter were limited to workers with mental retardation, physical disabilities, and severe mental illness. Practitioners might find that the CB interventions designed to enhance the job-related social skills of individuals with brain injuries, autism, LD, and other behavioral/emotional disorders, which were not discussed in detail, are effective in maintaining and advancing employment for those client groups as well. Other vulnerable clients also might benefit from the CB applications discussed in this chapter. For example, some of the strategies might assist low-income and ethnic/racial minority workers in attaining vocational goals by learning skills to enhance job performance, manage job behaviors independently, and interact with supervisors, co-workers, and/or customers in socially acceptable ways. Recent immigrants, some of whom might be unfamiliar with social customs and appropriate employment-related social interactions, might benefit from SST to advance their employment goals. Finally, clients with attention deficit disorder also might profit from CB interventions that increase on-task behaviors. Such applications also are areas for future research.

Freedom, Control, and Social Justice

Many of the interventions discussed in this chapter were conducted in integrated, competitive employment settings. As discussed by Tice (1994), the goals of supported work programs are consistent with an empowerment perspective and with social justice values. The programs provide opportunities for individuals with disabilities to work in community job settings, interact with able-bodied peers, and receive at least a minimum wage. Tice's research also suggests that integrated work settings can increase positive attitudes and behaviors of able-bodied workers toward their co-workers with disabilities. For example, able-bodied employees reported greater willingness to work with co-workers with disabilities and improved perceptions of the co-workers' abilities to learn new skills. Enhancing job and job-related social skills that result in maintaining employment, employment advancement, and transfer from a sheltered workshop to a competitive, integrated work setting also are outcomes consistent with empowerment and social justice.

A number of the interventions also are consistent with enhancing client freedom and control. Examples include using graduated prompting strategies, involving workers in setting their own production goals, and teaching self-management strategies (e.g., using visual prompts, recruiting reinforcement, problem solving, and self-monitoring, self-reinforcement, and self-instruction). Self-management strategies allow workers to increase control over their own environments, to perform work tasks more independently, and to adapt to changing circumstances without the constant need for prompting, correction, or reinforcement from others, such as supervisors or job coaches (Agran & Moore, 1994; Grossi & Heward, 1998).

Regardless of whether vulnerable clients participate in setting their own goals or use self-management strategies, other ethical and assessment issues are relevant from a social justice and empowerment perspective. For example, under what circumstances are prompting, using self-management skills (e.g., setting a timer), and reinforcing production rates and conforming social behaviors empowering or coercive? Those interventions might result in the maintenance of work that is unrewarding or in decreases in the client's well-being in other areas, such as increasing psychiatric symptoms; or they may serve the employer's, not the client's, best interests. These are ongoing assessment and ethical questions that practitioners and researchers can address through observation, client interviews, setting life goals with clients (and significant others), discussing intervention options, and weighing the benefits and costs of intervention and employment options.

Social Validity

Socially relevant goals and results. Evaluations of the CB interventions suggest a variety of methods that practitioners and researchers can use to ensure the social validity of job and job-related social behaviors targeted for change, as well as the ultimate intervention goals. Examples of methods for identifying socially relevant job behaviors include consultations with employers, supervisors, other workers, and the clients themselves. Surveys of relevant literature and conducting a task analysis based on observations of workers performing the identified job tasks are additional methods. Although the workers involved in the interventions reviewed in this chapter appeared to agree with the goal of enhancing their productivity, work quality, or job-related social behavior, treatment goals usually were determined by external work standards (e.g., those established by the supervisor or employer). Of course, if a client's goal is to maintain or advance in employment, work and social behavior must conform to some degree to these external standards.

Once a goal was established to increase productivity, work quality, or social skills, the evaluations frequently, but not always, used socially relevant measures of change. Socially relevant measures include comparing job performance with industrial or able-bodied worker standards and qualitative satisfaction evaluations of the workers' performance by supervisors, co-workers, and the workers themselves. However, as much as work might serve an important function in the lives of most individuals, many vulnerable individuals, particularly those with severe disabilities, such as schizophrenia, are unable to maintain the goal of full-time or even part-time employment (Tsang, 2003). This suggests the need for practitioners to engage clients in realistic goal setting, ongoing assessment, and, when necessary, adjusting vocational goals.

Evaluations of the CB interventions indicate that the majority of the workers increased their job performance, continued employment that was in jeopardy, received increases in salary and benefits, or acquired a better position. These all appear to be socially valid results. On the other hand, no study indicated whether the workers' enhanced work productivity, work quality, or related social behavior resulted in maintained or improved salaries or working hours that were sufficient to even meet poverty thresholds. Measures of workers' satisfaction with salary, benefits, and number of working hours would be important indicators of the success of these interventions to empower vulnerable workers. Finally, social conformity and increased work productivity and quality might not necessarily result in a better quality of life, regardless of economic benefit.

Socially relevant intervention procedures. None of the previously described CB applications were preceded by individual functional assessments. Individualized assessment and intervention are hallmarks of CB methods, and important components of supported work programs (McDonnell et al., 1989) and case management services provided in Welfare-to-Work programs (Perez-Johnson et al., 2000), and are necessary to determine relevant interventions. In their review of studies evaluating SST for adults with mental retardation in employment settings, Huang and Cuvo (1997) criticized researchers for not conducting a functional and ecological assessment of the work environment. Such assessments could identify relevant behaviors, reasons for particular maladaptive behaviors occurring under particular conditions, and naturally occurring cues and corrective consequences. That information could then be used to design appropriate interventions.

Despite the lack of individual assessment, the CB strategies discussed in this chapter suggest methods that practitioners and researchers might use to enhance the social relevance of their interventions. For example, appropriate role-play situations and responses for enhancing job-related social skills could be obtained from related literature and through interviews with clients, supervisors, employers, and other workers. When practitioners use CB interventions in work settings or expect clients to continue using them after formal intervention, they must assess the practicality and acceptability of the interventions from the perspective of the clients, employers, supervisors, and co-workers. For example, if training and/or continued use of the strategies interfere with ongoing activities of the worker or other employees (e.g., the use of verbal self-instructions and timers), they likely will be rejected. Many of the evaluations of the CB interventions reported positive feedback from the participants, co-workers, and supervisors on the suitability of, satisfaction with, preference for, and desire to continue the interventions. However, one worker reported that using a self-evaluation procedure to increase his work productivity was too stressful. This outcome suggests the need for researchers and practitioners to conduct ongoing assessments to determine whether the interventions are acceptable or result in negative outcomes.

To accommodate the special needs of some vulnerable workers, practitioners and researchers might adopt the adaptations that were made in the CB strategies discussed in this chapter. The adaptations, which primarily accommodate the cognitive limitations of workers with mental retardation, include using pictures and mounted items to demonstrate the relation between productivity and earnings and teaching workers abbreviated self-management statements (e.g., Now-Did-Next). Specially designed prompts such as photographs of the workers carrying out work tasks and a self-operated auditory prompting system are yet other examples. A variety of feedback systems also can be used to enhance job performance, such as specially designed production trays, graphic displays, counters and timers, self-monitoring checklists and production sheets, and colored tokens. More immediate instead of delayed monetary reinforcement also can be used to increase productivity.

Maintenance and generalization. Many of the evaluations of the previously described interventions that reported favorable results (e.g., continued employment or improved job performance or social skills) did not report whether the intervention gains were maintained. If maintenance was measured, follow-up data were gathered only after a short period (e.g., two weeks). A few of the evaluations indicated that the workers could not maintain their improved job productivity after formal intervention was withdrawn, suggesting the need for practitioners to ensure ongoing job support. Designing effective strategies to maintain enhanced job performance and job tenure is particularly important for many vulnerable workers. For example, research indicates that only one-half of the workers diagnosed with schizophrenia maintain their jobs for more than six months, even when they receive supported employment services (Kern et al., 2002).

The previously discussed interventions, as well as other research (e.g., Huang & Cuvo, 1997; Wacker et al., 1989), suggest that practitioners can maintain intervention gains by involving co-workers or supervisors in the training, using booster sessions, teaching self-management strategies, and, in some cases, providing ongoing external monitoring and prompting. For some vulnerable workers, particularly for workers receiving supported employment services, a reasonable goal might be to receive the fewest number of services necessary to maintain enhanced job performance or job-related social behaviors.

The majority of the interventions discussed in this chapter were applied in sheltered workshops or in competitive employment settings, which eliminated some of the problems related to transferring the skills from artificial to work settings. Job and job-related social skills that were taught in other settings did generalize to actual work sites after short-term intervention. However, whether skills learned in a sheltered workshop can transfer to competitive employment, or whether skills learned in one competitive job setting and context (e.g., with particular supervisors, co-workers, and work items) can transfer to other job duties and social situations, was rarely examined. The ability to transfer the skills to novel situations would be extremely important to maintaining employment. Finally, research suggests that practitioners can enhance the transfer and maintenance of intervention gains in job and job-related social skills by teaching clients self-management strategies (Grossi & Heward, 1998; Martin & Hrydowy, 1989). However, further research is necessary to determine the most effective self-management strategies to assist particular clients in maintaining and transferring their acquired skills.

This and the previous chapter presented multiple CB interventions designed to assist vulnerable workers in securing, maintaining, and advancing in employment, all reporting overall positive results. Despite this optimistic assessment, many vulnerable clients will be unable to reach these vocational goals. And even when vulnerable workers are able to successfully secure and maintain employment, many jobs do not provide sufficient income and benefits to satisfy even their basic needs. For this reason, practitioners must be aware of interventions that can assist vulnerable clients in accessing economic and related assistance from other sources. Chapter 9 discusses CB interventions that accomplish this goal.

ADDITIONAL READINGS AND RESOURCES

Agran, M., & Moore, S. C. (1994). *How to teach self-instruction of job skills.* Washington, DC: American Association on Mental Retardation.

Bond, G. R. (1992). Vocational rehabilitation. In R. P. Liberman (Ed.), *Handbook of psychiatric rehabilitation* (pp. 244–275). New York: Macmillan.

Bryson, G., Bell, M. D., Lysaker, P., & Zito, W. (1997). The work behavior inventory: A scale for the assessment of work behavior for people with severe mental illness. *Psychiatric Rehabilitation Journal, 20,* 47–55.

Calabrese, D. N., & Hawkins, R. P. (1988). Job-related social skills training with female prisoners. *Behavior Modification, 12,* 3–33.

Elksnin, N., & Elksnin, L. K. (2001). Adolescents with disabilities: The need for occupational social skills training. *Exceptionality, 9,* 91–105.

Goldman, B. (1989). Job search strategies for women on welfare. In S. Harlan & R. Steinberg (Eds.), *Job training for women* (pp. 389–413). Philadelphia: Temple University Press.

Martin, G. L. (1995). A staff manual to help developmentally disabled persons improve their work habits and productivity. *Behavior Modification, 19,* 325–338.

O'Reilly, M. F., & Chadsey-Rusch, J. (1992). Teaching a social skills problem-solving approach to workers with mental retardation: An analysis of generalization. *Education and Training in Mental Retardation and Developmental Disabilities, 27,* 324–334.

West, M. D., & Parent, W. S. (1992). Consumer choice and empowerment in supported employment services: Issues and strategies. *Journal of the Association for Persons with Severe Handicaps, 17,* 47–52.

Wong, S. E. (1996). Psychosis. In M. A. Mattaini & B. A. Thyer (Eds.), *Finding solutions to social problems: Behavioral strategies for change* (pp. 319–344). Washington, DC: American Psychological Association.

9 Accessing Public and Private Sources of Economic Resources

As discussed in chapter 7, poverty places adults, children, and youths at risk of multiple adverse health, mental health, educational, interpersonal, and social outcomes. Other vulnerable populations, including women, noncitizens, individuals with disabilities, and persons from some racial/ethnic minority backgrounds, are disproportionately poor. When vulnerable groups cannot secure or maintain employment, or when earnings from employment are insufficient to provide for their own and/or their families' basic needs, they must rely on assistance from other public and private sources. This chapter focuses on CB interventions that increase the knowledge and skills of economically disadvantaged clients to assist them in securing public and private economic related assistance.

Descriptions of the interventions are preceded by a brief discussion of the types and importance of public and private assistance for low-income individuals and families. A discussion of the CB interventions that assist vulnerable clients in accessing financial related resources from public benefits programs, members of their social support networks, and other community sources follows. The final section provides an analysis and critique of this chapter's content for practice and future research.

PUBLIC AND PRIVATE SOURCES OF ECONOMIC ASSISTANCE

Receipt of means-tested public benefits among low-income households is common (Mosley & Tiehen, 2004; Wu & Eamon, in press). Public benefits include welfare, housing and energy assistance, Supplemental Security Income (SSI), food stamps, Medicaid, the Earned Income Tax Credit (EITC), Special Supplemental Program for Women, Infants and Children (WIC), and school meals. Unfortunately, in recent decades, social policy changes have eroded social protection for economically vulnerable individuals and families. These changes include privatization, devolution, and decreases in program benefits (Marwell, 2004).

The trend in privatizing the federal government's responsibility to assist economically disadvantaged individuals and families has resulted in increased reliance on volunteer and private activity. Federal funds that are more likely to be allocated to the private sector, such as to nonprofit private agencies and organizations, infrequently provide direct economic assistance to low-income households. Devolution, the shifting of administrative decisions related to program participation from the federal government to lower levels of government, has given states increased discretion in designing and implementing their means-tested benefits programs. This flexibility has resulted in large variations in program eligibility requirements, benefits, and services. Finally, recent legislation, particularly the 1996 welfare reform act (PRWORA), has cut benefits and tightened eligibility for economically disadvantaged families with children. This legislation also has tightened program benefit eligibility for other vulnerable groups, such as immigrants and the disabled (Greenberg et al., 2002; Hacker, 2004; Lynn, 2002).

Many low-income households fail to receive public benefits even when they are eligible. The size of the potential benefit, inconvenience and costs (e.g., long lines, the application process, liquidating assets, and co-payments), social stigma, unawareness of available benefits, eligibility requirements, the appeals process, and lack of assertiveness skills are among the reasons for nonparticipation. For immigrants, language problems and concerns about their citizenship status can be additional barriers (Greenberg et al., 2002; Remler & Glied, 2003).

In addition to public benefits, economically disadvantaged households obtain assistance from charitable and nonprofit organizations, such as churches, food emergency providers, and other community groups, and from their social support networks. Private assistance can include cash, food, child care, housing, and clothing. Although such assistance can enhance well-being and ensure daily survival, low-income households tend to depend on public benefits to a greater degree than on private assistance (Danziger, Corcoran, Danziger, & Heflin, 2000; Hollar, 2003; Wu & Eamon, in press). In many cases, assistance from nonprofit groups or organizations is unavailable. When private assistance is available, lack of information, inadequate social skills, psychological factors, and the temporary and unreliable nature of the assistance might deter low-income individuals from accessing it (Ahluwalia, Dodds, & Baligh, 1998; Henly & Lyons, 2000).

Additional factors might prevent economically disadvantaged individuals from obtaining financial-related resources from their social support networks. Despite their heightened need and experiences with negative financial events (e.g, job loss), low-income individuals have the smallest and most economically disadvantaged social support networks. Thus, individuals with low income might not be able to mobilize the required assistance from their social support networks, despite the strong cultural value placed on social support among many vulnerable groups (McLeod & Kessler, 1990; Mickelson & Kubzansky, 2003).

Despite the limitations of public and private assistance among low-income populations, many low-income individuals and families must rely on or supplement their earnings with these types of assistance to meet their basic needs. CB interventions can assist vulnerable clients in accessing these important sources of economic-related assistance.

ASSISTING VULNERABLE POPULATIONS IN ACCESSING PUBLIC AND PRIVATE ASSISTANCE

The CB interventions discussed here assist individuals with few economic resources, including clients with severe mental illness, African American adolescents, youths with physical disabilities and behavioral/emotional disorders, and females, in accessing public and private economic-related assistance. Relatively few CB interventions have been designed to assist vulnerable clients in accessing these two types of assistance, and all but one of the interventions were described in previous chapters. Because those interventions include strategies for assisting vulnerable groups in accessing economic-related assistance from public and private sources, they are relevant to this chapter as well. The interventions primarily involve SST, including assertiveness training. PST and reinforcement also are used.

Adults with Severe Mental Illness

The social and independent living skills modules designed to increase the interpersonal problem-solving skills of clients with severe mental illness developed at the UCLA CRTRP also contain training on securing economic resources unrelated to employment (Liberman, Eckman, & Marder, 2001; see chapter 4 for a discussion of the basic components of the training modules and for ordering information). An example of a role-play scenario involves a recipient of disability benefits handling a situation in which she failed to receive her monthly check and is not being adequately assisted by a Social Security Office clerk (Liberman et al., 2001, p. 32).

Another group SST program described in chapter 5, which teaches social skills to clients diagnosed with chronic schizophrenia to assist them in coping more effectively with community situations, includes financial skills training (Brown & Munford, 1983). Examples of the financial skills involve talking with a social worker to locate economic resources and obtaining information from a local bank on opening a checking account. The skills are practiced on the hospital ward. Some of the tasks, such as obtaining information about financial resources, also are performed in the community. The clients' social skills increased after training, as indicated by evaluations of role plays and improved scores on the finances subtest of the Life Skills Inventory.

Minority Youths and Youths with Disabilities

Three SST programs that teach racial/ethnic minority adolescents and youths with physical, behavioral/emotional, and learning disabilities to set goals and recruit others to assist them in achieving the goals were developed by Fabricio Balcazar and his colleagues (Balcazar et al., 1991; Balcazar, Majors, et al.,1991; Balcazar et al.,1995) and described in chapter 6. Because some of the outcomes and training materials are related to accessing economic assistance, they are briefly discussed here.

After intervention, the youths participating in all three SST programs enhanced their social skills to recruit potential helpers. One indicator of this success was the increased number of social network members providing them with material assistance. One of the African American high school students set a goal to apply for college scholarships. After SST, the student obtained two college scholarships. Finally, the training materials used to teach adolescents with behavioral/emotional and learning problems to access potential helpers to assist them in achieving transitional goals include role plays for situations related to acquiring economic-related resources. The economic resources include scholarships and financial aid for college, health care, and housing.

Females with Low Income

Three other CB programs discussed in chapter 6 also are relevant to assisting low-income females in accessing economic-related assistance from public and private sources. The first program is designed to enhance the social support and psychological well-being of predominately poor, minority pregnant or parenting adolescents (Barth & Maxwell, 1985; Barth & Schinke, 1984; Barth et al., 1985). To accomplish these goals, the group SST teaches the adolescents help-seeking skills, which involves providing the adolescents with a handout prompting them to identify members of their social support networks who could provide various types of support (see Barth & Schinke, 1984, p. 529). The support includes child care, transportation, and money. After intervention, the adolescents participating in the CB program, compared to the comparison group, had stronger social support networks. At the four-month follow-up, they also had higher social support, as indicated by three of the four social support measures, including the "Asking for Aid Scale."

In the second program, a counselor uses a variety of reinforcers to increase the attendance of low-income women at self-help group meetings (Miller & Miller, 1970). The intervention can increase the women's economic or material resources in two ways. First, one of the main purposes of the meetings is to assist the women in resolving financial problems, particularly related to their welfare benefits. At the beginning of each meeting, the group leader goes through a checklist of welfare-related problems, which includes questions about whether the group members received their checks on time, received their medical card, and experienced any changes in their benefits. The group discusses problems revealed by the checklist or brought up by group members (including other economic-related problems) and suggests specific strategies for resolving the problems and for accessing community resources.

Second, the reinforcers provided for attendance are related to economic or material resources. The reinforcers include concrete goods (e.g., major appliances, furniture, clothing), services (e.g., assistance in negotiating complaints over welfare benefits, locating better housing, finding day camp scholarships), and information (e.g., available benefits from community social service agencies). The intervention dramatically increased attendance at the group meetings, and many of the fifty-two members received the economic-related reinforcers. However, with the exception of receiving the reinforcers, whether attendance at the self-help group meetings increased the economic well-being of the women was not measured.

The final CB program discussed in chapter 6, which also is relevant to this chapter, is the survival skills workshop developed for low-income, urban, and primarily minority women (Thurston, 1990; Thurston et al., 1984). Obtaining community resources is one of the several training themes of the workshop. During skills training, in addition to using material consistent with the training theme, workshop facilitators provide group members with a community resource list and assign homework related to the area of obtaining community resources. Although a large percentage of the women submitted proof that they completed the assignments and increased their scores on a survival skills knowledge test, whether the women increased their economic resources was not determined.

Linda Thurston and colleagues (Thurston, 1994) later developed materials for a Survival Skills for Women (SSW) program, which provides skills, knowledge, and support to assist women in succeeding in other training and educational programs and eventually becoming economically independent. The SSW has become incorporated into a number of state's welfare reform initiatives and has been expanded to include men and vulnerable youths. However, no peer reviewed evaluation of the programs could be located (see "Additional Readings and Resources" at the end of this chapter to obtain additional information on the programs and workshop materials).

Galinsky, Schopler, Safier, and Gambrill (1978) developed a model for an assertiveness training workshop to enhance the ability of public welfare clients to independently obtain community resources and services. No evaluation of the workshop was conducted, but because so few CB applications could be located that assist vulnerable groups in accessing economic-related assistance, the workshop is briefly described. The content of the six group sessions is consistent with traditional assertiveness training and includes the following treatment objectives:

1 Learn to distinguish between passive, aggressive, and assertive responses and identify problematic situations in which clients would like to be more assertive.
2 Learn assertiveness skills using role plays of previously prepared and client-identified problematic situations.
3 Learn nonverbal components of assertiveness (e.g., eye contact, body posture, facial expression).
4 Identify personal rights (e.g., the right to respect, express feelings and opinions, ask for information and make requests, say "no" without guilt) and situations in which assertiveness furthers the clients' best interests by weighing the benefits and risks of the behavior.
5 Learn methods to cope with possible negative reactions from others.
6 Learn to appropriately give and receive compliments.

After each session, group facilitators assign group members homework related to the content of the session. In subsequent sessions, homework assignments are reviewed, discussed, and rehearsed, as needed. Exercises and examples relevant to obtaining economic-related resources include handling a telephone disconnection, an inaccurately recorded appointment for food stamps, and being overbilled; returning a defective product; and asking a social worker about a housing allowance.

ANALYSIS AND CRITIQUE FOR PRACTICE AND RESEARCH

Because individuals living in poverty are a vulnerable group, and poverty rates among other vulnerable populations are disproportionately high, securing public and private financial and related assistance is especially important. Economically disadvantaged populations can obtain financial assistance, including tax credits, college financial aid, SSI, TANF, and other cash assistance, and economic-related resources, such as health insurance, food, child care, and housing, from government benefits programs and/or private sources (e.g., nonprofit agencies, churches, educational systems, members of social support networks). Relatively few CB interventions that assist vulnerable clients in obtaining such assistance have been developed and evaluated. Many vulnerable individuals must depend on case managers or other helping professionals to assist them in locating and accessing relevant economic resources. If individuals with low income do not receive such assistance, they might fail to receive the economic resources to which they are entitled or could obtain, because they lack the relevant information, resources, or skills. Because all but one of the interventions reviewed in this chapter were included in previous chapters, this section is brief. Only a critique of the effectiveness of the interventions and suggestions for other CB applications to assist vulnerable populations in securing economic-related resources are provided.

Evaluations of the CB interventions are limited by the use of nonexperimental methods. Even when random assignment was used (e.g., Brown & Munford, 1983), the researchers did not determine whether participants in the SST or comparison group actually obtained financial resources. Therefore, whether the interventions can increase the economic resources of African American youths, youths with disabilities, adults with severe mental illness, and females with low income remains a topic for future research. Regardless of the current status of research in this area, the interventions reviewed in this chapter, and other interventions discussed in the previous two chapters (e.g., the Job Club method), suggest that practitioners and agencies might use a number of CB strategies to teach vulnerable clients the knowledge and skills necessary to access nonemployment-related economic resources.

The interventions could provide information on public benefits programs and other sources of economic-related assistance. The information could include explanations of public benefits programs and eligibility requirements, agency and organizational names, phone numbers, addresses, and, for government programs, information on appeals processes and for obtaining legal assistance when benefits are unjustifiably denied. Other interventions might provide instruction and assistance in filling out the necessary application forms and access to other resources, such as telephones and computers with Internet connections. Locating individuals who can assist with transportation and communication problems, such as for non-English speakers and individuals with physical or sensory impairments, also could be appropriate interventions.

Some agencies (e.g., DuPage Foundation on Human Services Reform, RealBenefits, and Community Service Society of New York) have developed comprehensive training materials to increase case workers' knowledge of available public benefits programs and the appeals process to assist clients in obtaining the benefits to which they are entitled (see "Additional Readings and Resources" at the end of this chapter for contact information for these agencies). Making such knowledge directly available to potential recipients of public assistance might be more empowering for vulnerable populations. For example, the Community Service Society Internet site (http://www.cssny.org/pbrc/tools.html#applications) provides information on public benefits programs and online applications to assist potential recipients in applying for a variety such benefits. Agencies and researchers also might develop, evaluate, and offer programs teaching clients relevant skills and knowledge and, whenever possible, making the applications available online. The online materials also can be made available to any person who has access to an Internet connection. As a result, vulnerable populations would be less dependent on social workers and other social service staff.

In addition to providing relevant information, instruction, and needed assistance, other CB interventions could be developed and evaluated to assist clients with few economic resources in accessing economic-related resources from public and private sources. SST, including assertiveness training, might be relevant for clients who lack social skills for making the necessary phone calls and office visits, asking relevant questions, addressing misunderstandings, and seeking administrative redress or legal assistance when benefits are denied. Graduated exposure therapy might be useful for clients with social anxiety, and cognitive restructuring might assist clients whose thoughts or beliefs about accepting economic assistance are barriers to their applying. SST, exposure therapy, and cognitive restructuring also might be applicable to clients who have difficulties in accessing economic-related resources from members of their social support networks. Finally, PST might assist clients in evaluating the benefits and costs (e.g., negative psychological reactions and incurred obligations) of requesting and accepting assistance from different public and private sources.

The described and proposed CB interventions might be applied in multiple settings, such as mental health, school, health care, child welfare, vocational, community action, and immigrant services, and could be conducted with individuals or in groups. Given the importance of social support networks in accessing job leads and obtaining other job-seeking assistance (e.g., transportation), conducting interventions in groups might be particularly effective in assisting vulnerable clients in accessing economic-related resources. Vulnerable clients who lack relevant knowledge, social skills, or other resources, or face psychological barriers preventing them from acquiring economic-related resources, might benefit from the suggested CB interventions. These suggestions also provide areas for future research.

Summary

The three chapters of part III described multiple CB interventions that can empower vulnerable populations by assisting them in acquiring and increasing economic resources. CB methods can assist vulnerable groups in gaining employment by teaching job-seeking skills; in maintaining and advancing in employment by increasing on-the-job productivity and improving work quality and related social skills; and in accessing economic resources from members of social support networks, other private sources, and public benefits programs by increasing relevant knowledge and social skills.

Because the CB programs described in parts II and III assist vulnerable populations in increasing social and economic resources, they are consistent with an empowerment perspective. The majority of the applications discussed in these chapters, however, have three important limitations. First, assessments were not conducted to ensure that participants had the skills necessary to be active decision makers when setting social and vocational goals. Second, if participants lacked skills or opportunities to be active decision makers, the interventions rarely assisted them in acquiring the relevant skills or assisted others in making opportunities available. Finally, the interventions rarely taught relevant knowledge and self-advocacy skills to address denial of personal and legal rights. CB interventions designed to specifically address these shortcomings and related outcomes are discussed in part IV.

ADDITIONAL READINGS AND RESOURCES

Community Service Society of New York, 105 East 22nd Street, New York, NY 10010. Available at http://www.cssny.org/index.html

DuPage Federation on Human Services Reform, 146 West Roosevelt Rd., Villa Park, IL 60181. Available at http://www.dupagefederation.org/

RealBenefits, 30 Winter St., Boston, MA 02108. Available at http://www.realbenefits.org/

Survival Skills Education & Development, 436 Spring Garden Street, Greensboro, NC 27401. Available at http://www.ssed.org/

Thurston, L. (1994). *Survival skills for women: Facilitator manual & materials.* Manhattan, KS: Survival Skills Education and Development.

PART

FOUR

Increasing Self-Determination

10 Enhancing Personal Control and Input into Decision Making

Although the definition of self-determination and the circumstances under which it can be exercised have been debated and applied differently during various historical periods, social work as a profession has long recognized the right of all human beings to self-determination (Freedberg, 1989; Rothman, 1989). Clients' right to self-determination, including the right to establish their own treatment goals, is reflected in the NASW (1999) Code of Ethics. The right of self-determination of people with disabilities is included in NASW's (2000) policy statement on this topic, which recommends self-advocacy training to assist clients with disabilities in becoming socially integrated. Federal law also recognizes the importance of exercising self-determination for individuals with disabilities. For example, the Individuals with Disabilities Education Act (IDEA) Amendments of 1997 (PL 105–17) require that schools invite students with disabilities who are at least fourteen years old to participate in their Individual Education Programs (IEPs) and transition planning conferences. In addition, these students must provide input into establishing their educational goals (Test et al., 2004).

The three chapters of part IV describe CB interventions that empower vulnerable populations by teaching them knowledge, skills, and other strategies to (1) enhance personal control and input into decision making in academic, home, and work settings; (2) increase choice making in routine activities, including recreation/leisure, work, eating, and self-care, and in the longer-term decision of selecting a community residence; and (3) secure legal rights, such as civil and disability accommodation rights and the right to refuse unwanted or unprotected sexual behavior.

The CB interventions previously discussed in parts II and III also can facilitate the self-determination of vulnerable populations. For example, acquiring social, recreational/leisure, and employment skills, as well as the necessary skills to recruit assistance and obtain economic resources, can expand clients' options. Enhancing other skills such as problem solving can assist clients in assessing and choosing among alternatives. Rearranging and enriching physical environments also can provide increased opportunities for choice making. The CB interventions described in part IV, however, are unique. The interventions specifically focus on teaching self-determination and related skills, such as choice making and self-advocacy, intended to facilitate individuals' ability to make their own choices, set their own goals, and secure their personal and legal rights.

The concept of self-determination, the reasons for restricted self-determination among vulnerable populations, and the importance of enhancing self-determined behavior are discussed next. A description of CB interventions that assist students and clients with physical, learning, cognitive, mental health, and multiple disabilities in learning and using self-determined skills to exert more control over and input into personal decision making follows. The final section contains an analysis of the interventions, including applications for practice and research.

SELF-DETERMINATION OF VULNERABLE POPULATIONS

Scholars from other professions, including psychology, education, and rehabilitation, who have developed many of the CB interventions described in part IV, as well as disability rights advocates, also recognize the basic right to exercise self-determined behavior and its importance for vulnerable groups. From the multiple definitions of self-determination, Field (1996) identifies three common elements—freedom, choice, and control—which also are central elements of empowerment definitions. As Field and other scholars (e.g., Durlak, Rose, & Bursuck, 1994; Rothman, 1989; Snyder, 2002) contend, exercising self-determination implies that individuals have the freedom to identify and to choose among options contingent on their personal characteristics, including abilities, values, and preferences, without undue external interference or influence from others. To optimally exercise self-determination, an individual also must have particular knowledge, abilities, skills, and attitudes, many of which can be enhanced by the CB interventions discussed in this chapter. For example, a person must have knowledge of the available options, and the ability to define personal goals, identify and choose among options, and communicate choices. A person also must have the skills and attitudes, such as self-management, assertiveness, self-advocacy, and self-efficacy, needed to achieve established goals.

External factors, such as availability of resources, laws, service mandates, the social control function of organizations and agencies, and conflicts with other professional values, restrict self-determination for all clients (Rothman, 1989). The self-determination of vulnerable populations, however, is frequently unnecessarily constrained compared with other groups. For example, individuals with disabilities believe that they have little control over their lives, and research supports this perception. Family members, caretakers, service providers, educators, and other professionals frequently provide few opportunities for individuals with disabilities to express preferences, to be actively involved in educational and vocational planning, and to set personal goals (Agran, Blanchard, & Wehmeyer, 2000).

Compared with other groups, the special characteristics of some vulnerable populations place more limits on their ability to learn and exercise self-determined behavior. For example, the ability to identify goals and options to attain the goals, plan, communicate with others, initiate behavior, or respond flexibly to a variety of conditions is often compromised for individuals with mental retardation, LD, severe mental illness, and some physical disabilities (Field, 1996; Liberman & Kopelowicz, 2002). As demonstrated by evaluations of the interventions described in this chapter, lack of relevant knowledge and skills is also among the factors that can limit self-determined behavior. For example, individuals with disabilities frequently lack knowledge or an understanding of their disability, their legal and personal rights, and the skills necessary to set and achieve goals, make and communicate choices, and advocate on their own behalf. Unfortunately, for many individuals with disabilities, few opportunities are available to learn the relevant knowledge and skills.

Societal attitudes and values, frequently reflected in social policies, programs, and the behavior of family members, helping professionals, educators, and support staff, also impede vulnerable groups from learning and performing self-determined behavior. For example, others unnecessarily make and carry out choices for individuals with disabilities. These individuals believe that persons with disabilities need protection, cannot learn the skills for self-determined behavior, and will make poor choices or choose options in conflict with their educational or rehabilitation goals (Linhorst & Eckert, 2003; Sievert, Cuvo, & Davis, 1988). Even social workers have been criticized in health and rehabilitation settings for not adjusting their traditional helping roles to accommodate the self-determination movement (Beaulaurier & Taylor, 2001). Individual autonomy also can be constrained to increase efficiency and to avoid conflict (Kondrat, 1995). For example, staff and family members might prefer making and carrying out decisions for children, youths, and adults with disabilities, because the alternative, negotiating with and assisting them in making and carrying out their own decisions, can increase time demands and conflict.

Failing to teach self-determination skills or to provide opportunities for using them denies individuals with disabilities their right to make choices and to control their own lives to the extent possible. Restricting self-determined behavior can result in other negative consequences as well. Overdependence on family members, professionals, and support staff can decrease the likelihood that clients with disabilities will adapt to community life and live as independently as possible (Cooper & Browder, 2001). Limited choice making and control over one's environment also can decrease life quality, lead to learned helplessness, and contribute to behaviors such as aggression, self-injury, or noncompliance. Researchers have interpreted these behaviors as clients' attempts to escape participation in undesirable activities or the control of others (Bambara, Koger, Katzer, & Davenport, 1995). Enhancing self-determination is fundamental to empowering vulnerable populations, and increasing freedom, control, and choice is related to numerous positive outcomes. The outcomes include a better quality of life, higher levels of self-esteem and self-efficacy, and improved performance in education, communication, socialization, employment, independent living, leisure/recreation, and self-care (Agran et al., 2000; Browder, Cooper, & Lehigh, 1998; Field, 1996; Hicks-Coolick & Kurtz, 1997; Kearney, Bergan, & McKnight, 1998; Wehmeyer & Palmer, 2003).

The next section describes CB interventions that empower youths with disabilities (e.g., mental retardation, LD, emotional/behavioral disorders, and physical and multiple disabilities), as well as adults with severe mental illness, by assisting them in learning and using a variety of self-determination skills. The skills assist vulnerable youths and adults in assuming more control over the decisions made about their lives in their schools, places of employment, homes, and communities.

ENHANCING CONTROL OVER PERSONAL DECISION MAKING

The CB interventions discussed here are divided into two main groups. Interventions that teach self-determination skills to students with disabilities to enhance their control over personal decision making and to effectively participate in their educational conferences are described first. A description of CB programs designed to teach students with disabilities and clients with severe mental illness to establish and attain their personal goals follows.

Decision Making in Multiple Areas and Participating in Educational Conferences

The three programs described in this section, which assist students with disabilities in learning and using self-determined behavior, incorporate a variety of CB interventions. The interventions include PST, guided simulation, and SST techniques, including instruction, practice in setting and carrying out personal goals, identifying and practicing verbal and nonverbal communication and listening skills, and role-playing situations with passive, aggressive, and assertive responses.

Researchers evaluated the programs using a pretest-posttest design (Abery, Rudrud, Arndt, Schauben, & Eggebeen, 1995); a single-system, multiple-probe design (Van Reusen, Bos, Schumaker, & Deshler, 1994); and a multiple-baseline design across skill areas (Snyder, 2002). One evaluation employed three research designs, which involved assigning students to two intervention groups and a comparison group (Lancaster, Schumaker, & Deshler, 2002). The researchers then used a multiple-probe design across all of the participants, a posttest comparison group design comparing the performance of the experimental and comparison groups, and a pretest-posttest comparison group design that compared the performance of the two experimental groups.

Students with mental retardation. Abery and his colleagues (1995) designed and evaluated a CB program to enhance the self-determination of high school students with mild to moderate mental retardation. The program, which includes a ten-module competency-building component for the students and an eight-module education component and a support component for their families, was developed through information obtained from three main sources. The sources included focus groups; consisting of individuals with disabilities, their parents, and educators serving students with disabilities; current research related to self-determination; and collaboration with teachers from a variety of school districts.

The ten topics covered by the student module are self-awareness, self-esteem, personal control, personal values, goal setting, communicating assertively, making choices, self-regulation, problem solving, and self-advocacy. The intervention sessions are designed to provide opportunities for students to identify personal characteristics from which they can draw on to gain greater control over their lives, develop personal goals, enhance self-determination, obtain knowledge about relevant community resources, and acquire a better understanding of their own rights and responsibilities. With the exception of the first group session, facilitators summarize and review the main concepts and skills presented in the previous session, and they discuss homework assignments that require students to apply the previously learned skills in natural settings. The group facilitators then present the main concepts and skills relevant to the topic of the current session, followed by group discussion, learning experiences, and homework assignments. CB interventions used in the student module include PST, practice in setting and carrying out personal goals, rehearsing verbal and nonverbal communication and listening skills, and role-playing situations with passive, aggressive, and assertive responses.

Practitioners implement the family support component in the homes of the students. During the sessions, practitioners educate the family on the concept and importance of self-determination, and they provide practical methods that family members might use to support the youths in developing and practicing self-determined behavior. Examples of the family topics are planning the student's future, balancing self-determination and family values, promoting choice making, supporting problem solving, achieving personal goals, encouraging self-advocacy, and developing links between home and community. The topics are taught through instruction, role playing, guided simulations, discussion, and sharing of personal experiences (see Abery et al., 1994, in "Additional Readings and Resources" at the end of this chapter to obtain the training modules).

Parents participating in the evaluation of the program rated significant improvements in their youths' (N = 18) overall self-determination skills, as well as in specific skills related to choice making, self-regulation, problem solving, and personal advocacy over a three-month period. After intervention, the parents reported significant increases in providing opportunities for their adolescents to assume more control within the family and over their own health-care issues. Parents also reported observing their youths attempting to make more of the decisions offered to them. No changes in self-determination skills were observed in the school or in the work settings for employed students.

Students with developmental, learning, and physical disabilities and emotional/behavioral disorders. The primary goal of the three CB interventions discussed here, the Self-Advocacy Strategy, the Interactive Hypermedia Program, and the Self-Directed IEP Program, is to assist students with disabilities in becoming active participants in their educational conferences. Snyder (2002) also argues that teaching students with disabilities the skills needed to effectively participate in their own educational conferences is an important step in learning to assert their goals, interests, and preferences in other areas of their lives.

The Self-Advocacy Strategy is a motivational and self-determination program designed to prepare high school and middle school students with disabilities for participating in their education and transition planning meetings (Test & Neale, 2004). This self-advocacy program consists of five steps, which are taught using instructional and SST techniques that follow lessons provided in an instructor's handbook (see Van Reusen et al., 1994, in "Additional Readings and Resources" at the end of this chapter to obtain the handbook). The acronym I-PLAN is used to facilitate teaching the following five steps.

1. "Inventory." Students list their strengths, areas of needed improvement, education and transition goals, required accommodations, and learning preferences. This information is placed on the students' inventory sheets, which are taken with them to their IEP meetings.
2. "Provide Your Inventory Information." Students learn to provide the previously identified information during their meetings.
3. "Listen and Respond." Students learn to listen to others' statements or questions and to respond appropriately.

4 "Ask Questions." Students learn to ask appropriate questions to obtain relevant information.
5 "Name Your Goals." Students learn to communicate personal goals and to suggest actions to attain the goals.

After intervention, the four eighth-grade students involved in the program's evaluation (two African Americans; two whites), none of whom had previously attended an IEP meeting, attended their meetings and improved their response scores. The response scores measured the quality of the students' contributions, and the skills generalized to their actual IEP meetings. The students increased their self-determination scores after intervention, but the increases were not statistically significant from baseline measures. Finally, the students favorably evaluated the degree to which the program assisted them in preparing for and participating in their IEP meetings.

The Self-Advocacy Strategy also has been incorporated into an Interactive Hypermedia Program (IHP), which teaches communication and I-PLAN self-determination skills to high school students with disabilities (Lancaster et al., 2002). The IHP is presented on a CD and includes video and audio segments, text, graphics, and animation and provides students with individualized feedback. The strategies are designed to assist students in preparing for and participating in any type of educational conference. The program teaches five communication skills, called SHARE behaviors: **s**itting erectly, **h**aving a pleasant tone of voice, **a**ctivating thinking, **r**elaxing, and **e**ngaging in eye contact. This content is followed by instruction on the five steps of I-PLAN (as described in the previous intervention). Approximately one hour of live instruction also is incorporated into the program, which involves a practitioner providing an explanation of the program, examining the students' understanding of the content, answering questions, and facilitating role plays. The students also participate in a simulated educational conference. Prior to the students' IEP conference, a practitioner meets individually with the students to review the conference procedures, prompt them to use their acquired skills, answer any questions, and give the students their personal inventory.

The students with LD, behavior disorders, or health impairments volunteering to participate in the program evaluation (N = 22) were given a choice to be included either in an intervention or in a comparison group receiving no instruction. The students who chose an intervention group then were randomly assigned to live instruction or to the IHP. The IHP combined with practitioner involvement was just as effective in teaching the skills as live instruction (content was identical, but paper based). Students in the intervention groups were more proficient at sharing relevant IEP information, including their strengths, weaknesses, learning and testing preferences, and goals, compared with students in the comparison group. Students' ratings of their satisfaction with their conferences were higher for the intervention groups, but the difference was not statistically significant. Surveys completed by teachers and parents attending the educational conferences, however, supported the superior performance of students in the experimental groups in preparedness, responding to and asking questions, and articulating their goals, learning preferences, and effective learning activities.

This third program, the Self-Directed IEP (developed by J. E. Martin & colleagues, 1993a; 1993b; evaluated by Snyder, 2002), teaches adolescent students with disabilities to lead their own IEP meetings. The self-directed program, which incorporates SST techniques, consists of eleven sessions. Interventions include a video presentation providing an overview of the instructional package and depicting a student running his own IEP meeting. Practitioners give workbook assignments on a variety of topics. The topics include identifying personal goals; reviewing past goals, performance, and action needed to meet the identified goals; identifying methods to obtain feedback from IEP team members, appropriate questions, and compromising skills; and asking for needed support. A practitioner also assists the students in completing scripts for their IEP meeting, discusses expected behavior, and provides vocabulary instruction. Sessions focus on students developing skills in four main areas: introducing others at their IEP meetings, reviewing their past IEP goals, discussing their future goals, and closing their meetings. Finally, a simulated IEP meeting is conducted for each student, using a prepared script (see Snyder, 2002, appendixes C and D, for a more detailed description of the sessions and the simulated IEP meeting script).

Five students (two Latinos, two whites, and one African American) with a diagnosis of mild mental retardation and a behavioral disorder participated in the program evaluation. All of the students substantially increased their skills in the four main areas after intervention. Ratings of videotaped simulated and actual IEP meetings also demonstrated improved skills. Finally, the students rated their overall satisfaction with the program and its results as high.

Establishing and Attaining Personal Goals

Two CB programs designed to enhance the self-determination of students with disabilities by teaching them skills to establish and achieve their personal goals are described first. The final program assists clients with severe mental illness in establishing and achieving personal goals. All three programs use SST and methods to transfer the acquired skills to natural settings (e.g., homework assignments and eliciting cooperation from teachers and significant others). Other CB interventions included in the programs are reinforcement, prompts (picture and cue cards), and self-management strategies, such as problem solving, self-instruction, self-monitoring, and self-evaluation. The programs were evaluated using multiple-baseline designs, a pretest-posttest design, and simple descriptive statistics.

Students with developmental, learning, and physical disabilities and emotional/behavioral disorders. Agran and his colleagues (2000) developed a "Self-Determined Learning Model of Instruction" (SDLMI) to teach middle school and high school students with disabilities to establish their own goals, to take steps to achieve their goals, and to adjust the goals and action steps as needed (see Mithaug, Wehmeyer, Agran, Martin, & Palmer, 1998, in "Additional Readings and Resources" at the end of this chapter for a more detailed description of the program). With the assistance of a practitioner, students identify and select skills for improvement related to work, social interactions, education, or community living. Following directions, improving job performance, personal hygiene, budgeting, computer use, and arranging transportation are examples of skill areas. When applicable, such as for work-related skills, relevant individuals (e.g., work supervisors) assist in identifying the skills. Practitioners use three instructional phases, each presenting a problem that must be solved, and four questions that students pose and answer to resolve the problem, to teach the model. During the first phase, students identify goals by answering the following four questions.

1 "What do I want to learn?"
2 "What do I know about it now?"
3 "What must change for me to learn what I don't know?"
4 "What can I do to make this happen?" (Agran et al., 2000, p. 358)

In the second phase, students identify plans to meet the goals by answering the following four questions.

1 "What can I do to learn what I don't know?"
2 "What could keep me from taking action?"
3 "What can I do to remove these barriers?"
4 "When will I take action?"

The practitioner provides the students with worksheets designed to assist them in learning the first two phases of the model. The practitioner also teaches the students to identify and learn specific CB strategies that they can use to implement their self-selected goals. Examples of strategies include self-instruction, self-monitoring, self-evaluation, problem solving, and picture cues. As the students implement their action plans and use their self-directed learning strategies, they are taught to apply four questions in the third phase of the model. The four questions, which assist the students in revising their goals or action plans as needed, follow.

1 "What actions have I taken?"
2 "What barriers have been removed?"

3 "What has changed about what I don't know?"
4 "Do I know what I want to know?"

The practitioner reads the questions; clarifies their meaning if necessary; and after students answer the questions, provides praise and corrective feedback as appropriate.

A multiple-baseline design across three student groups demonstrated a marked increase in student performance of the identified skills after intervention for all but two of the nineteen participants. The participants had one disability (LD or mental retardation) or a combination of LD or mental retardation and another physical or sensory disability. The majority of the students maintained their improved performance after formal intervention ended. Teacher ratings before and after intervention indicated that 89% of the students' goals were attained at or above the expected level of outcome. Teachers also perceived that the students enjoyed the process and having responsibility for their own decisions and actions. All of the students reported that the program increased their skill proficiency and independence, and they enjoyed the problem-solving process.

Agran and colleagues (Agran, Blanchard, Wehmeyer, & Hughes, 2002) also adapted the SDLMI to accommodate middle school students with mild to moderate mental retardation, autism, and multiple disabilities. In this program, practitioners assist students in selecting their goals then use SST techniques to teach students the problem-solving process by asking and answering the following questions.

1 "What is the problem?"
2 "What can I do about it?"
3 After implementing the chosen solution, "Did that fix the problem?"
4 "Did I meet my goal?" (p. 283)

The practitioner provides the students with cue cards to further assist them in learning the problem-solving process and to prompt them if they need assistance in remembering the steps. The practitioner also encourages the students at the beginning of each class period to follow the problem-solving steps, and the classroom teacher provides opportunities for the students to apply the steps to achieve their goals in the classroom. Examples of student goals are to follow directions and contribute to the class. All four students participating in the evaluation met or exceeded their goals after intervention, and they performed their identified behaviors above the levels expected by their teachers. The students reported that the intervention assisted them in learning to problem solve, improving their identified skills, and enhancing positive feelings about themselves. The behaviors were maintained for up to two weeks.

Researchers also adapted the SDLMI to meet the cognitive and developmental level of early elementary school students (ages 5–9 years) receiving educational supports for mental retardation and LD (Palmer & Wehmeyer, 2003) and middle school students with mental retardation and LD (Palmer, Wehmeyer, Gipson, & Agran, 2004). Evaluations indicate similar positive results.

This second main program, Take Action, teaches high school students with mild to moderate mental retardation to attain their IEP goals. The program was developed by Huber-Marshall et al. (1999) and later evaluated (German, Martin, Marshall, & Sale, 2000). Practitioners can teach the program using one of two formats—long-term and daily goal attainment. The first format contains eight lessons teaching students to break their long-term goals into well-defined short-term steps that can be accomplished within a week. The students then establish a plan to achieve their goals by answering six questions related to six main steps.

1 Standard: "What will I be satisfied with?"
2 Feedback: "How will I get feedback on my performance?"
3 Motivation: "Why do I want to do this?"
4 Strategy: "What method will I use?"
5 Support: "What help do I need?"
6 Schedule: "When will I do it?" (Huber-Marshall et al., 1999, p. 30)

The format for attaining daily goals involves only the final three steps, which teach students to evaluate and to adjust their plans on a daily, instead of a weekly, basis. In teaching this format, the practitioner constructs for each student thirty daily goal cards containing various tasks that the student can perform but cannot perform adequately. Students then select three of the daily goals taken from their IEPs, into which they had input. Two examples of goals are finding the want-ad section in the daily newspaper and completing five tasks in a row without a prompt. The practitioner teaches the Take Action process using an instructional package, which involves four lessons. The lessons involve the students performing the following behaviors.

1 Complete a set of activities to learn the four steps of the process: plan, act, evaluate, and adjust.
2 Watch a video depicting high school students using the process to attain their goals, after which the practitioner teaches the steps of strategy, support, and schedule.
3 Review sample plans, practice writing plans, and write plans to achieve the students' own goals.
4 Learn evaluation strategies to determine whether the developed strategy, support, and scheduled activity achieved the goals. If the goals are not accomplished, learn to adjust the plans.

After completing the four sessions, students practice using Take Action to attain their daily goals for up to six days. As the students complete and carry out their action plans, the practitioner provides prompts and feedback. At the end of the day, the practitioner also provides support, instruction, and feedback as students complete the evaluation and adjust their tasks. After formal intervention ends, the students select three daily goals from their cards and complete their plan forms (the practitioner can assist in writing the plan). At the end of the day, the practitioner verbally praises the students for any goals achieved.

The multiple-baseline design used to evaluate the daily goal attainment format demonstrated that all participants (N = 6) increased the number of daily goals attained. During baseline, the number of goals the students attained ranged from zero to two. Ten days after intervention the majority of the students attained all three of their goals. The students reported that the program taught them strategies to achieve their goals without feeling "stupid." Student goal attainment also was related to enhanced perceptions of themselves and to increased confidence in making choices.

Adults with severe mental illness. The "Personal Effectiveness for Successful Living" (PESL) program is a CB intervention that teaches clients with severe mental illness to be "their own case managers" (Liberman & Kopelowicz, 2002). For more than thirty years, this program has been implemented in a variety of treatment settings throughout the world, including community mental health centers, private practices, psychiatric hospitals, and veterans' medical centers.

The PESL program, which can be conducted with individuals, families, or groups, uses SST to teach clients to set goals, engage in problem solving, learn appropriate verbal and nonverbal behavior, and complete community-based homework assignments. Clients are reminded of the communication and problem-solving skills through information placed on wall posters or easels. The clinician provides clients with video feedback, which highlights role plays depicting the clients engaging in appropriate communication skills. Clients also are given homework in the form of a reminder card, which contains the date, the assignment, and prompts to use the acquired nonverbal communication behaviors (e.g., eye contact, appropriate tone of voice and facial expression, and communicating with the goal in mind).

During the sessions, the clinician assists clients in articulating their personal long-term goal as positive goals, then identifying specific actions that, if successfully completed, would bring them closer to attaining their goals. For example, if a client chooses the goal of increasing his number of friends, a series of action goals leading to this long-term goal might be "attend a Bible class where there would be others who share my interest in religion" or "call a friend from high school with whom I've stayed in contact and invite him to join me for coffee or a movie." During the skills training sessions, the clinician also uses the acronym SMART (**s**pecific, **m**eaningful, **a**ttainable, **r**ealistic, and **t**ransfer) to assist clients in setting specific, incremental goals. First, clients answer the following three questions to develop specific goals.

1 "What is the goal?"
2 "With whom do I need to interact to achieve the goal?"
3 "When and where will this interaction likely take place?" (p. 1377)

Second, clients link goals to a longer-term personal goal. Third, each goal must be attainable—neither too difficult nor too easy to accomplish. Fourth, the goal should be realistic. That is, the goal should be consistent with the clients' rights and responsibilities and with improving their social functioning, while building on the clients' current strengths and resources. Finally, the clinician mobilizes community-based case managers and members of the clients' social support networks to promote transfer of the skills from the treatment setting into their daily lives (see UCLA CRTRP in "Additional Readings and Resources" at the end of this chapter for information on obtaining the "Personal Effectiveness" clinical manual).

Liberman and Kopelowicz (2002) reviewed the goals of seventy-nine clients who participated in PESL groups led by various professionals in different types of treatment settings. The researchers identified a total of 123 personal goals, which involved 658 specific behavioral assignments; 72% of the assignments were satisfactorily implemented. The clients also reported successfully achieving 63% of their overall personal goals. The results, however, varied. Clients with more thought disorder and psychiatric symptoms achieved fewer goals, while clients with stable or remitted symptoms achieved the greatest number of goals. Clients establishing highly motivating long-term goals (e.g., restoring a driver's license, maintaining child custody) also were more successful in achieving their goals. Unfortunately, neither baseline measures nor other evaluations of the PESL program were reported.

ANALYSIS AND CRITIQUE FOR PRACTICE AND RESEARCH

This chapter described CB interventions designed to empower vulnerable populations, including students with mental retardation, LD, emotional/behavioral disorders, and physical and multiple disabilities, and adults with severe mental illness, by teaching them knowledge, skills, and strategies to gain more control over their lives. A variety of CB methods are used, sometimes in combination with other instructional techniques, to assist students and clients with disabilities in learning and engaging in self-determined behavior. The methods include SST, problem solving, prompting, self-instruction, self-evaluation, self-monitoring, and practicing the skills in natural settings. With the exception of the PESL program for clients with severe mental illness, the interventions were conducted within or in conjunction with the school system. Although the interventions have direct application for school and mental health social workers, none were developed or evaluated by social workers. Given the importance of self-determination as a basic value guiding social work practice, particularly for vulnerable populations, this is surprising and suggests areas for future social work research.

Effectiveness and Additional Applications

Evaluations of the previously described CB interventions suggest that they can provide vulnerable children, adolescents, and adults with relevant skills and increased opportunities to exert more control over their lives. Despite these optimistic results, the evaluations have a number of limitations. Researchers primarily used nonexperimental designs, and the evaluation of the PESL program simply reported percentages of completed assignments and goals attained by the clients. In the evaluation that randomly assigned students to two different intervention groups (the IHP or traditional instruction), the students first chose whether to join an intervention or a comparison group. Thus, self-selection might have biased the favorable results found in the intervention groups. In addition, participants sometimes were selected based on characteristics that were not representative of all the individuals in a particular population. For example, German et al. (2000) selected students who had excellent school attendance to participate in the Take Action program.

Further, not all students or clients improved on the outcome measures, and some evaluations indicated that intervention was more successful for clients with particular characteristics. For example, in the PESL program that assists clients with severe mental illness in setting and attaining their own goals, clients with stable or remitted psychiatric symptoms were more likely to succeed. Other studies demonstrated that participants improved only in certain settings, and no changes were made on important outcome measures (e.g., a self-determination scale).

The findings and methodological shortcomings of the research evaluating the interventions preclude drawing firm conclusions about their effectiveness or applicability to particular clients. Nonetheless, the evaluations suggest that some youths and adults with disabilities can learn a variety of self-determination skills to set and attain their own goals, actively participate in school conferences, and increase input into the decisions made about their lives. Recent reviews of studies evaluating CB interventions that teach vulnerable populations (primarily students with LD and mental retardation) self-determination skills drew similar conclusions (Algozzine, Browder, Karvonen, Test, & Wood, 2001; Test et al., 2004).

Although the interventions discussed in this chapter have direct application in mental health and school settings, they might be applicable to other vulnerable clients and in other areas of social work practice. Federal law also recognizes the importance of adults with disabilities exercising self-determination. Similar to the amendments to the IDA, which require students with disabilities to participate in their IEPs and transition planning meetings, legislation (e.g., Rehabilitation Act Amendments of 1992 and 1998) also encourages the self-determination of adults with disabilities. The law recognizes the rights of adults with disabilities to participate in the development of their individual rehabilitation plans, to live independently, to make choices, and to be integrated into all aspects (e.g., political, economic, and social) of American society (Field, 1996; Test et al., 2004). The previously discussed interventions that enhance the skills of students with disabilities to actively participate in their educational conferences and to set and achieve their own goals also might be used or adapted to enhance the self-determined behavior of adults with similar disabilities.

The interventions also might be applicable when individual assessment indicates that skill development and/or more opportunities to make decisions are necessary to increase client control in specific environments or over specific areas of their lives. Additional social work practice areas include health care, physical and vocational rehabilitation, and child welfare. Other vulnerable clients, such as the economically disadvantaged and ethnic/racial and sexual minorities, also might benefit from interventions that increase self-determination skills.

Freedom, Control, and Social Justice

All of the interventions discussed in this chapter focus on enhancing individual control and freedom. The interventions teach clients to set and achieve their own goals and to actively participate in educational conferences and in other decisions made about their lives. These outcomes also are consistent with social justice.

Although all of the CB interventions are standardized, they incorporate methods to enhance participants' freedom, input, and control over the intervention process. For example, students with disabilities identify their own strengths, limitations, needed accommodations, educational preferences, and goals. Students with disabilities and clients with severe mental illness are provided opportunities to practice setting, communicating, and carrying out their own goals and making their own decisions in a variety of settings. Making decisions and setting goals, of course, are constrained in many ways. For example, within school systems, students might be limited to goals consistent with those established at a previous educational conference. Finally, the intervention programs use a variety of self-management strategies, including problem solving, self-instruction, self-monitoring, and self-evaluation, which can enhance individual control. Some students with mental retardation who participated in the Take Action program, which teaches self-management strategies to attain personal goals, reported that they learned the skills without feeling stupid. This response suggests that CB procedures can respect the abilities of students with learning difficulties, which also is consistent with social justice.

Social Validity

Socially relevant goals and results. The goals of the CB interventions discussed in this chapter include increasing self-determination and related scales, which were completed by parents, teachers, and students; parents increasing opportunities for their children to make decisions about their lives; and youths attempting to make more of their own decisions. Other examples of intervention goals are enhancing students' participation skills and contributions to their IEP conferences, such as sharing important information and the number of goals contributed. In other evaluations, outcome measures included the number of goals that were set and achieved by the students or clients. These intervention goals all are consistent with the socially valued concept of self-determination. However, limitations exist. For example, an intervention goal for actually including the students' contributions into the IEPs was not established.

Practitioners and researchers might adopt other methods from the previously discussed CB interventions to ensure that their goals are desirable, acceptable, viable, and meaningful to those involved in the interventions. For example, student goals can be negotiated with teachers and can be consistent with the students' previously established IEPs into which they had input. Practitioners can enhance the social relevance of intervention goals for clients with severe mental illness by assisting them in choosing meaningful, attainable, and realistic personal goals.

Evaluations of the interventions suggest that many of the participants enhanced their self-determination, as indicated by increases in attempting to make more of their own decisions, in the type and number of contributions to their IEP conferences, and achieving individually set goals. However, these intervention gains are not necessarily socially relevant to the students or clients. For example, did the students' enhanced performance at their educational conferences result in any meaningful difference in the students' educational experience? Even though they were not always favorable, some of the intervention evaluations provide methods to determine the social relevance of intervention gains. Students can rate whether participating in the intervention assisted them in preparing for or enhanced their satisfaction with their educational conferences. Students also can provide feedback on whether they experienced other favorable outcomes, such as enhanced self-perceptions and self-confidence in making choices, as a result of participating in the intervention. Teachers can complete preintervention and postintervention ratings of the expected level of the outcomes of students' goals and report on improvements in other socially relevant indicators (e.g., academic and behavioral performance).

None of the evaluations of the interventions reported investigating unfavorable results of the interventions. Negative results might include increased conflict between educators and students, or between parents and their children, after youths are encouraged to set their own goals and assume more control over their lives. Conflict likely would occur when individuals choose goals and/or make decisions that are inconsistent with family, school, or agency expectations or values or are perceived to be in conflict with the individual's best interests. Neither did the evaluations determine whether negative consequences, such as disappointment, sadness, and demoralization, resulted when participants failed to achieve their desired goals. These possible outcomes suggest the need for practitioners and researchers to discuss and prepare clients and involved others to cope with any anticipated unfavorable outcomes.

Socially relevant intervention procedures. None of the CB interventions discussed in this chapter conducted individual functional assessments. The intervention developers appeared to assume that a lack of skills, and in some cases a lack of opportunity, was the maintaining antecedent of the participants' failure to exert more control over their lives. Other possible maintaining conditions, such as a negative evaluation of one's abilities, fear of or actual negative consequences after attempting to assume more control, value or cultural conflicts, or a lack of resources, were not examined. Practitioners need to conduct an individual functional assessment to identify these types of maintaining conditions that could suggest more relevant interventions.

Despite the lack of attention to individualized assessments, developers of the CB interventions discussed in this chapter used other techniques to enhance the social relevance of their interventions, which can inform practice and future research. Information gathered from focus groups (e.g., individuals with disabilities, their parents, and educators), research on self-determination and related topics, and collaboration with other professionals and specialists serving similar populations can identify socially relevant tasks and responses targeted by the intervention materials. Providing opportunities for participants to practice the skills in the context of their own lives and assisting families in balancing the youths' self-determination with family values are other examples of strategies to enhance the acceptability and feasibility of the interventions.

Practitioners and researchers also can make interventions more acceptable and feasible by accommodating the special needs of the participants. The use of acronyms (e.g., I-PLAN and SMART) and breaking down the problem-solving process into simpler steps can assist clients with cognitive or psychiatric disabilities in remembering the problem-solving and other skills-building processes. Obtaining teachers' cooperation to provide opportunities for the identified behaviors to be exhibited, providing daily prompts and feedback, and constructing daily goal cards also can assist students with cognitive limitations in performing the identified skills. Placing information on wall posters and easels and giving homework assignments in the form of reminder cards are additional techniques practitioners might use to assist clients with severe mental illness in learning the skills and applying them to situations in their own lives.

Even if interventions are successful in attaining a socially valid goal, if they are to be continued in school or other settings, they must be acceptable to participants, staff, and other professionals who implement them. Practitioners, researchers, and administrators might adopt methods to measure the acceptability of a CB intervention from evaluations of the previously described interventions. The strategies include students rating their satisfaction with and enjoyment of the intervention process and teachers observing students' reactions to the interventions (e.g., their enjoyment and willingness to participate). Teachers' intentions to continue using the intervention are another indication of the acceptability and feasibility of the intervention procedures. However, the time involved in carrying out the interventions might be a major barrier to their acceptability. For example, the classroom-based self-determination program developed by Abery et al. (1995) involves twenty-four-weekly sessions of approximately ninety minutes each over a twenty-four-week period. As the researchers acknowledge, teachers and other school staff, who frequently are overworked and struggling to teach required curricula and to cope with problems interfering with students' academic achievement, might lack the time to teach and monitor additional skills and outcomes. The evaluation of the IHP suggests that developing computer software to assist students in learning self-determination skills might be a viable alternative. Finally, availability of IHP software and standardized manuals to implement the previously discussed interventions can decrease the cost and time involved in extensive training and program development.

Maintenance and generalization. The previously described interventions and evaluations are consistent with frequent criticisms of CB methods designed to enhance vulnerable students' self-determination skills and of the evaluating research (Abery et al., 1995; Test et al., 2004). First, the interventions do not plan for maintenance or transfer of the acquired skills to other natural contexts, including community, home, work, and higher education settings. Second, the evaluations do not assess long-term maintenance or generalization of the skills. With two exceptions, the interventions discussed in this chapter also do not involve individuals in other settings, such as parents, caretakers, and employment supervisors.

The first exception, the PESL program, assigns case managers and mobilizes natural supports (e.g., family members) to promote transfer of the skills into the daily lives of clients with severe mental illness. Abery and his colleagues' (1995) multicomponent program that enhances the self-determination skills of students with mental retardation is the only school-based program involving the student's family. Interestingly, that evaluation found that only within the context of the home (not in the school or work setting) in which family members were actively involved in the intervention did students enhance their self-determination. This finding suggests the need for practitioners to involve relevant individuals from multiple settings. Practitioners also could assess and, if necessary, intervene in relevant settings to ensure opportunities, resources, and reinforcing consequences are present to assist vulnerable clients in assuming more control over their lives. The latter suggestion is supported by comments from the focus groups conducted by Abery and his colleagues. The participants identified the attitudes of society and professionals serving youths with disabilities as barriers to self-determination.

Evaluations of the interventions discussed in this chapter suggest two other important yet neglected issues that can inform practice and future development of CB interventions to assist clients in maintaining their self-determination skills and transferring them to multiple natural settings. First, when significant others, such as teachers, assisted students in performing the skills (e.g., by prompting and specifically providing opportunities), whether the students were able to maintain the skills in absence of such assistance was not determined. If students and clients cannot maintain the intervention gains without assistance, strategies must be used to ensure that needed support continues. Second, unless practitioners discuss and prepare clients for possible negative feelings (e.g., disappointment from not attaining personal goals) and negative reactions from others (e.g., rejection of their decision), clients are likely to fail to maintain and/or transfer their acquired skills to other settings, situations, and individuals.

This summary and analysis pose many unanswered questions but suggest practitioners can use CB interventions to increase self-determined behavior of vulnerable students and clients. Also noted were unique opportunities for social work researchers to design and evaluate CB interventions to enhance the self-determination of vulnerable populations.

The next chapter continues the description and evaluation of CB strategies that increase self-determined behavior of vulnerable groups. The interventions empower vulnerable clients by teaching them choice-making skills and providing opportunities for choice making in routine activities, such as recreation/leisure, work, eating, and self-care, and in the longer-term decision of selecting a community residence.

ADDITIONAL READINGS AND RESOURCES

Abery, B., Arndt, K., Greger, P., Tetu, L., Eggebeen, A., Barosko, et al. (1994). *Self-determination for youth with disabilities: A family education curriculum.* Institute on Community Integration, University of Minnesota, 102 Pattee Hall, 150 Pillsbury Drive SE, Minneapolis, MN 55455. Ordering information can be found at http://www.ici.umn.edu/products/curricula.html#self

Agran, M. (1997). *Student-directed learning: Teaching self-determination skills.* Pacific Grove, CA: Brooks/Cole.

Algozzine, B., Browder, D., Karvonen, M., Test, D. W., & Wood, W. M. (2001). Effects of interventions to promote self-determination for individuals with disabilities. *Review of Educational Research, 71,* 219–277.

Field, S., Martin, J., Miller, R., Ward, M., & Wehmeyer, M. (1998). *A practical guide for teaching self-determination.* Reston, VA: Council for Exceptional Children.

Karvonen, M., Test, D. W., Wood, W. M., Browder, D., & Algozzine, B. (2004). Putting self-determination into practice. *Exceptional Children, 71,* 23–41.

Martin, J. E., Marshal, L. H., Maxson, L. L., & Jerman, P. (1993a). *Student workbook: Self-directed IEP.* Colorado Springs: University of Colorado at Colorado Springs.

Martin, J. E., Marshal, L. H., Maxson, L. L., & Jerman, P. (1993b). *Teacher's manual for the self-directed IEP video and workbook.* Colorado Springs: University of Colorado at Colorado Springs.

Mithaug, D. E., Wehmeyer, M., Agran, M., Martin, J. E., & Palmer, S. (1998). The self-determined learning model of teaching: Engaging students to solve their learning problems. In M. Wehmeyer & D. J. Sand (Eds.), *Making it happen: Student involvement in educational planning, decision-making and instruction* (pp. 299–328). Baltimore: Paul Brookes.

Sands, D. J., & Wehmeyer, M. L. (Eds.). (1996). *Self-determination across the life span: Independence and choice for people with disabilities.* Baltimore: Paul Brookes.

UCLA Center for Research on Treatment and Rehabilitation of Psychosis, West LA VA Medical Center, 11301 Wilshire Blvd., Los Angeles, CA 90073. Ordering information for the "Personal Effectiveness" clinical manual is available at http://www.mentalhealth.ucla.edu/projects/irc/index.html

Van Reusen, A. K., Bos, C. S., Schumaker, J. B., & Deshler, D. D. (1994). *The self-advocacy strategy.* Lawrence, KS: Edge Enterprises.

Wehmeyer, M. L., Agran, M., & Hughes, C. (1998). *Teaching self-determination to youth with disabilities: Basic skills for successful transition.* Baltimore: Paul Brookes.

Wehmeyer, M. L., & Garner, N. W. (2003). The impact of personal characteristics of people with intellectual and developmental disability on self-determination and autonomous functioning. *Journal of Applied Research in Intellectual Disabilities, 16,* 255–265.

11 Increasing Choice Making in Daily and Long-Term Decisions

Most adults exercise self-determination by making multiple short- and long-term decisions about their lives. Daily or more routine choices include when to get up and go to bed, what to wear and eat, in which recreational or leisure activity to participate, and how to perform aspects of daily chores and jobs. Long-term choices include where to live, with whom to live, and a variety of educational and vocational decisions (Faw, Davis, & Peck, 1996). Although choices of children and adolescents generally are more restricted than those of adults, they exercise self-determination by making many of the same types of decisions.

Choice is a common element in definitions of self-determination and is fundamental to empowerment. Shevin and Klein (1984) define "choosing" for individuals with disabilities as "the act of an individual's selection of a preferred alternative from among several familiar options" (p. 160). Unfortunately, some vulnerable populations, particularly those with specific types of disabilities, frequently lack effective choice-making skills, the ability to adequately communicate choices, and opportunities to make routine and longer-term choices that the majority of us take for granted (Agran et al., 2000; Bambara et al., 1995).

This chapter presents CB interventions that empower clients with mental retardation and physical and multiple disabilities to more effectively make and communicate their choices. The interventions engage caretakers and staff in identifying and offering choices to clients and in assisting clients in learning choice-making skills. The interventions also are designed to increase clients' choice making in routine activities, such as recreational/leisure, work, eating, and self-care, and in the longer term decision of selecting a community residence. An analysis of the interventions, including a brief summary and practice and research implications, is provided as the final section.

RECREATIONAL AND LEISURE ACTIVITY

Recreational/leisure time is, by definition, time that is spent as one chooses. Identifying preferences, having preferences available, making choices, and sustaining involvement in an activity with minimal outside intervention all are necessary for vulnerable individuals to engage in meaningful recreational/leisure activity in their schools, communities, and homes (Nietupski et al., 1986). This section describes behavioral interventions that assist individuals with mental retardation, as well as others with combinations of physical and learning disabilities, in communicating preferences and making choices in recreational, leisure, and play activity.

The interventions described here include using preference assessments and a variety of strategies to assist vulnerable clients in making and communicating their choices, including choice charts, activity books and cards, a microswitch communication system, and badges. Multiple behavioral strategies such as physical, gestural, verbal, and picture prompting; modeling; role plays; an errorless teaching procedure; and social reinforcement also assist clients in learning choice-making skills. In two of the behavioral programs, peers with no disabilities are involved in the interventions. All of the interventions were evaluated using multiple-baseline designs.

Individuals with Mental Retardation

The main goal of this behavioral intervention is to increase the ability of adolescents with moderate to severe mental retardation to choose, self-initiate, and sustain recreational/leisure activity during a free activity period in a school or other relevant setting (Nietupski et al., 1986). The practitioner begins by constructing a choice chart designating activities that each youth appears to enjoy based on the observations of others. For youths with no reading ability, a "picture choice chart" containing four or five pictures of available activities is constructed. For other youths, names of the recreational/leisure activities, such as board and video games, magazines, and puzzles, are printed on the choice charts. The practitioner periodically updates the choice charts to add and remove activities in which the adolescents show little or no interest.

During intervention, which can be conducted during leisure times in the adolescents' school or in other locations (e.g., a community domestic living training site or group home), the adolescents are given the opportunity to select a leisure activity from their choice chart. After making a selection, the practitioner verbally praises the youths. If the adolescents fail to make a choice, the practitioner physically and verbally prompts them to make a selection and to obtain the necessary materials. After beginning the activity, if the youths participate appropriately, the practitioner uses verbal praise; if the adolescents inappropriately engage in the activity, the practitioner verbally prompts appropriate participation. If the prompt is ineffective, the practitioner models participation, which is followed by a physical prompt as needed.

Evaluation of the intervention, which took place in a school setting, demonstrated that the three participants rarely failed to make a choice when given the opportunity. The participants also substantially increased the amount of time they engaged in leisure activity with no outside involvement. The improvements were maintained from one to four weeks later. School staff found the procedures acceptable and adopted them for use with other students. A behavioral intervention discussed in chapter 5 also is relevant here (Hughes et al., 2004). The intervention taught adolescent students with mental retardation and other support needs to choose a recreational activity and ask another student to participate during PE classes.

Bambara and Ager (1992) designed a behavioral intervention to teach adults with moderate mental retardation to choose, schedule, and initiate leisure activity. The activities, which are chosen based on interviews of clients and staff, can be conducted in the home (e.g., caring for plants, listening to music, phoning friends, watching a favorite TV show) or in the community (e.g., traveling to a local store, restaurant, or mall and visiting friends or family). A commercially available activity book and cards (manufactured by Attainment Corporation) are used to teach the clients to choose and schedule the activities. The book contains pages of clear plastic pockets to display activity cards, with the days of the week (and relevant pictures for clients who are unable to read) depicted at the top of each page. The activity cards contain pictures, words, or a combination of both, depending on the client's reading ability. Cards for activities requiring some type of support or assistance contain prompts to remind the clients to set up assistance prior to scheduling the activity. For example, a picture of a car prompts the clients to arrange transportation to visit family.

Skills training is used to teach the clients to self-schedule the activities, which involves selecting an activity card for each day of the week, scheduling the cards by placing them in the appropriate slots, and seeking staff support for the cards indicating required assistance. Staff also prompt the clients to use their activity books daily and to self-initiate their selected activities (e.g., "Get your book" or "Look at your activities"). Each evening, the staff review the day's scheduled activities, and praise any engagement in leisure activity. If the clients do not engage in a scheduled activity, the staff discuss the activity but communicate no disapproval. After intervention, the prompts and nightly reviews are withdrawn, but staff continue to meet weekly with the clients while they schedule their leisure activities.

The three clients participating in the evaluation, who were receiving supported community living services, all learned to independently self-schedule their leisure activity. The skills were maintained six to eight months after intervention. The intervention also resulted in substantial increases in the frequency and diversity of the clients' self-directed leisure activity, which were maintained between nine and twenty weeks following formal intervention.

Behavioral interventions also can teach adults with severe mental retardation and limited means of communication (i.e., they can only verbalize a few words) to choose a setting for engaging in particular leisure activities (Browder et al., 1998). In this intervention, the practitioner selects two activities for each client in which he or she has previously engaged, has never refused participation, and can perform on a regular basis in two settings (e.g., in an adult day center and in another community setting). For example, one activity might be looking at magazines, which can be done in an adult day center, as well as in a local library. The practitioner then teaches the clients to choose one of two objects representing the activity in the two settings. For the magazine activity, the object representing the center might be a magazine subscription card, and the community object a library card. An errorless teaching procedure, which incorporates time delay, is then used to teach the clients to choose one of the two objects.

During the first session, the practitioner uses a combination of an immediate gestural and physical prompt. For example, the practitioner says, "Show me what you need for looking at magazines *here*," while pointing to the magazine subscription card with the client's left hand and guiding the client to pick up the magazine subscription card with his or her right hand. The practitioner praises the client for selecting the item, and the client is taken to the activity. During the second session, the gestural prompt is given immediately, and after a five-second delay, the gesture is followed by physical guidance. If the client selects the wrong object, the practitioner responds, "No, you need this one," then physically guides the client to select the correct item, which is followed by praise. The client is taken to the corresponding setting. During subsequent sessions, the practitioner waits for five seconds before providing the prompts. After the client can successfully distinguish between the two settings, the two objects representing the two settings are simultaneously displayed, and the client is asked, "Where do you want to go?" After picking up one of the objects, the client is escorted to the activity setting.

Evaluation of the intervention demonstrated that the clients (N = 3) learned to select the object representing the respective setting, clearly exhibited preferences, and made no errors. For example, if clients chose the activity in the day center, they did not prepare to leave with other clients going to community activities. As Browder et al. (1998) observed, their evaluation demonstrates that when the appropriate materials and intervention are available, even individuals with severe disabilities can express and make choices in the area of recreational activity.

Individuals with Multiple Disabilities

Kennedy and Haring (1993) developed this behavioral intervention to teach students (ages five to twenty years) with profound, multiple physical and developmental disabilities to use a microswitch communication system to request a change in recreational activity in integrated public schools. The intervention is designed for individuals who have limited mobility and can communicate only through facial expression, various sounds, and head nods. The intervention begins with a recreational activity preference assessment for each student, which determines the activities to be used in conjunction with the microswitch communication system. During the assessment, a variety of familiar activities and recreational objects, such as a windup toy, keyboard, jigsaw puzzle, computer game, talking book, and music, are placed on a lapboard or table in front of each student. During one session for four days, the practitioner appropriately uses the material or object and prompts the students to engage with the object (i.e., touch or face it). The percentage of time that the students engage in each activity is recorded (see Kennedy & Haring, 1993, pp. 65–66 for more details of the procedure), and the items with the highest and lowest levels of student engagement are kept.

The practitioner then teaches the students to press a microswitch on a tape recorder that activates a prerecorded message of a peer making several requests to change the activity (e.g., "Let's try something else"). The students are presented with an item and prompted to look at or touch the item, and the interaction continues until the students press the microswitch or discontinue engagement for five continuous seconds. If the students discontinue engagement, the item is removed, and they are physically prompted to press the microswitch (i.e., the students' arm/hand is moved to activate the switch). If students press the switch themselves, the item is removed and replaced by another item. After the students learn to activate the switch, same-age peers without disabilities are recruited to interact with them using the microswitch during recess or a break time.

Three of the four students involved in the evaluation used the microswitch to request changes in the object or activity during most of the available opportunities, and engagement with the recreational items increased after intervention. The students' use of the microswitch communication system also generalized to social interactions with the students' able-bodied peers, and two of the students were more engaged in interactions when they chose when to change the item. However, one student was more engaged when a peer chose when to change the activity, and the fourth student indicated no preference. Finally, the evaluation indicated that children and youths with profound and multiple disabilities clearly have preferences for specific objects or activities, but ongoing assessment is necessary because preferences can change over time.

The final behavioral intervention discussed in this section assists nonverbal early adolescent students with severe, multiple disabilities (e.g., profound mental retardation, a seizure disorder, or cerebral palsy) in choosing and initiating activities when playing in an integrated school setting (Jolly, Test, & Spooner, 1993). The intervention is particularly empowering. Similar to the intervention discussed in chapter 5 and cited in the previous section (Hughes et al., 2004), this intervention teaches the students to choose both a playmate and a play activity. The intervention begins with the construction of badges with photographs of activities the students with disabilities enjoy, which are attached to the students' wheelchairs. The practitioner then conducts role plays including the students with disabilities, school staff (e.g., a teacher and teacher assistant), and a student without a disability. During the role plays, the practitioner uses a hierarchy of least-to-most intrusive prompts to teach the students with disabilities to approach another person, pull off a badge, and hold it out toward the selected individual. The selected person then retrieves the activity and plays with the student. After the students with disabilities learn to independently use the badges, they are taken to a free-time play area. The practitioner explains to the students without disabilities that their friends have a new way of telling them what they want to do. The two students with disabilities involved in the evaluation increased their initiations of play activity, but no increases in sustained interactions between them and their peers without disabilities were observed.

ROUTINE AND DAILY ACTIVITIES

The behavioral interventions discussed in this section are particularly relevant to enhancing the self-determination of individuals with severe and multiple disabilities. The interventions increase choice making in daily activities, including household routines, self-care, dressing, eating, and work. As discussed in the beginning of this chapter, individuals with disabilities frequently have little choice in such routine aspects of their lives, which most individuals take for granted. Several interventions designed to increase the choices of clients performing daily activities in their place of residence are described first, followed by techniques that determine job task preferences and provide workers with a choice of job tasks or of methods to perform their jobs. The interventions include prompting, SST, and a self-monitoring strategy. Two of the behavioral programs involve peers with no disabilities, and several of the interventions specifically teach staff in residential group homes to assess and/or provide choices to clients. Single-system or multiple-baseline designs were used to evaluate all of the interventions.

Individuals with Mental Retardation

This case study demonstrates the use of behavioral methods that provided Al, a 50-year-old group home resident, with choice opportunities within daily routines (Bambara et al., 1995). Al was diagnosed as severely developmentally disabled, had been institutionalized for more than thirty-two years, and communicated in one- to four-word phrases that staff rarely could understand. Although he could complete most steps of household and self-care routines independently, Al often required prompting before initiating the next step in the routine. Unfortunately, the prompting frequently was followed by Al's refusal to comply and display of inappropriate behavior, such as screaming, aggression, and property destruction. As a result, Al's participation in self-care, household, and community activities steadily declined. Before intervention, a functional analysis that was conducted determined that Al was more likely to exhibit aggressive or refusal behavior when he was directly told what to do. Al was less likely to exhibit such behavior when he was asked or given a choice regarding when and what to do.

After Al's preferred routines were identified as dusting, vacuuming, and making a dessert, the tasks of each routine were identified, then modified to provide some type of choice (e.g., in materials, locations, and time). For example, two tasks for the vacuuming routine were "takes vacuum to room" and "plugs vacuum in outlet," and Al was given the corresponding choices "between two rooms" and "between two outlets" (see Bambara et al., 1995, pp. 189–190 for the choices within each routine). With the assistance of a scripted choice prompt, staff prompted Al to perform each step of the routines. When prompting the vacuuming routine, for example, staff asked Al if he would like to take the vacuum to the office or to the living room.

The A-B-A-B reversal design assessed the effects of providing Al with choices across the three different preferred routines and on the frequency of his inappropriate behavior and task initiations. During baselines, when staff offered Al no choice, task initiations were near or at zero for each activity, and the number of inappropriate behaviors was high. After staff implemented the choice condition for each routine, Al increased his task initiations and decreased his inappropriate behavior. Al also appeared to be happier (i.e., smiling and joking with others) as he performed the routines after being offered a choice.

A similar behavioral intervention provided choice-making opportunities within and between three activities in an educational setting for a 15-year-old female student with a severe intellectual disability (Dibley & Lim, 1999). The activities were meal times (morning tea and lunch), toileting, and listening to a tape player during music period. After intervention, the student's task initiations increased, and her serious disruptive behaviors decreased.

Parsons and Reid (1990) developed strategies to assess the food and drink preferences of adolescents and adults with profound mental retardation, to teach them choice-making skills, and to teach staff to apply the procedures in residential facilities. During the preference assessment, the staff select pairs of food or drink items that are available in the client's residence or are considered common choices for persons without a disability to make during meals or snack time. Examples of choices are drinking coffee black versus with cream/sugar, eating applesauce versus pudding for dessert, and eating corn chips versus banana slices for snack. During the assessment procedures, which also teach the clients to make choices, the staff tell the clients that they will be given a choice between food and drink options, and then they are given a small sample of both choices for a food/drink option. Next, samples of the two choices for each option are placed in front of the clients, and they are instructed to choose one. Assessment continues until at least one preferred item within a choice is identified for each client (see Parsons & Reid, 1990, pp. 185–186 for complete details of the assessment). The practitioner teaches the procedures to the residential facilities' staff using SST.

All of the clients (N = 14) involved in the evaluation expressed clear preferences for food and drink items during the assessment, and the majority of the choices generalized to their normal meal and snack times. Staff members (N = 5) learned to conduct the behavioral assessment procedures with some supervision. The evaluation also determined that before assessment the staff did not accurately identify the clients' food and drink preferences. This is an important finding, as providing meal preferences is an important goal of service providers working with this vulnerable population (Parsons & Reid, 1990). The choice procedures also are practical, as they can be taught to residential staff.

Individuals with Multiple Disabilities

Salmento and Bambara (2000) also demonstrated that a staff training program (developed by Brown, Belz, Corsi, & Wenig, 1993) can teach staff working in community-based residential homes to present choice opportunities in daily routines to adults with profound mental retardation and severe physical disabilities (e.g., seizures, cerebral palsy, scoliosis). Staff training involves three main phases. First, supervisors hold a consultation meeting with the staff to discuss the importance of choice making for the residents. The supervisors then present and discuss choices that the residents can make in three different areas. Areas include a choice of (1) tasks between or within activities; (2) whether, with whom, where, and when to participate in the activity; and (3) when to terminate the activity. Supervisors then assist staff members in identifying several choice opportunities for various routines. For example, choice opportunities for a dressing routine include choices between two items (e.g., between two shirts, pants, socks, deodorants), either/or choices (e.g., "Do you want to wear perfume or not?"), and choices of order (e.g., "Do you want to put your shirt on first or your pants on first?").

Second, supervisors use SST to teach the staff to use a sequence to present the identified choice opportunities and to respond to the clients' choices during the clients' daily dressing and grooming routines. The residents indicate preferences through idiosyncratic responses, such as body movements, facial expressions, and pointing. The clients' gestures are validated as indicating preference by procedures developed by Reid, Parsons, and Green (1991). The sequence is listed in table 11.1

During the third phase of the program, supervisors provide performance feedback to staff. Evaluation of the intervention demonstrated that during baseline the four staff, all of whom had high school educations, provided residents with no choice opportunities, and the four residents made no choices. After intervention, the number of choices staff offered the residents increased, as did the number of choices the residents made. Session choice means ranged from 4.3 to 10.2. Increases in the choice-offering and choice-making behaviors were maintained one to three months later. The behaviors transferred to lunch activities with one of the same residents, and to dressing and grooming activities with another resident not involved in the evaluation.

Cooper and Browder (2001) designed another behavioral program to enhance client choice making that involves group home staff. The program assists staff in learning the skills for teaching adults with severe disabilities (e.g., severe to profound mental retardation and dual diagnoses of mental retardation and mental illness) to make food choices and other choices while visiting community fast-food restaurants. The intervention also meets the needs of clients who are nonverbal and can only communicate through

---

Table 11.1. Sequence for Providing Choice Opportunities

1. *Present and describe both options*. Describe the two options, making sure that the resident can see the options; for clothing, rub the item against the resident's arm.
2. *Offer first option*. Ask the resident whether he or she wants to wear or use the first item by showing it to the resident. Then wait 5 seconds for the resident to move voluntarily toward the item or to reject the item by moving away from it.
3. *Offer second option* (same as 2, but use second item).
4. *Reoffer options*. If the choice selection is unclear (the resident does not clearly approach or reject the item), repeat steps 2 and 3. If no choice is made, select and give an option to the resident.
5. *Provide choice*. If one of the items is clearly selected (resident approaches one option and rejects the other), give the item to the resident and praise him or her.
6. *Repair*. If the resident appears unhappy with the choice, acknowledge the mistake (e.g., "Oh, you changed your mind") and prompt the resident to approach the other item. Then provide the other item.
7. *Repeat*. Repeat the sequence for the next choice opportunity in the identified routine.

Note. From "Teaching Staff Members to Provide Choice Opportunities for Adults with Multiple Disabilities," by M. Salmento & L. M. Bambara, 2000, *Journal of Positive Behavior Interventions, 2,* p. 16. Copyright 2000 by PRO-ED, Inc. Adapted with permission.

objects, pictures, or idiosyncratic behavior. Staff learn to teach the clients five choice options during each restaurant visit: selecting a door to enter the restaurant, a food item, condiments, a seat, and a door to leave the restaurant. Table 11.2 demonstrates the procedure the supervisor uses to assist staff in teaching the residents to choose between two food or drink items (see Cooper & Browder, 2001, pp. 5–7 for the intervention steps for all choices).

The supervisor uses SST to teach the staff the skills for teaching the choice-making behaviors to the clients. Staff also are taught to self-monitor their own performance by using a checklist of the procedures as they are carried out. In addition, the supervisor observes the staff performing the relevant behaviors at the community restaurants and provides them with performance feedback.

Before intervention, the four staff involved in the evaluation provided few opportunities for the clients ($N = 8$) to make choices. Instead, the staff frequently used intrusive prompts or performed the behaviors for the clients.

Table 11.2. Offering Choice and Prompting Performance

Offering Choice	Performance Step	Prompting Performance
Zero Delay: Point to each photo while also asking "Which one do you want?" while guiding the learner's hand between the two options.	Pick up photo and hand it to the cashier.	*Wait 5 seconds* for the learner to hand the photo to the cashier.
Five-second delay: Wait 5 seconds then point to each photo while also asking, "Which one do you want?" while guiding the learner's hand between the two options.		*Specific Verbal:* Say "Hand the photo to the cashier," then wait another 5 seconds. If the learner does not respond, use the next prompt.
		Specific Verbal & Gesture: Say "Hand the photo to the cashier" while also pointing to the cashier. If the learner does not respond in 5 seconds, use the next prompt.
		Physical Guidance: Gently take the learner's hand and assist him or her in handing the photo to the cashier.

Note. From "Preparing Staff to Enhance Active Participation of Adults with Severe Disabilities by Offering Choice and Prompting Performance During a Community Purchasing Activity," by K. J. Cooper & D. M. Browder, 2001, *Research in Developmental Disabilities, 22,* p. 5. Copyright 2001 by Elsevier Science Ltd. Adapted with permission.

After training, staff offered an average of five choices out of the five choice opportunities and transferred the intervention to different settings and to clients not involved in the evaluation. After training, the clients increased their choice-making skills, as well as the number of choices they made while eating at fast-food restaurants. The staff interactions and clients' choice behaviors were maintained at follow-up approximately two to fifteen weeks after intervention.

These next two behavioral interventions, developed by Reid, Parsons, and their colleagues (Parsons, Reid, Reynolds, & Bumgarner, 1990; Reid, Parsons, Green, & Browning, 2001) provide workers with disabilities with more choices in and control over their work environments. In the first intervention, behavioral methods assess work preferences and assist workers with multiple disabilities (moderate to severe mental retardation, inability to verbally communicate, seizure disorder, and/or visual impairment) in choosing job tasks in their employment setting. First, the job activity is broken down into specific tasks. For example, for assembling plaques, five job tasks are placing, staining, wiping, sanding, and gluing. The worker's job preferences are determined by presenting various combinations of the tasks and asking the worker to choose among them. At least one high-preference task (i.e., selected during at least 70% of pairings) and one low-preference task (i.e., selected during no more than 30% of pairings) are identified for each worker. Based on this assessment, three choice-related alternatives are then given to each worker. That is, the worker chooses a work task, is assigned a preferred task, or is assigned a nonpreferred task. The four workers participating in the evaluation of the intervention demonstrated clear preferences for particular job tasks. When they were assigned to work on their preferred tasks, the workers attended to the job tasks approximately twice as long as compared with when they were assigned to work on a nonpreferred task.

This second behavioral intervention was designed to increase the choice making of supported work employees with severe developmental and physical disabilities who communicate only through gesturing or brief vocalizations. The choice is between working more independently and working with the assistance of a job coach. For each worker, assistive devices are developed for the job tasks. For example, a task in a small publishing company might be collating pages, and an adaptive device might be designed to hold stacks of pages in separate compartments. The job coach then gives the workers a choice between using the assistive device, which gives them much more independence, and declining to use the device, which results in the job coach providing various forms of assistance. The assistance might include manipulating the work materials and giving directions, physical prompts, praise, and feedback. During the choice intervention, the job coach places the necessary materials with or without the assistive device on either side of the worker's table. The worker then is asked to choose to do the job with or without the assistive device by pointing to either set of materials. The three workers involved in the evaluation chose the independence-enhancing device in at least 83% of the choice opportunities.

COMMUNITY RESIDENCE

The two CB programs described here teach skills to clients with dual diagnoses (mental retardation and a mental illness) to evaluate and choose a community residence. Participating in choosing their own residence is particularly important for individuals with disabilities. First, choosing a residence is one of the most important decisions most adults make. Second, social policy supporting integration of individuals with disabilities into the community suggests the need to assist these individuals in maximizing their input into and control over their residential decisions (Faw et al., 1996). The programs use SST, self-management techniques, and intervention materials adapted for the cognitive levels of the clients. Both programs were evaluated using multiple-baseline designs.

This CB program assists institutionalized adults diagnosed with mild mental retardation and a mental illness in choosing a community residence based on their own preferences (Foxx, Faw, Taylor, Davis, & Fulia, 1993). In order to identify appropriate questions for clients to ask about residential options, the researchers developed a survey using items from other questionnaires related to the satisfaction and independence experienced by individuals with mental retardation residing in the community. The relevance of the survey items was further evaluated by professional and support staff from group homes considered potential residential placements for clients. Based on these ratings, two fifteen-question sets were developed to assess client preferences. One set contains the questions most frequently rated as most important, and the other contains the questions most often identified as unimportant. The clients take the combined thirty-item preference test to identify their ten strongest preferences. For each preference area, pictures illustrate contrasting lifestyle options. For example, two photographs are used to offer clients options to engage in personal hygiene activities in private or with others. One photograph depicts an empty bathroom with one shower and toilet, while the other depicts two clothed residents occupying a bathroom. After the pictures are explained, the practitioner asks the clients to indicate which option they would prefer in their place of residence.

The clients are then taught to obtain information on their preferences by asking questions to the guides showing them the group homes and to report their findings to their social workers. In order to accomplish this, clients are given lifestyle preference photo albums that assist them in asking questions related to their preferences and in recording and reporting information based on the guide's answers. Each photo album page contains a picture representing a lifestyle preference (e.g., an individual smoking in the home), a corresponding question (e.g., "Am I allowed to smoke in the home?"), and three boxes labeled "yes," "no," and "maybe." Practitioners use group SST to teach clients the skills for asking the questions, eliciting the three possible responses, recording the responses, and self-managing the process. To self-manage the question-asking process, group facilitators teach the clients to place a paperclip on each album page and to remove it after asking the question on the respective page. After asking the final question, the clients check for any remaining paperclips.

Evaluation of the program demonstrated that the clients ($N = 6$) consistently selected the same options, indicating that they had community living lifestyle preferences and were able to express them. After intervention, the clients increased their lifestyle preference questioning and reporting. The behaviors generalized to actual group home tours conducted by home staff and to interviews conducted by the clients' regular social workers. Assessments completed on five of the six clients available for follow-up indicated that their skills were maintained six to eight weeks later. After the study, the placement model was adopted by the inpatient facility in which the evaluation took place.

Faw et al. (1996) added a worksheet to the previously described residential choice program to assist institutionalized clients with similar diagnoses in evaluating their overall preference for each group home. The bottom half of the worksheet depicts a picture of a home and a sidewalk containing twenty squares that end at the front door. The second ten squares of the sidewalk (those closest to the home) are shaded. The previously selected preference questions appear on the top half of the worksheet, and next to each question the clients mark the "yes," "no," and "maybe" responses. A visual prompt is placed next to each response, indicating a specified number of squares for the client to cross off the sidewalk. Two squares are next to "yes"; one square is next to "maybe;" and no squares are next to "no." On the bottom of the worksheet appears the question, "Based on this information, would this group home be a good place for you to live?" with printed "yes" and "no" responses. If clients cross off any of the sidewalk's shaded squares (which indicates that the clients checked either a "yes" or a "maybe" to over half of their preference questions), they are to answer "yes" to the decision question.

SST is used to teach the skills needed to obtain information regarding their preferences while touring community group homes, to report the information to their social workers, and to evaluate the homes based on the information obtained. All four clients involved in the evaluation of the revised program demonstrated substantial increases in their ability to ask the questions, report information to their social workers, and evaluate the homes. The skills were maintained up to a month later for three of the four clients.

ANALYSIS AND CRITIQUE FOR PRACTICE AND RESEARCH

This chapter presented CB interventions designed to empower vulnerable populations by assisting them in identifying preferences and in increasing their choice making. Vulnerable populations include individuals with mental retardation and multiple disabilities (e.g., combinations of mental illness, physical disabilities, and visual impairments). Choices in daily and routine activity, such as leisure/recreation, work, self-care, and meals, as well as in the more long-term decision of a community residence, are facilitated. SST, prompting, self-monitoring strategies, and reinforcement are frequently used interventions. Evaluations of the CB methods indicate that even individuals with severe disabilities have preferences; their preferences can be determined, and they can and do make choices when offered and given the means to do so. Higher-functioning clients can take an even more active role in evaluating and providing input into long-term and important decisions, such as their community residence. The interventions can be used by practitioners in a variety of school, institutional, residential, and other community settings and can be taught to staff providing services to vulnerable clients.

Effectiveness and Additional Applications

Despite the encouraging results of the evaluations of the previously discussed CB interventions, all suffer methodological shortcomings. None of the studies used random assignment, sample sizes were small and generally homogeneous, and the treatment packages used various combinations of interventions. The use of these research methods precludes drawing any conclusions about the effectiveness of the interventions or determining which of them might be more effective for increasing choice making. Clearly, further research in the area of teaching vulnerable clients choice-making skills in routine and longer-term life decisions is needed. As with many of the interventions reviewed in this book, not all clients benefitted to the same degree, suggesting the need for initial and ongoing individual assessments.

Although methodological limitations exist, the interventions suggest that practitioners can assist clients with disabilities in identifying preferences, learning choice-making skills, and making other types of choices in school, rehabilitation, vocational, and residential settings. For example, clients could choose among teaching methods, physical rehabilitation and other treatment options, activity partners or roommates, working conditions, and a variety of purchase decisions, such as clothing and recreational and leisure materials. Faw et al. (1996) also suggested that the decision-making model designed to assist clients with mild mental retardation and a psychiatric diagnosis in evaluating residential preferences might be applied to other major life decisions, such as selecting a job. Their intervention, as well as some of the other interventions previously described, might be applicable to or adapted for other vulnerable populations, such as clients with severe mental illness or elderly clients with cognitive deficits. For example, Parsons, Harper, Jensen, and Reid (1997) developed a method for evaluating the leisure choice-making skills of older adults with severe disabilities. Their method might be used by practitioners and staff to assist elderly clients in choosing among leisure activities. Evaluating CB applications that teach choice making to vulnerable populations in other areas of their lives, to staff who provide services to these clients, and to family members who provide caregiving are areas of future research.

Freedom, Control, and Social Justice

Increasing choice (for those who desire to make choices) enhances freedom, increases individual control, and is consistent with a social justice perspective. The main objective of the interventions described in this chapter is to increase choice making in some aspect of the lives of vulnerable clients. Of course, the choices offered are constrained by a variety of factors. The availability of options, such as the number and type of residential group homes and the activities present and accessible in residential, community, and school settings, certainly are restricted. Organizational policies and other constraints, such as educational mandates, job tasks available and amenable to choice, safety of clients and others, and clients' abilities, also are constraining factors.

Whether the interventions, particularly those involving individuals with severe disabilities, are actually empowering is not always easily determined. Using verbal prompts to assist clients in making a choice among several items, or physical prompts to sustain a student's participation in a chosen activity, might enhance choice making among several items or sustain involvement in an enjoyable activity. However, if individuals would rather choose to decline engagement in any of the activities, those interventions might not increase their freedom and control. On the other hand, if participating in some leisure activity is required in a particular setting, such as in the school, identifying preferred choices, teaching choice-making skills, and sustaining a chosen activity without ongoing supervision can enhance freedom and control. Those issues challenge practitioners and researchers to develop and use methods that ensure clients' freedom and control actually are enhanced. An example of such a method is group home staff discussing with clients when a scheduled activity is not implemented, but showing no disapproval of the client's decision to decline participation in the activity.

Several of the CB strategies might be adopted by practitioners to enhance client control of or input into the intervention process. These include teaching a variety of self-management techniques, such as self-selection and self-scheduling of leisure activities and using paperclips to self-monitor asking relevant questions related to residential choice. Practitioners also can use graduated prompting strategies that recognize and build on clients' skills and various strategies to individualize the interventions. Examples of the latter are discussed in the following section on socially relevant intervention procedures.

Social Validity

Socially relevant goals and results. The goals of the CB interventions described in this chapter emphasize the importance that social workers, counselors, other helping professionals, educators, and other members of society place on the right of individuals to make their own choices. Being able to identify, communicate, and choose among options is necessary for self-determined behavior. Achieving those goals is particularly relevant for individuals with mental retardation and combinations of severe disabilities, who frequently have limited opportunities to learn, communicate, and exercise choice-making behaviors. Drawing from studies supporting the social significance of particular types of choices offered to clients, such as the choice of residence and food items at meals, is another method to establish the social validity of treatment goals.

The interventions also provide examples of setting goals consistent with the client's cognitive and physical abilities. Neglected, however, is developing methods to establish whether the choice-making goal is meaningful or desirable from the perspective of the client. For example, is choosing between two items of clothing meaningful to individuals with profound mental retardation? In Kennedy and Haring's (1993) evaluation, one student preferred allowing a peer to make a choice of a recreational activity for him and another was indifferent to making such a choice. Practitioners should not assume that choice-making goals are appropriate for all clients or in all situations.

The majority of the clients participating in the interventions indicated clear preferences for particular choice options and chose among available options when they were offered. These outcomes suggest that the intervention results were socially valid. The social relevance of treatment results also can be established by measuring other aspects of the clients' lives that are enhanced by increased choice making. Examples include increases in self-initiating, sustaining, and engaging in a diversity of leisure/recreational and other routine activity; decreases in inappropriate behavior; and increases in attention to job tasks and job independence. Another method that practitioners and researchers might use to assess whether treatment gains are meaningful to clients with severe mental retardation is suggested by observations of Al. Al appeared to be happier (judged by facial expressions and joking) when performing routines that involved some choice.

No other evaluations of participants or significant others were conducted to determine whether the increased choice making enhanced the quality of clients' lives in work, school, or community settings. Although the clients participating in the CB programs that teach skills to choose a community residence were able to obtain relevant information; report the information to their social workers; and, in one of the programs, evaluate the information, they did not actually choose a residence. Therefore, whether learning and using the skills resulted in socially valid results, such as increasing clients' satisfaction with their residence or sustaining community placement, is unknown.

The previous observations suggest the need for future research to determine the degree to which increasing particular kinds of choice making enhances the quality of life for vulnerable populations. In some cases, even negative consequences might result. For example, if a selected residential option was not available (e.g., the vacancy was filled by the time the decision was made), clients might experience negative emotional consequences, such as anger and disappointment. Those emotions might result in lower levels of adjustment and reduced satisfaction with residing in a less desirable residence, compared with placement in a residence when no choice was provided. Unfortunately, none of the evaluations of the interventions described in this chapter reported determining whether unsatisfactory results occurred as a result of the interventions. Researchers and practitioners should anticipate and plan for such consequences.

Socially relevant intervention procedures. Although the CB interventions reviewed in this chapter assessed clients' choice preferences, only one study (Bambara et al., 1995) conducted a functional assessment of the target behavior (refusal and disruptive behavior when asked to perform common routines) before intervention. No functional assessments were conducted to determine the maintaining conditions of choice behaviors before any of the interventions were implemented. Practitioners should determine whether other maintaining conditions besides a skills deficit, such as environmental opportunities and punishing consequences (e.g., aversive reactions to an appropriate request), may be maintaining low levels of choice behavior. As previously discussed, choices available to any individual, particularly vulnerable clients, are constrained for a variety of reasons. However, a thorough assessment of a client's capabilities, the available options, and other maintaining conditions might suggest additional client accommodations that must be made, indicate more options could be made available and offered, and identify significant others (e.g., parents, staff, teachers, and other professionals) who need to be involved in the intervention process.

After a treatment goal is established to increase the choice making of clients in a specific area, practitioners might use some of the methods described in this chapter to identify options and present meaningful choices to their clients. Methods include observing the client engaging in relevant activities, interviewing staff and clients, measuring the length of time clients engage in various activities, and asking clients to select among paired alternatives. Other examples of enhancing the social relevance of the interventions are reflected in the development of the intervention materials that assist clients in making a decision about their residence. Relevant choice options are identified from survey information and ratings from other clients, staff, and professionals. The residential options are depicted in pictures, and clients choose the options that are most important to them, which serves as the basis for asking questions regarding a potential residence.

The interventions also demonstrate a variety of accommodations and adaptations that practitioners might use to address the special needs of their clients, thereby enhancing the acceptability and feasibility of the interventions. Examples include the use of picture choice charts, specially designed activity books and cards, photographs depicting choice options, a microswitch communication system for requesting a change in leisure/recreational activity, and assistive work devices. Lifestyle preference photo albums provide multiple examples of special accommodations that can increase the social relevance of the intervention to assist clients with cognitive limitations in selecting a community residence. The accommodations include photos of residential options, specific questions to ask tour guides, boxes to record responses, paperclips to self-monitor asking all relevant questions, and a specially designed worksheet to assist in evaluating residential options.

Despite efforts to develop socially relevant interventions, none of the evaluations formally evaluated whether the interventions were acceptable to clients, agency administrators, or staff. In some cases, the acceptability and feasibility of the interventions might be assumed because they were successfully used in natural environments. For example, choice options were provided to clients in residential settings and while in fast-food restaurants. Reports of the institution or organization adopting the program is another indication of the acceptability, desirability, and feasability of the interventions. For example, the inpatient facility for dual diagnosed clients adopted the lifestyle preference photo album to assist patients in choosing their community residence.

Salmento and Bambara (2000), however, observed several staff problems when choice opportunities were implemented in the routines of residents with severe, multiple disabilities that are relevant to agency staff and supervisors. One of the staff members offered the clients few choice opportunities, and offering clients choices can increase staff time and effort. For example, some staff members experienced difficulty in waiting five seconds for the resident's choice response. The researchers suggested that to increase staff's acceptance and use of the procedures, supervisors might need to modify job descriptions, make choice offering a job responsibility that is reinforced, and provide booster sessions, when necessary.

Other researchers who evaluated the interventions discussed in this chapter acknowledge that the time involved and expertise required to assess choice preferences, develop intervention materials, and implement the interventions are likely to be barriers to large-scale adoption of the methods. Reid et al. (2001), for example, cautioned that developing assistive devices, assessing choices, and arranging work environments to present choices might not be possible or acceptable in all work settings. Faw and his colleagues (1996) also noted that implementing the decision-making model to assist clients in evaluating residential options is time consuming and requires expertise. They suggested that this complex procedure might be used only for decisions in which choices are expected to be relatively stable and have long-term consequences, such as choosing a residence and employment.

Maintenance and generalization. Evaluations of the previously described CB interventions vary in the degree to which they examined whether the choice and related behaviors were maintained after formal intervention (from no measure to approximately five months), and whether the acquired skills transferred to other choice situations and environments. Given the severe disabilities of many of the participants involved in the evaluations, and the specially designed materials and methods used for choice making, materials and methods likely would need to be adapted for choice situations significantly different from those described in the interventions. In addition, if choice behaviors are to be maintained even in the environment in which they were taught, some type of continued intervention and support would be necessary. For example, staff would need to be trained to offer and prompt pictorial, card, verbal, and recorded choices. Even among clients who learned to use their activity book and cards to schedule leisure/recreational activities, group home staff continued to meet with them weekly while they scheduled the activities. Staff also provided other forms of support.

When maintenance of clients' choice-making behaviors is dependent on staff involvement, ongoing evaluation and booster sessions are sure to be needed. In addition, client preferences are likely to change over time, as new interests develop and clients become bored with particular eating or leisure/recreational activities. If choice making is to be maintained, staff and significant others must be able to periodically assess relevant choice options. Finally, practitioners can learn from the evaluation by Jolly et al. (1993), which determined that even though the students with disabilities used their badges to increase choosing a play partner and activity, sustained interactions with peers did not result. The researchers suggested a variety of reasons for this disappointing finding. They include differences in skills, mobility, interests, and communication ability between the students with disabilities and their nondisabled peers. One or more additional interventions, such as positive reinforcement, might sustain such interactions. Some type of ongoing intervention also might be needed to maintain the choice-initiating behaviors. Otherwise, the nondisabled peers might begin to ignore even the initiations of the peers with disabilities, thus decreasing or eliminating these acquired behaviors.

Although a few of the evaluations determined that the enhanced choice-making skills transferred to similar environments (e.g., to other community fast-food restaurants), none of the interventions used strategies to transfer the skills from one type of setting to another (e.g., from school to home). If interventions are to be used with future clients, in different settings, and by staff, family members, or significant others, they must be easily adaptable to a variety of situations and acceptable to involved individuals, and those individuals must also be included in the intervention process.

Despite ongoing challenges of establishing the effectiveness of the interventions and the social validity of goals, treatment results, and interventions, and maintenance and generalization of treatment gains, this chapter suggests that CB strategies can increase the choice making of clients with disabilities. The next and final chapter of part IV describes CB interventions that empower vulnerable groups by assisting them in securing their legal and personal rights, such as disability accommodations and the right to refuse participation in unwanted or unsafe sexual behavior.

ADDITIONAL READINGS AND RESOURCES

Belfiore, P. J., Browder, D. M., & Mace, C. (1994). Assessing choice making and preference in adults with profound mental retardation across community and center-based settings. *Journal of Behavioral Education, 4,* 217–225.

Cannella, H. I., O'Reilly, M. F., & Lancioni, G. E. (2005). Choice and preference assessment research with people with severe to profound developmental disabilities: A review of the literature. *Research in Developmental Disabilities, 26,* 1–15.

Dyer, K., Dunlap, G., & Winterling, V. (1990). Effects of choice making on the serious problem behaviors of students with severe handicaps. *Journal of Applied Behavior Analysis, 23,* 515–524.

Kearney, C. A., & McKnight, T. J. (1997). Preference, choice, and persons with disabilities: A synopsis of assessments, interventions, and future directions. *Clinical Psychology Review, 17,* 217–238.

Lancioni, G. E., O'Reilly, M. F., & Emerson, E. (1996). A review of choice research with people with severe and profound developmental disabilities. *Research in Developmental Disabilities, 17,* 391–411.

Lohrmann-O'Rourke, S., & Browder, D. M. (1998). Empirically based methods to assess the preferences of individuals with severe disabilities. *American Journal on Mental Retardation, 103,* 146–161.

Moes, D. R. (1998). Integrating choice-making opportunities within teacher-assigned academic tasks to facilitate the performance of children with autism. *Journal of the Association for Persons with Severe Handicaps, 23,* 319–328.

Parsons, M. B., Harper, V. N., Jensen, J. M., & Reid, D. H. (1997). Assisting older adults with severe disabilities in expressing leisure preferences: A protocol for determining choice-making skills. *Research in Developmental Disabilities, 18,* 113–126.

Reid, D. H., & Parsons, M. B. (1991). Making choice a routine part of mealtimes for persons with profound mental retardation. *Behavioral Residential Treatment, 6,* 249–261.

Sigafoos, J., Couzens, D., Roberts, D., Phillips, C., & Goodison, K. (1996). Teaching requests for food and drink to children with multiple disabilities in a graphic communication mode. *Journal of Developmental and Physical Disabilities, 8,* 247–261.

Sigafoos, J., Roberts, D., Couzens, D., & Kerr, M. (1994). Providing opportunities for choice-making and turn-taking to adults with multiple disabilities. *Journal of Developmental and Physical Disabilities, 5,* 297–310.

12 Securing Legal and Personal Rights

Self-advocacy—the ability to assert one's rights—is essential to self-determination and empowerment. Self-advocacy is closely related to freedom, choice, and control, which are central to all definitions of self-determination (Field, 1996). Cunconan-Lahr and Brotherson (1996) define self-advocacy as individuals speaking or acting on their own behalf in order to make personal change, to improve their quality of life, or to address inequities. Disability rights activists encourage persons with disabilities to act on their own behalf instead of relying on others, such as professionals and family members. Self-advocacy also has played a fundamental role in social activist movements, from early labor and civil rights through the more recent disabilities and gay rights movements (Hayden & Nelis, 2002).

The self-determination or self-advocacy movement has been characterized as one of the most important influences in the fields of rehabilitation and special education (Algozzine et al., 2001). The importance of teaching clients with disabilities self-advocacy skills also is reflected in NASW's (2000) policy statement, "People with Disabilities." As the interventions in this chapter demonstrate, learning self-determined skills, such as asserting or advocating one's right to refuse engagement in sexual or unsafe sexual behavior, also can empower females and sexual minorities by promoting a sense of owning and making healthful choices about their own bodies (Levine et al., 1993).

Assertiveness training and related interventions (e.g., self-advocacy training) are commonly used to teach clients to secure and maintain their rights without infringing on the rights of others. Assertiveness training can assist clients in behaving more assertively when expressing their desires, opinions, and feelings, making requests, refusing unreasonable requests, asking for what they are entitled to, and standing up for specific rights (Alberti & Emmons, 2001). Situations in which persons can assert their rights might involve relatively minor issues, such as the right to receive the correct meal ordered at a restaurant, as well as more serious types of issues. This chapter discusses CB interventions that assist vulnerable populations in securing rights of a more serious nature.

The first section of this chapter describes CB interventions that empower vulnerable populations by assisting them in securing their legal rights, including civil rights and disability accommodation rights in work and educational settings. CB programs that assist vulnerable populations in refusing to engage in unwanted or unsafe sexual behavior are presented next. The chapter ends with an assessment of the interventions, including a brief summary and discussion of effectiveness, additional applications, and issues of social justice, freedom and control, and social validity.

SECURING LEGAL RIGHTS

Individuals with disabilities frequently lack knowledge of their legal rights. When their rights are violated, they commonly have few skills for advocating on their own behalf and for securing the assistance of others. If vulnerable clients lack relevant knowledge and skills, they may be at risk of losing their civil rights, of achieving few personal goals, and of experiencing less-than-desirable educational and vocational outcomes. For example, among employees with visual impairments, perceived barriers to work site accessibility and to performance of essential work activities can lower levels of job mastery and job satisfaction (Rumrill, 1999).

The CB interventions described in this section teach individuals with disabilities (i.e., physical, developmental, learning, and mental health disabilities, visual impairments, and chronic illness) about their disabilities, their legal rights, and skills for advocating on their own behalf. The interventions target three categories of legal rights—general rights, workplace accommodations, and educational accommodations. With one exception, all of the research evaluating the interventions determined only whether the interventions enhanced knowledge and skill development. Studies of interventions designed to assist vulnerable populations in securing their legal rights generally do not measure whether the increased knowledge and skills result in participants actually securing their rights. For this reason, only CB interventions that have research support for increasing participants' relevant knowledge and/or self-advocacy skills can be included here.

Three of the CB programs described in chapter 10 also teach self-advocacy skills to public school students with disabilities in the context of assisting them in enhancing self-determination. These skills include a competency-building program that increases self-determined behavior in a variety of settings (Abery et al., 1995) and the Self-Advocacy Strategy and the Self-Directed IEP Program, which teach students to become active participants in their educational conferences. Readers interested in CB interventions designed to enhance the self-advocacy skills of public school students with disabilities to achieve those goals are referred to chapter 10.

The CB interventions discussed in this section rely heavily on SST (instruction, modeling, role plays, feedback, and a variety of practice strategies). Other interventions include discrimination training, prompting, social reinforcement, problem solving, and homework assignments. The interventions were evaluated using a multiple-baseline design, random assignment, and informal feedback. One program was not evaluated.

General Legal Rights

This is a discrimination and SST program designed to teach self-advocacy skills to adults with disabilities to assist them in securing their legal rights (Sievert et al., 1988). Disabilities include cerebral palsy, speech impairments, mild mental retardation, LD, and mental health disorders. By reviewing the disability rights literature, the researchers identified thirty legal rights. In the intervention, the rights are further divided into four general categories, and the requirements that must be met for exercising each right are stipulated. The four rights categories and an example of each right follow (see table 1, Sievert et al., 1988, p. 301, for other examples).

1 Personal rights (e.g., the right to marry and to vote)
2 Community rights (e.g., the right to get a job and to housing)
3 Human services rights (e.g., the right to receive and to terminate services)
4 Consumer rights (e.g., the right to buy safe products and to have action taken on complaints)

During training, the practitioner uses a pair of scenarios for each right, one depicting a nonviolation and the other depicting a violation. Nonviolation scenarios describe requests that are justifiably denied. For example, a person fails to meet a requirement, such as getting a blood test when applying for a marriage license. The violation scenarios illustrate the denial of a person's request without justification. For example, the right had no condition or the person met all the necessary conditions for a conditional right, such as meeting all requirements for a marriage license.

Discrimination training teaches the clients to discriminate among the four different categories of legal rights to which they are entitled, as well as the conditions they must meet before obtaining the particular right. During the training, the practitioner defines the rights, then the clients practice naming the rights and identifying whether the developed scenarios depict rights violations. The practitioner provides praise for correct responses and a sequence of prompts for nonresponse and incorrect responses. The sequence of prompts proceeds with a nonspecific prompt (e.g., "Look closely at the scenario. Did you meet all the conditions?"), followed by a specific verbal instruction (e.g., "You did not meet all the conditions; therefore, it is not a violation of your rights"); if the client still does not respond appropriately, the practitioner verbally models the correct response.

To respond to rights violations, the practitioner teaches a three-step procedure, which is based on the consumer complaint process literature. The content of this training was validated by the director of an agency providing information and legal assistance to persons with disabilities and by experienced service providers. First, the clients assert their rights to the person who violated them (e.g., a case manager). Second, if the person does not resolve the problem, the clients complain to the person in the next higher level of authority (e.g., a supervisor). Third, if the problem is not resolved, the clients seek assistance from a community advocacy agency. To assist the clients in seeking assistance, the practitioner provides a directory of telephone numbers of relevant agencies frequently used by individuals with disabilities. SST is used to teach clients specific responses for the three-step procedure. Responses include the following.

1. Assert one's rights (e.g., "You have no right to_____")
2. Explain why one's rights were violated, including stating the conditions that were met (e.g., "I paid the fee, passed the tests, and filled out all the necessary forms")
3. Complain to the supervisor or advocacy agency personnel, including a description of what already was done to resolve the problem (e.g., "I talked to the sales clerk and his supervisor, and neither of them would help me")

SST involves the practitioner providing instruction on the relevant skills and giving clients a "redressing rights violations checklist" based on the identified responses. Clients also view a videotape demonstrating role plays of strategies to redress rights violations in situations involving the four types of rights. While the clients view the video, they use the checklist to check each response as it occurs on the video. Finally, the clients rehearse the skills.

The multiple-baseline design indicated that the eight participating clients, who were receiving services from a rehabilitation facility, substantially increased their ability to recognize and identify legal rights and appropriately respond to rights violations as a result of the intervention. The latter skills were evaluated in classroom and community role plays. Except for one client, the skills generalized to the community role plays. At the three-month follow-up, all three clients maintained their acquired skills.

Workplace Accommodations

Visual impairments. Rumrill (1999) developed a social competence/self-advocacy individual training program to assist clients with visual impairments in increasing their knowledge of the ADA Title 1, initiating requests for on-the-job accommodations, and enhancing their self-efficacy. The evaluation of this program was unique. It determined whether the clients enhanced their skills and knowledge, as well as whether they actually secured their workplace accommodation rights.

The practitioner begins by assisting the clients in identifying barriers in four work areas: work site accessibility, job accommodations and modifications, job mastery, and job satisfaction. Clients then rank their top three barriers in order of importance, suggest a reasonable accommodation for each, and identify resources to assist in implementing the accommodations. The practitioner also gives the clients a handout providing information on ADA's Title I provisions and presenting a collaborative win-win procedure for requesting, discussing, and implementing reasonable accommodations with employers (see Roessler, Rumrill, Battersby, & Garnette, 1996, in "Additional Readings and Resources" to obtain the publication). The publication is offered to clients in various formats, including large print, Braille, and audiotape.

The practitioner discusses the information in the brochure and models a request for a reasonable accommodation using the collaborative approach described in the brochure. Based on clients' individual situations, appropriate modifications to the presentation are made, and the clients practice making a request for an accommodation, with the practitioner assuming the role of employer. Behavioral rehearsal is followed by corrective feedback, then by further refinement and practice of appropriate verbal and nonverbal skills. The clients also practice engaging the employer (played by the practitioner) in a problem-solving process to determine the most cost-effective way to implement the accommodation. Finally, the practitioner assists the clients in developing a list that contains four items.

1 The identified accommodation needs
2 The manner (including verbal and nonverbal behaviors) the clients will use to approach the employer about their needs
3 Specific accommodations that would assist the clients in performing the job duties and a rationale for each
4 Resources that could assist in identifying and implementing cost-effective accommodations

At the end of the session, the practitioner prompts the clients to request an accommodation review from their employers and to apply the acquired skills. A follow-up session is held eight weeks later to monitor progress.

Forty-six volunteers (primarily whites, but including four African Americans and two Latinos) who were visually impaired and employed in a variety of occupations, ranging in nature from professional to manual, participated in the evaluation. The volunteers were matched on relevant characteristics (e.g., age, gender, and degree of visual impairment) then randomly assigned to a control or intervention group. Data gathered sixteen weeks after intervention determined that participants in the intervention group, compared with the control group, were more knowledgeable of ADA's Title I and demonstrated increased self-efficacy in performing the acquired skills. Even more important, participants in the intervention group were more likely to have requested an employer review of their accommodation needs, to have met with their employer to discuss the accommodations, and to have the accommodations implemented.

Chronic health conditions. Learning relevant skills for requesting workplace accommodations also is a topic of one of the four modules described by Petrides et al. (1995). The CB group intervention assists individuals in coping more effectively with type 1 diabetes and is described more fully in "Meeting Medical and Emergency Needs" in chapter 6. The "coping with special working situations" module uses instruction, discussion, modeling, and role plays to assist group members in learning to refuse unreasonable demands of co-workers or supervisors and to request appropriate accommodations. Accommodations include work schedule changes to accommodate doctors' visits and meal and diet requirements. Effectiveness of the group intervention was not evaluated.

Educational Accommodations

The next three CB programs were developed to assist students with learning, physical, and combinations of disabilities in understanding and securing their educational accommodation rights in postsecondary educational settings.

Durlak and his colleagues (1994) developed and evaluated a self-determination skills program for high school students with LD and a combination of LD and a behavioral/emotional disability. The purpose of the program is to assist the students in making a successful transition to postsecondary education. The program targets seven self-awareness and self-advocacy tasks, which were determined by a review of research identifying the characteristics of students with LD that predict a successful transition to educational settings after high school. The tasks were further validated with the assistance of an expert panel, including coordinators of special needs programs and LD specialists at colleges and universities. The tasks include the following.

1 Ask an instructor to clarify lecture material.
2 Disclose the LD to an instructor.

3. Schedule an appointment with an instructor to discuss needs and/or accommodations.
4. Ask an instructor if class lectures can be recorded with a tape recorder.
5. Obtain instructor approval for another student to take notes or to copy another classmate's notes.
6. Request assistance from a librarian.
7. Arrange an appointment with an outside resource person to request academic assistance.

Group facilitators then use SST to teach the relevant skills for each step of the identified tasks, which were previously identified by a task analysis. The steps for clarifying lecture material in class are presented in table 12.1.

Table 12.1. Steps for Clarifying Lecture Material

1. During class, raise your hand as soon as something is not clear, or shortly thereafter. Be specific: "I don't understand the statement you just made about _____" or "Could you please explain what that means?"
2. If you think you will need more time for the teacher's answer, *write down* the unclear material, or put a big red question mark by your notes, then approach the teacher after class.
3. Say, "Do you have a minute to explain _____?" or "I did not understand _____" or "What does _____ mean?"
4. Write down the teacher's response.
5. Thank the teacher for assistance.

Note. From "Preparing High School Students with Learning Disabilities for the Transition to Post-Secondary Education: Teaching the Skills of Self-Determination," by C. M. Durlak, E. Rose, & W. D. Bursuck, 1994, *Journal of Learning Disabilities, 27*, p. 55. Copyright 1994 by PRO-ED, Inc. Adapted with permission.

After the students master the tasks in session, they practice them in their high schools. Faculty and staff are asked to respond to the students' requests and interactions normally and to indicate on the students' small checklists that the tasks were performed. As indicated by a multiple-baseline design across tasks, the eight students involved in the program's evaluation (all were white, with the exception of one Latino student) learned the skills for the seven tasks. The skills were maintained one week later. Although the majority of the students carried out the assignments, none of the self-report and teacher rating scales assessing changes in self-awareness, self-advocacy, self-concept, and assertiveness were significantly different after intervention.

These final two CB programs designed to assist students in securing educational accommodations are conducted with university students. This first program is a seven-session summer transition program that teaches self-advocacy skills to students with LD (Brinckerhoff, 1994). During the first five sessions of the seminar, the students are given handouts, view videos, and receive instruction on and discuss the main topics of the seminar. The main topics include the following.

1. Understanding LD
2. Students' legal rights
3. Overview of self-advocacy and the roles of support staff
4. Determining which accommodations might be most helpful and strategies for discussing specific needs and accommodations with instructors
5. Dependence issues related to students' reliance on parents to resolve their problems, rather than advocating on their own behalf

In the fifth session, group facilitators use group problem solving to assist the students in identifying ways in which effective self-advocacy might have better handled past situations that became embarrassing as a result of parental involvement. In the final two sessions, students participate in role-play situations providing an opportunity to practice self-advocacy and negotiation skills. The negotiation skills include the following.

1. Facing the other person
2. Maintaining eye contact
3. Using appropriate nonverbal and listening behaviors
4. Requesting an accommodation
5. Stating the rationale for the request
6. Thanking the other person if an agreement is reached or proposing a compromise in the case of a disagreement

The group facilitators also provide examples of accommodations for resolving educational problems in four main areas.

1. Reading (e.g., ask to have textbooks taped; ask for extra time to complete reading assignments)
2. Math (e.g., work with a peer tutor; ask the instructor for concrete examples)
3. Organizational (e.g., ask for directions to be repeated when needed; schedule an appointment with the instructor to obtain clarification of the course material)
4. Writing (e.g., ask for proofreading assistance; ask to tape record lectures)

To assist in learning this process, students are taught the I-PLAN components during the sixth session (see chapter 10 for description of the components). Finally, the students apply their newly acquired self-advocacy and negotiation skills to real-life situations by arranging a meeting with the instructor of the course they are currently attending. During the meeting, students describe their LD and identify accommodations that might be required in the class. Although no formal evaluation of the seminar was conducted, faculty members' informal feedback indicated that the students appropriately asked for classroom and testing accommodations using a non-confrontational style. Students also reported that the seminar increased their independence and self-confidence.

Palmer and Roessler (2000) designed and evaluated an eight-hour Self-Advocacy and Conflict Resolution Training that teaches college students with disabilities self-advocacy and conflict resolution skills for implementing their educational accommodation rights. In the first of the two modules, instructors teach self-advocacy and communication skills. The training focuses on the following seventeen behaviors, which research has identified as predicting successful self-advocacy for classroom accommodations.

1. Greeting the instructor
2. Introducing oneself
3. Referring to a specific class
4. Identifying one's disability status
5. Explaining the way the disability can compromise academic achievement
6. Stating any previously secured accommodations
7. Explaining the benefits of those accommodations
8. Making a request for an accommodation
9. Identifying resources and ways they can help
10. Explaining what the student will do
11. Asking for an agreement
12. Affirming the agreement
13. Restating the agreed on accommodations
14. Clarifying the student's role
15. Clarifying the instructor's role
16. Closing the meeting with a positive statement
17. Expressing appreciation to the instructor

Following a brief introduction to academic barriers, accommodations, and the request process, the students observe as instructors model the seventeen skills involved in effective self-advocacy. The students then practice requesting accommodations with the instructors, one another, faculty members, and other staff.

In the second module, instructors teach the students negotiation skills for resolving conflicts in a variety of situations. Students observe as a live model uses the conflict resolution skills in seven different areas: specifying the conflict issues, reflecting, mutualizing, collaborating, inventing, selecting, and summarizing. The students then practice the skills in role plays. In addition to the general training, students are given a pamphlet providing additional information specific to their college. The pamphlet identifies their rights for academic accommodations, their responsibilities, strategies for requesting and implementing the accommodations, and policies and procedures for resolving any disagreements.

Fifty students (68% white; 16% Native Americans, the second largest ethnic group) from six- two- and four-year colleges participated in the evaluation. The students who had a variety of disabilities (primarily LD and physical disabilities) were randomly assigned to a treatment or control group within each college. The experimental groups exceeded the control groups on acquiring self-advocacy and conflict resolution skills, general knowledge of rights and responsibilities for academic accommodations, self-efficacy related to accommodation requests and conflict resolution, and social competence.

RIGHT TO REFUSE UNWANTED AND UNPROTECTED SEXUAL BEHAVIOR

The self-determined behavior of asserting one's right to refuse engagement in sexual or unprotected sexual behavior can be constrained among vulnerable populations for a variety reasons. Vulnerable persons might lack sexual knowledge, an understanding of safe sex practices and related high-risk behavior, and the skills necessary to assert their desires. Other factors, including cultural values and expectations, beliefs, fear of retaliation or other negative consequences, dependence on others for economic survival, social isolation, and societal attitudes and values, also can deter self-determined behavior related to sexual activity.

Cultural values of some women, particularly women of color, might prevent them from appearing knowledgeable about sex or asserting their right to refuse participation in sexual behavior or in unsafe sexual behavior (Hobfoll, Jackson, Lavin, Britton, & Shepherd, 1994). Female adolescents might engage in unwanted sex because they cannot assert their right to refuse, they desire to please or satisfy their boyfriends, or they believe that engaging in sex is expected (Schinke, 1982). Fear of retaliation or other negative consequences also can be a barrier to self-determined sexual behavior. Many females believe that refusing sex or unprotected sex will negatively affect their relationship with their partners, incur their partners' anger, or result in feelings of embarrassment or guilt (Barth, Middleton, & Wagman, 1989). Self-efficacy beliefs (e.g., that behavior can be changed and the outcome will be favorable) also are frequently low among vulnerable populations (Abery et al., 1995; Hunter & Schaecher, 1994).

Economic circumstances also can influence an individual's decision to engage in sex or unsafe sexual activity even when he or she desires to refrain from such behavior. For example, poverty might constrain one from purchasing contraception. Because some women with low income are dependent on men for money, housing, or emotional support, they might find asserting their right to refuse to engage in sex or high-risk sexual behavior to be very difficult (Nyamathi, Flaskerud, Keenan, & Leake, 1998; St. Lawrence, Wilson, Eldridge, Brasfield, & O'Bannon, 2001). Homeless individuals, including gay men or persons diagnosed with a severe mental illness, might feel compelled to exchange sex for money, food, and lodging (Hunter & Schaecher, 1994; Johnson-Masotti, Pinkerton, Kelly, & Stevenson, 2000). Engaging in high-risk or unwanted sexual behavior might not even be perceived by many vulnerable groups as a significant threat compared with the many social and physical risks, such as poverty and homelessness, that confront them daily (Harris, Bausell, Scott, Hetherington, & Kavanagh, 1998)

Stigmitization of sexual minority status also can result in social isolation. Social isolation, in turn, can lead to few sources of social support and an absence of role models for asserting and negotiating rights to refuse sexual activity or to have protected sex among gay, lesbian, and bisexual individuals. As a result of emotional and social isolation, gay males frequently seek other gay men in the streets and bars, settings that encourage sexual contact but make it difficult to negotiate safer sex. Gay and lesbian racial/ethnic minorities face even more difficulties in building social support because of homophobia in their ethnic communities, racism in the gay and lesbian community, and attitudes and discrimination in the broader society (Hunter & Schaecher, 1994). As is the case with heterosexual females, fear of rejection or other negative consequences might influence the decisions of sexual minorities to engage in unwanted sex or high-risk sexual activity.

Societal values and attitudes, such as the morality of abstaining from premarital sex and same-sex activity, also are reflected in sex education programs, which can only add to the previously discussed problems. For example, if sex education programs do not provide relevant education and skills-building activities, vulnerable youths, particularly sexual minorities, might have few other opportunities to gain knowledge of high-risk sexual behavior and the skills for exerting their right to decline engagement in such activity. In addition, sex education programs that do provide the necessary education and skills training are frequently based solely on a heterosexual model (Hunter & Schaecher, 1994).

Failing to assert one's right to refuse engagement in undesirable or high-risk sexual activity can result in serious consequences, such as unwanted pregnancies, abortions, and sexually transmitted diseases, including human immunodeficiency virus (HIV) infection. Adolescent pregnancy rates and incidents of STDs are particularly high among individuals with low income and African Americans. HIV infection also occurs disproportionately among gay/bisexual men (particularly young African Americans and Latinos), ethnic/racial minority adolescents and females, and individuals who are poor, use alcohol and drugs, and are diagnosed with a severe mental illness

(Coates, 1990; Hobfoll et al., 1994; Hovell et al., 1998; Johnson-Masotti et al., 2000).

This section describes CB interventions that empower vulnerable populations by teaching them relevant knowledge and skills to assert their right to refrain from unwanted or unsafe sexual activity. Vulnerable populations include females, racial/ethnic and sexual minorities, and individuals with low income, severe mental illness, and dual diagnoses. The first two programs are designed to prevent unwanted pregnancies and STDs; the remaining interventions are designed to prevent HIV infection. In pursuit of these goals, the interventions achieve other outcomes, including increasing sexual knowledge, enhancing skills for asserting one's right to refuse engagement in sex or high-risk sexual activity, reducing unprotected or other high-risk sexual behavior, and increasing protected sex.

All of the CB interventions discussed use SST techniques to teach a variety of social skills, such as assertiveness and negotiating sex or safer sexual behavior, and/or skills training to teach effective contraceptive use. Although all of the programs use SST, they combine other CB interventions in a variety of ways. The interventions include providing basic sexual and contraceptive knowledge, prompting and motivational strategies, identifying and coping with antecedent risk conditions, problem solving, cognitive rehearsal, cognitive restructuring, aversive conditioning, self-instructional training, social reinforcement, contractual agreements, and homework assignments. Various relapse prevention strategies also are incorporated into the programs. The interventions discussed here also are particularly sensitive to the needs and cultures of vulnerable populations, including women with low income and African Americans. With the exception of one CB program (Artz et al., 2005), all of the interventions were evaluated using traditional experimental methods in which participants were randomly assigned to a control or some type of comparison group.

Females

This section describes five CB programs for adolescent and adult females primarily from low socioeconomic backgrounds. This first intervention, a fourteen-group session knowledge and social skills building program, is designed to prevent teenage pregnancy and to be conducted within the public school system (Schinke, Blythe, & Gilchrist, 1981; Gilchrist & Schinke, 1983). The sessions begin with the group facilitators providing an overview of the program and basic instruction on reproduction and contraceptive methods. The basic steps of problem solving are then introduced, after which group members apply the process to their own life decisions in areas such as dating, sexual behavior, and birth control. SST is then used to teach group members verbal and nonverbal communication skills to assist them in discussing birth control, negotiating the purchase of contraception, requesting necessary information, and refusing unacceptable demands. As the students practice the skills, the group facilitators, as well as other group members, provide instruction, coaching, and feedback.

Cognitive rehearsal also is used in the program. After the group facilitators guide the youths through relaxation exercises, the students are asked to imagine a partner and a situation in which it is possible that they may engage in sex. The students are then instructed to imagine using their acquired social skills to discuss with their partners the possibility of having sex and their desire to use birth control. In a subsequent homework assignment, the students are asked to write out their imagined dialogue, which is later role played. The youths are given additional homework assignments, and they contract to use their acquired knowledge and skills outside of the sessions. Examples of homework assignments include obtaining information on birth control from community sources, pricing contraceptives at local drug stores, discussing birth control with current dating partners, and requesting opinions about sex from parents and other persons involved in the youths' lives (e.g., clergy and counselors). The students' experiences carrying out the assignments are discussed in subsequent group meetings.

The students (N = 36) involved in the evaluation (both males and females) were randomly assigned to an intervention or control group. Students participating in the intervention had better postintervention test scores on sexual knowledge, interpersonal problem solving, and ratings of videotaped role-play interactions, compared with the control group. The role plays involved responding to social pressure and requesting that partners share responsibility for birth control and sexual decisions. At a six-month follow-up, the students in the intervention group also reported using birth control more frequently and having fewer instances of intercourse without contraception. Feedback on the usefulness of the program from the adolescents, as well as from their teachers and parents, was very favorable (Schinke et al., 1981). Gilchrist and Schinke (1983) also evaluated a similar CB program for adolescent students that can be implemented with large groups (more than twenty members).

This second CB intervention is a one-hour program designed to promote the use of the female condom (a prophylactic that is inserted like a diaphragm) for adult women attending a STD clinic (Artz et al., 2005). In addition to preventing STDs, a major rationale for teaching the women to use the female condom is to give them, instead of their male partners, more control over the decision to use protection during sexual intercourse. The program was developed and modified using information from the literature on the female condom and from interviews with experts (e.g., health professionals), focus groups with women, and qualitative interviews with women and their male partners.

The CB program, which is administered to clients individually, begins with the client viewing a testimonial-style video. In the video, women discuss their perceptions of using the female condom, and they provide information that enhances awareness of STD risk and the need for protection. An instructor then discusses the advantages and demonstrates the use of the female condom, and the woman practices using it with an anatomic model. Using SST, the instructor also teaches the woman methods to cope with common problems, skills to promote use of the female condom to the woman's sex partner, and problem-solving skills to cope with potential problems. The woman signs an agreement to use the female (or a male) condom every time she has sex until the next visit. The woman also is given an opportunity to practice inserting the female condom, after which she receives feedback on correct placement (the article provides detailed scripts to teach the various skill components). At the end of the session, the woman is given a free supply of her chosen method of contraception and informational brochures for herself. The woman also is provided with methods to introduce the female condom to her male partner, including humorous condom cards and a video to show to her partner before trying the contraceptive device. As determined by a pretest-posttest design, the use of condoms (both male and female) increased significantly among the participants (N = 1,159 predominately African American women) after intervention. The women also continued to use some type of protection at a high rate during the six-month follow-up. The female condom was used at least once by 79% of the women, and the majority of those women used the contraceptive device multiple times.

The three CB group interventions discussed next are HIV and AIDS prevention programs designed for socioeconomically disadvantaged female adolescents and adults. Kelly and his colleagues (1994) developed such a program to assist women with low income in asserting their right to refuse unwanted or unprotected sexual activity. The group sessions provide information on HIV risk and behaviors that increase and decrease risk of infection. Skills are taught using SST, which involves role plays of initiating a discussion of AIDS concerns and condom use with a potential partner and resisting pressure to engage in unwanted or unprotected sex. The group facilitators demonstrate correct condom use, after which the women practice the behaviors with phallic models. The group facilitators also assist the women in identifying circumstances that triggered past high-risk sexual behavior, such as drinking, drug use, loneliness, and involvement in coercive or unequal sexual relationships. After this activity, the group is then taught a problem-solving process that assists the women in developing alternative strategies to cope with the identified antecedent conditions.

Because research supports the benefits of social support for promoting behavioral change (e.g., it can assist women in coping with their male partners' resistance and in buffering the stress from the multiple other life stressors they frequently face), group social support also is enhanced. For example, the facilitators encourage the women to share strategies that they have used to handle past high-risk sexual situations. The women also are assisted in building a consensus that denying men sex unless they use condoms is legitimate. Finally, the women are encouraged to identify the benefits of engaging low-risk behavior, such as protecting their children from AIDS and personally controlling their own sexual decisions.

The women participating in the program evaluation were attending urban health clinics (N = 197; 87% were African American) and were randomly assigned to the CB intervention or to a comparison group. At the three-month follow-up, as judged by AIDS educators' ratings of taped role plays, the intervention group exhibited enhanced communication and negotiation skills in postponing sex until a condom was obtained and in refusing sex without a condom. Women in the intervention group also reported a decline in unprotected sexual intercourse and an increase in condom use. No changes were made in the comparison group.

This second AIDS prevention program was designed for low-income ethnic/racial minority pregnant women (Hobfoll et al., 1994; a comprehensive description of the program is provided in Levine et al., 1993). The sessions are conducted interactively using four videotapes featuring actors from similar backgrounds as the women. The taped segments illustrate assertiveness (e.g., refusing sex without a condom) and negotiation, planning, and other relevant skills that reduce risk of infection (e.g., cleaning drug paraphernalia). After viewing the tapes, the women discuss and role-play the situations. Group facilitators encourage the women to apply the skills to their own lives, share their personal experiences, and work together on finding realistic and useful solutions to the identified problems related to AIDS prevention. Culturally diverse staff provide role models with whom the women can identify and enhance mastery of the curriculum by reinforcing the women's use of the skills and their successes. Group facilitators also communicate the expectation that the women will be successful.

For more private behavior, such as using a condom during intercourse, women are taught cognitive rehearsal. During the procedure, the women imagine themselves problem solving a situation that they choose or one that is described to them (e.g., the woman is ready to have sex without a condom). Afterward, group members discuss the situations, make suggestions on methods to better handle the situations, and provide support to one another. Group facilitators also use aversive conditioning to increase the women's sense of vulnerability. In this procedure, women imagine a scene in which they engage in a high-risk behavior resulting in an aversive outcome (e.g., having sex without a condom and becoming HIV infected). To enhance a sense of mastery, women also imagine a situation in which a low-risk or healthy behavior results in a positive outcome (e.g., refraining from illicit drug use and giving birth to a healthy baby). Relapse prevention is the topic of the final session. Group facilitators engage the women in discussion, role play, and cognitive rehearsal to assist them in identifying and planning for possible obstacles to their continued and increased use of healthy behaviors.

While conducting the interventions, group facilitators pay special attention to enhancing the women's social support, building on their sense of community, and responding to the economic, gender, and cultural contexts of the women's lives. The importance of behavioral change for the women individually and their unborn children, family, and ethnic group are emphasized. The program pays for babysitting and transportation costs. When mothers cannot find appropriate child care, the children are cared for at the program site. Because economic circumstances can influence women's daily decision making, the program recognizes and supports educational and career aspirations that might improve their economic well-being. For example, group facilitators attempt to schedule group meetings during times that do not interfere with school or work obligations, and they include strategies for achieving education and employment goals in discussions and role plays. Topics of discussion also include power relationships between men and women, particularly as they relate to economic hardship, the disproportionate number of African American females to African American males, and the meaning of sex as experienced by different racial/ethnic groups.

This AIDS prevention intervention was evaluated through the random assignment of 206 single, pregnant low-income young women (57% African American, 40% white, and 3% other ethnic origin) seeking obstetrical care at inner-city clinics to an intervention group or two control groups (a health information and no-treatment group). The AIDS prevention group performed better than the two control groups in increasing frequency of safer sex behavior, purchases of condoms and spermicide, and discussions of AIDS-related behavior with their partners. Pharmacy reports of the women obtaining condoms also were higher for the AIDS prevention and health group, compared to the nonintervention group. Most of the improvements were maintained six months later.

Carey et al. (2000) evaluated this final HIV-risk reduction (HIV-RR) intervention for women with low income, which was based on an information-motivation-behavioral skills model for socioeconomically disadvantaged urban adolescent and adult females. The HIV-RR program is conducted in small groups using a prepared manual developed from information obtained from a variety of sources, including survey data and focus groups (intervention procedures are provided in Carey et al., 1997). Group facilitators use motivational interviewing strategies to enhance motivation for change. The strategies include directly communicating the goal of reducing HIV infection risk while using a nonjudgmental and empathic style. This style encourages the women to choose risk-reduction behaviors consistent with their own values and relationships and in the context of their own lives. The facilitators provide HIV transmission and prevention education and assist the women in identifying self-motivational statements.

Presenting and discussing a videotaped interview of a local woman infected with HIV and providing group members with personalized feedback on their HIV risk based on a preintervention survey also increase risk sensitization. SST is used to teach self-management and sexual assertiveness skills. Specific skills include purchasing and using condoms, identifying high-risk situations (e.g., substance use), altering cognitions related to behavior change (e.g., countering negative attitudes toward condom use), and negotiating condom use with partners. Group facilitators also assist the women in developing action plans. That is, the facilitators elicit risk-reduction strategies from the women and present the demonstrated skills as options the women might find useful.

The adolescents and women (predominately African American) participating in the evaluation of the HIV-RR program (N = 102) were randomly assigned to an intervention or a health-promotion control group. Postintervention and follow-up data (twelve weeks after intervention) determined that women in the HIV-RR program strengthened their intentions to engage in risk-reduction behaviors to a greater degree, compared with the control group. After receiving the HIV-RR intervention, women who expressed weaker intentions to carry out the risk-prevention behaviors increased their use of condoms, talked more with their partners about condom use and HIV testing, and were more likely to refuse unprotected sex.

African American Youths

This is a comprehensive eight-week CB program designed to reduce the risk of HIV infection specifically among low-income African American adolescents (St. Lawrence et al., 1995). The CB program begins with AIDS education, followed by a second session discussing sexual decisions and values. To clarify values and generate discussion on related sexual topics, group facilitators show a specially prepared videotape for African American youths. Related topics for discussion include adolescents' vulnerability to AIDS; attitudes toward safer sex, condoms, and abstinence; and obtaining social support for their personal values from friends and family. During the third session, group facilitators use a penile model to teach the adolescents the correct use of condoms. The facilitators also teach the youths cognitive restructuring to recognize and dispute beliefs leading to high-risk sexual behaviors and to replace the beliefs with statements leading to safer behaviors, for example, "If he won't use a condom, then he doesn't really care about me." In the fourth session, group facilitators teach communication and assertiveness skills in three different contexts: (1) having an advanced discussion about condoms with a sexual partner, (2) standing up to pressure to engage in unprotected sexual activity, and (3) sharing information with peers on reducing HIV risk. Using assertion training techniques, group facilitators teach the youths to refuse or to acknowledge their partner's desire to have unprotected sex while firmly stating and providing a rationale for their position and suggesting a safer alternative. After role-playing similar situations (based on information obtained from focus groups of high school students) and receiving feedback, the youths discuss their comfort using the skills when encountering similar situations. Group facilitators encourage the adolescents to practice the skills in relevant situations they encounter in their actual lives.

During the fifth session, a "Rap Team" discusses their own HIV infection with the adolescents. The purpose of the discussion is to raise awareness of the adolescents' own risk and perceptions of vulnerability. In subsequent sessions, the youths identify past situations in which they yielded to peer pressure and then anticipate future difficult situations. For the identified situations, the adolescents engage in problem solving to clarify the problem and develop specific strategies to reduce their risk. Adolescents also share their successful strategies with group members, which are then discussed and practiced. An example is a "condom and a quarter" card, which contains a condom in case youths decide to engage in sexual intercourse, and a quarter to call someone to pick them up if they decide to leave a risky situation. Providing the youths with peer coping models and strengthening their beliefs that they can successfully implement risk-reduction strategies are the main objectives of the final session. In order to achieve these objectives, group facilitators ask the adolescents to identify the most helpful aspects of the program and the personal changes they have made as a result of participating.

This program was evaluated through the random assignment of low-income African American adolescents ($N = 246$) to the CB group intervention or an educational program. The skills-building group increased self-efficacy ratings, rates of condom-protected intercourse, and behavioral skills related to handling coercive and high-risk situations and reduced rates of unprotected sex to a greater extent than the comparison group. The enhanced risk-reduction behaviors also were maintained at a higher rate one year later for the CB group. The participants rated their satisfaction with the CB program a mean of 6.8 on a seven-point scale (7 = very high).

Sexual Minorities

This is a twelve-week CB program designed to assist gay men with a history of frequent AIDS high-risk behavior, which is defined as unprotected anal or oral intercourse and oral/anal contact (Kelly, St. Lawrence, Hood, & Brasfield, 1989). The program contains the same basic components as the CB programs previously described for females and racial/ethnic minorities (see Kelly et al., 1994; St. Lawrence et al., 1995). That is, the program provides education, communication and assertiveness skills training and assists group members in developing strategies to cope with situations that trigger high-risk sexual behavior. Only the interventions unique to this CB program are described in the next two paragraphs.

After group members identify past and potential situations in which they have engaged or could engage in high-risk sexual behavior and the antecedent conditions of the risky behavior (e.g., mood, substance use, and setting), group facilitators teach a self-management strategy that involves identifying and practicing three main types of self-statements.

1 I can develop safer practices (e.g., "I can change risky sex practices").
2 I can reduce anxiety by engaging in safer behaviors (e.g., "I will feel much better tomorrow if I don't do anything risky tonight").
3 Reducing risk-taking behavior is worthy of praise (e.g., "I am proud that I didn't do anything high in risk this week").

Sexual assertion training also is taught in three types of situations. The situations are related to (1) initiating a discussion of the men's commitment to low-risk behavior with potential sexual partners, (2) resisting pressure to engage in high-risk behavior, and (3) declining immediate sexual propositions from individuals with whom the men would prefer to only have a social relationship. Group facilitators also teach the men problem-solving strategies to identify options that can enhance social support. Options include engaging in social dating prior to initiating sexual activity, expressing affection initially in nonsexual ways, and participating in gay community activities that reinforce self-respect and healthy behavior.

The program was evaluated through the random assignment of 104 white, Latino, and African American gay men to the CB intervention or a wait-list control group. At the four- and eight-month follow-ups, the men in the experimental group had reduced their frequency of unprotected anal intercourse and increased condom use during intercourse, relative to the control group. Ratings of videotaped role plays also demonstrated that only men in the intervention group increased their skills for handling casual propositions, refusing pressure to engage in unwanted sexual activity, and using safer sex practices. The CB program participants rated the value of the program a mean of 9.8 on a ten-point scale (10 = very valuable) and 8.9 for the degree to which the program assisted them personally in reducing AIDS risk.

A group CB program also was developed for bisexual and gay men who are at high risk for HIV infection (Roffman et al., 1997). Similar to other CB programs discussed in this section, this seventeen-session intervention incorporates multiple CB interventions. Early sessions focus on establishing group cohesion, HIV education, enhancing motivation, and setting goals. During the middle phase of the intervention, group facilitators assist group members in identifying antecedents to their risky behavior and in developing coping strategies to reduce risk. Coping skills training teaches group members to reduce high-risk behavior by enhancing their assertiveness and listening skills and by using self-talk, positive and negative imagery, and a variety of behavioral strategies, including avoiding risky situations, substituting positive behaviors for high-risk behaviors, and terminating sexual activity when it is no longer safe. The group members discuss both successes and problems they experience. During the final stages of the program, strategies are identified to maintain the safer behaviors, such as using social support, maintaining a healthy lifestyle, enhancing self-esteem, and encouraging norms for safer sexual behavior. The participants (N = 159) were matched and assigned to the intervention or a wait-list control group. Three months after intervention, the men participating in the group intervention were less likely to engage in unprotected sexual behavior compared with men in the control group. The intervention group also scored higher on several other outcome measures (e.g., satisfaction with social supports, sexual self-efficacy). However, the intervention appeared to be more effective for homosexual versus bisexual men.

The final CB program described here also was developed to reduce the HIV risk of homosexual and bisexual men but focuses on African Americans (Peterson et al., 1996). The training materials, including videotapes, games, and role plays, were pretested for accuracy and cultural relevance for African American homosexual and bisexual men. The intervention begins with the group facilitators, who are African American homosexual males, reinforcing the men's self-identity as members of both a minority sexual and racial group. Showing and discussing segments of the video *Tongues United* featuring African American homosexual men, reinforces this dual identity. Group members then discuss their feelings and experiences related to being members of both minority groups and the ways in which their minority status affects HIV risk. Group facilitators educate group members on AIDS risk by using activities (AIDS Jeopardy Game and Condom Games) that increase knowledge of risk-reduction behavior and effective use of condoms. Assertiveness training is then used to enhance the men's skills for negotiating low-risk sexual activities and refusing high-risk behaviors with current and future sexual partners. Finally, the men share strategies they have used for reducing risk and make a group commitment to change their risk behaviors.

African American homosexual and bisexual men (N = 318) were randomly assigned to one of three groups—a single-session experimental group, a three-session experimental group, or a control group. Both experimental interventions included strategies to develop self-identity and social support, AIDS-risk education, and self-management and assertion training. The men attending the three sessions had greatly reduced their frequency of unprotected anal intercourse at the twelve-month (from 46% to 20%) and eighteen-month (from 45% to 20%) follow-up periods, while the single-session group reduced unprotected intercourse only slightly. The control group made no changes in risk behavior.

Individuals with Severe Mental Illness

Kelly and his colleagues (Kalichman, Sikkema, Kelly, & Bulto, 1995) developed a four-session CB program to prevent HIV infection for low-income multiracial/ethnic clients receiving services from public mental health clinics in an inner-city area. Because the interventions are very similar to the previously discussed program developed for socioeconomically disadvantaged female adolescents and adults (see Kelly et al., 1994), the interventions are not described again. To evaluate the program, clients (N = 53) were randomly assigned to the AIDS prevention program or a wait-list control group. Compared with the comparison group, clients participating in the intervention were more likely to have decreased incidents of unprotected sexual intercourse and an increased percentage of condom use during sexual intercourse. The behavioral changes were maintained at a two-month follow-up.

Kelly et al. (1997) also compared three CB programs to prevent HIV infection for clients with severe mental illness. The programs included a single AIDS education session, a seven-session CB HIV risk-reduction group intervention, and a similar CB intervention that teaches clients to act as risk-reduction advocates with their friends. The single session provides education about AIDS and risk, describes high-risk practices, and provides information on risk-reduction strategies. The content of the CB group intervention is similar to the intervention previously discussed for socioeconomically disadvantaged female adolescents and adults (see Kelly et al., 1994). The advocacy training uses SST techniques to teach clients to effectively communicate AIDS and health information to others. Health information includes the importance of identifying the threat of AIDS, correcting misconceptions about AIDS, recommending strategies to reduce risk of infection, and emphasizing the importance and practicality of making behavioral change. Finally, clients agree to initiate conversations with their friends and to share their recently gained knowledge on avoiding HIV/AIDS risk. Clients (N = 104) were randomly assigned to one of the programs. Three months after intervention, all clients exhibited change in some risk-related characteristics, such as social norms for and perceived barriers to condom use and sexual risk behaviors. However, only clients receiving the CB intervention with advocacy training reduced their frequency of engaging in unprotected sexual activity.

This ten-session group assertiveness training program designed to reduce HIV risk for women with severe mental illness (Weinhardt, Carey, Carey, & Verdecias, 1998) also has components similar to the CB programs previously described. The components include education on HIV-related issues, raising awareness of risk to enhance the women's motivation for reducing risk behaviors, and assertiveness training to teach the women to discuss and negotiate condom use and other HIV-preventive behaviors with resistant partners and to refuse to engage in unsafe sexual behavior. During the final sessions, group facilitators encourage the women to apply the skills to their own lives, and the facilitators review and reinforce the acquired skills. Female outpatient mental health clients (N = 20) were randomly assigned to the intervention or a wait-list control group. Compared with the control group, the women in the intervention group increased their assertiveness skills, which were maintained at the two- and four-month follow-ups. At the two-month follow-up, frequency of condom-protected intercourse increased, but there was no statistically significant difference between the intervention and control groups at the four-month follow-up. The women rated the intervention as very interesting (mean = 3.9 on a four-point scale), but somewhat embarrassing (mean = 2.1).

This final CB group intervention is designed to reduce HIV infection among low-income adults with dual diagnoses of substance abuse and severe mental illness (Hanson, Cancel, & Rolon, 1994). The content of the nine-session education, self-management, and sexual-assertion training is similar to previously discussed programs, such as those evaluated by Kelly and his colleagues. The influence of substance abuse on high-risk sexual behavior, however, is specifically addressed during several of the sessions. For example, group facilitators link risky sexual practices to substance use by asking members to share ways in which substance abuse can increase the likelihood of their initiating sex with a stranger and giving in to a partner's pressure to engage in unprotected sex. Group members also discuss and practice strategies to refuse drugs and to avoid situations in which they have engaged in unsafe sexual practices in the past. The program was evaluated with a sample of thirty clients with low income (all but eight were African American) attending an inner-city day treatment program. Compared with a wait-list control group, clients in the intervention group were more likely to use condoms and to be more assertive during sexual encounters and less likely to engage in high-risk sexual behaviors. The behaviors were maintained at the two-week follow-up.

ANALYSIS AND CRITIQUE FOR PRACTICE AND RESEARCH

The first group of interventions described in this chapter use a variety of CB strategies that can empower persons with physical, learning, and mental health disabilities and visual impairments by increasing their ability to secure their legal rights. Legal rights include civil and general rights, such as the right to marry, to housing, to services, and to purchase safe products, as well as the right to educational and work accommodations for individuals with disabilities. All of the programs use SST (including assertiveness training), which is frequently combined with other interventions, such as PST, discrimination training, prompting strategies, and homework assignments. The interventions are applicable to social workers and other helping professionals providing services to clients in rehabilitation, health, mental health, and educational settings, and other community settings, such as social action agencies.

The main goals of the second group of interventions are to prevent unwanted pregnancies, HIV infection, and other STDs. In order to achieve these goals, the interventions assist vulnerable populations in asserting their right to refuse to engage in unwanted, unprotected, and other high-risk sexual behavior. The programs involve multiple types of CB interventions that can be used to assist vulnerable clients in asserting their sexual rights. The programs provide instruction on topics such as sexuality, contraception, and risk, safer, and assertive behaviors and use SST, including assertion training. Other interventions include PST, cognitive rehearsal, aversive conditioning, cognitive restructuring, recognizing and changing antecedent conditions, homework assignments, and relapse prevention. The interventions are designed for adolescent females, women with low income, racial/ethnic minorities, gay/bisexual men, and clients with severe mental illness and dual diagnoses. Practitioners might find these interventions applicable in a variety of mental health, health-care, school, group home, and social action agency settings.

Effectiveness and Additional Applications

The CB programs described in the first intervention section of this chapter, which assist vulnerable clients and students in learning and obtaining their legal rights, were evaluated with multiple-baseline designs, random assignment, and summaries of informal participant feedback. The intervention designed to assist patients with diabetes to request workplace accommodations was not evaluated. Although the programs were designed for individuals with a variety of physical, learning, and mental health disabilities, given the nature of the instructional materials and skills needed to self-advocate, the interventions would not be suitable for clients with severe cognitive deficits or exhibiting severe psychiatric symptoms. The evaluations that were conducted on this group of CB interventions suggest that many vulnerable clients can learn their legal rights and can advocate on their own behalf. However, the majority of the research designs were nonexperimental, and the programs used different combinations of interventions. Thus, drawing firm conclusions about the efficacy of the programs or determining which combinations of interventions is effective for particular clients cannot be done.

Despite the shortcomings in the evaluations, practitioners might find the interventions effective for assisting clients with disabilities in securing their legal rights. The interventions also might be applicable to other vulnerable clients and for assisting clients with disabilities and other vulnerabilities in securing other legal rights. The programs also suggest opportunities for researchers to develop and evaluate similar applications. For example, legal rights can be related to employment, housing, and other types of discrimination or workplace harassment based on race/ethnicity, age, gender, or sexual orientation. CB interventions might assist immigrants in understanding and advocating for their immigration rights and assist immigrants and other clients with low income or disabilities in understanding and advocating for their rights when applying for government benefits (e.g., TANF, food stamps, SSI, and Social Security Disability). CB programs also might be designed to teach vulnerable clients involved with the child welfare system; residing in nursing homes or in health care, mental health, or rehabilitation facilities; or receiving services in these areas the relevant knowledge and skills to advocate for their rights (e.g., to certain types of treatment or to refuse treatment).

In contrast to the research that evaluated the CB interventions designed to assist clients in securing their legal rights, all but one of the evaluations of the second group of programs randomly assigned participants to a CB intervention group or to some type of comparison or control group. With few exceptions, the CB program, compared with other interventions or a nonintervention group, was more effective in increasing participants' relevant knowledge, enhancing skills for refusing unwanted sexual activity, increasing protected sex, and decreasing related high-risk behavior. In contrast to other evaluations of the interventions described in part IV, sample sizes of the evaluations discussed in this section were relatively large. In many of the evaluations, samples also were heterogeneous with respect to race/ethnicity. However, the researchers did not determine whether the effectiveness of the interventions varied by the racial/ethnic identity of the participants. As was the case for other CB interventions presented in this book, the interventions were not equally effective for all outcome measures or for all participants or groups of participants (e.g., bisexual vs. gay men).

All but one of the CB programs that assist vulnerable clients in asserting their right to refuse to engage in unwanted or unprotected sexual behavior are conducted in groups, which can provide a number of advantages. Among these are having available peers to provide social support, coping models, and role-play partners; to share strategies; and to develop a shared sense of community, culture, and norms for sexual behavior. Group work also is cost effective, as multiple clients can simultaneously participate. Despite these advantages, many clients might feel uncomfortable engaging in some of the group activities, such as role-playing sexually assertive behaviors and practicing using condoms with phallic models.

The second group of interventions did not include vulnerable populations such as lesbians and bisexual females or individuals with mental retardation and other types of disabilities. Many lesbian adolescents use alcohol and drugs and have sex with older women and with young gay and heterosexual men, experiences that likely increase the chance that lesbian youths will engage in unwanted or high-risk sexual behavior (Hunter & Schaecher, 1994). Hunter and Schaecher describe a variety of programs that have incorporated CB strategies to assist vulnerable adolescents, including lesbian and homosexual youths, in refusing to engage in unwanted or high-risk sexual behavior. The programs are offered in schools (including an after-school program), street outreach, and various community agencies. However, no evaluations of the programs were provided.

Foxx, McMorrow, Storey, and Rogers (1984) developed a SST program to teach social/sexual skills to adults with mild to moderate mental retardation. Social confrontation is one of the six skills group facilitators teach the clients by using a board game and specially designed cards. One of the situations depicted on a card is a woman being touched by a stranger at a party. Although the evaluation determined that the intervention enhanced social/sexual skills, whether the clients specifically enhanced their ability to assert their right to decline unwanted sexual advances is unclear. This program, as well as other previously described interventions, might be applicable or modified to assist individuals with mental retardation in asserting their right to refuse unwanted or unsafe sexual activity. Researchers also might develop and evaluate CB programs accommodating the special needs of other vulnerable groups, such as those with physical disabilities and communicative difficulties.

The Freedom Self-Advocacy Curriculum is an example of a program that incorporates CB methods into three workshops designed to teach attitudes, knowledge, and skills to assist mental health consumers in advocating their rights. This program is notable because, compared with the programs discussed in this chapter, it involves a broader set of both personal and legal rights. Examples of legal rights include the right to social program benefits, to nondiscriminatory housing, to provide advance directives for treatment, to view one's records, and to refuse treatment in absence of a court order. The right to be in a nonabusive environment (e.g., not being the recipient of derogatory comments or teasing based on characteristics such as being poor, having a disability, minority sexual orientation, race/ethnicity, or culture), to set one's own priorities and goals, and to be treated with dignity and respect are examples of personal rights. Workshop facilitators use a variety of techniques, such as providing instruction, information, and legal and government resources, and teaching assertion and problem-solving skills. Unfortunately, no evaluation of the program could be located (see the National Mental Health Consumers' Self-Help Clearinghouse in "Additional Readings and Resources" at the end of this chapter to obtain the training manuals). Designing and evaluating effective CB interventions that assist vulnerable populations in advocating a broader range of legal and personal rights in educational, rehabilitation, mental health, health, and work settings provides many opportunities for future research.

Other researchers (Hovell et al., 1994) argue that if individual-level CB interventions are to be effective in reducing engagement in high-risk and unwanted sexual behavior, they must be accompanied by broader social environmental assessment and intervention. Environmental influences include the family (e.g., presence of appropriate models of sexual behavior and parent-youth discussion of sexual issues); public schools (e.g., access to condoms, sex education content, and communication between the school and family); peers (e.g., support for safer sexual practices); media (e.g., depiction of models practicing safer sexual behaviors); and government policy and community (e.g., establishing ordinances for public restrooms to have condom machines and tax breaks for media producers for depicting models practicing safer sexual behavior). Broader social environmental assessment and intervention also are likely necessary to enhance the effectiveness of CB interventions designed to assist vulnerable clients in securing their legal rights. These observations suggest the need for practitioners assisting clients in securing their personal and legal rights to assess and change, when possible, a broader set of maintaining conditions. The observations also suggest areas of future social work research.

Freedom, Control, and Social Justice

The CB interventions described in this chapter promote social justice and enhance the freedom and control of vulnerable groups. Assisting vulnerable clients in acquiring knowledge and skills to secure their legal and personal rights, including civil and disability accommodation rights and the right to refuse unwanted and unprotected sexual activity, certainly is consistent with social justice. Although all of the CB programs involve standardized procedures, the goal of assisting vulnerable populations in securing their personal and legal rights is consistent with enhancing personal freedom and control. In addition, many of the evaluations of the interventions provide evidence that after intervention vulnerable individuals can assert more control over important aspects of their lives. Even when researchers failed to evaluate whether acquiring the relevant knowledge and skills actually resulted in participants securing their rights, the intervention gains can provide vulnerable clients with increased freedom to choose to self-advocate in the future.

The flexibility of the CB interventions varies, but practitioners might adopt the methods that accommodate client input and control over the intervention process. An example is assisting clients in choosing their own work barriers and reasonable accommodations. Additional methods that increase client input into the standardized procedures are discussed in the section on socially relevant intervention procedures. Mastering CB techniques such as problem solving, cognitive rehearsal, self-statements, and cognitive restructuring also provides opportunities for individualizing standardized procedures and for client control. The sequence of prompts that assists participants in determining when rights violations occur allows clients to exhibit their knowledge before instruction. Group facilitators also can facilitate group members' input into and control over various aspects of the group process. For example, practitioners can encourage group members to share experiences and work together to identify realistic and useful responses to their own life situations.

Social Validity

Socially relevant goals and results. The instrumental goals of the first group of previously described CB interventions include learning to recognize legal rights violations, gaining knowledge of legal rights related to academic and work accommodations, learning self-advocacy and conflict resolution skills, and enhancing self-efficacy and social competence. The ultimate goals of most interest—self-advocating and securing one's rights—were established and measured in only one study. Rumrill (1999) determined whether participants with disabilities requested an employer review of their work accommodation needs, met with their employers to discuss the accommodations, and had the accommodations implemented.

Researchers supported the social significance of their intermediate and ultimate intervention goals by providing a variety of rationales and citing relevant research. For example, understanding one's legal rights and mastering self-advocacy skills are prerequisites for individuals to successfully advocate for their legal rights. The social relevance of assisting workers and students with disabilities in obtaining necessary accommodations also is supported by research, which indicates that the accommodations are associated with successful and satisfactory job and academic performance. Securing individual legal rights also is socially valued, as indicated by current civil and disabilities rights laws.

A variety of instrumental outcomes were measured in the CB programs described in the second group of interventions. The goals include acquiring sexual knowledge and a variety of skills, such as resisting social pressure, refusing to engage in unwanted and unprotected sexual activity and other high-risk behavior, and discussing and negotiating responsibility for issues such as birth control. The ultimate goals of refusing unwanted and unprotected sexual activity and of increasing safer sexual practices also were assessed. Researchers established the social relevance of their instrumental goals in several ways. For example, individuals must have accurate knowledge about sex and contraceptives to make informed decisions about engaging in protected sex. Research also supports the relation between consenting to unwanted and unsafe sexual behavior and social pressure, using alcohol/drugs, and lacking the requisite assertive or negotiation skills. The ultimate goals of refusing to engage in unwanted or unprotected sexual activity and increasing protected sex also have social importance because of the STDs (including HIV) and unwanted pregnancies that might otherwise result. However, intervention goals such as using a condom or a female negotiating sexual practices with a male may not be acceptable to all clients because of cultural or religious beliefs.

Whether participants' intervention gains in the instrumental or ultimate measures of the previously described programs were relevant or meaningful is frequently difficult to determine. This is particularly the case for increases in advocacy, negotiation, and assertiveness skills measured by role plays. Although the social relevance of the skill enhancement was sometimes judged by "experts" or validated scales, only one of the evaluations in the first group of interventions determined whether the participants used their acquired skills to advocate on their own behalf and to secure their rights. Of course, whether clients self-advocate and secure certain types of rights is difficult to measure, especially in the short term. Many rights violations (e.g., denial of the right to marry) probably occur relatively infrequently, especially in small samples. Long-term follow-up studies on larger samples are needed to determine whether the CB applications described in this chapter accomplish more than simply increase knowledge and skills and change attitudes.

Even Rumrill's (1999) evaluation, which determined that workers in the intervention group were more likely to request and receive accommodations, did not evaluate whether participants perceived that the accommodations actually improved their work performance or satisfaction with their jobs. Although no formal evaluation of effectiveness was conducted on the university-based summer transition program for students with LD, Brinckerhoff (1994) reported two indicators of socially relevant results. Faculty reported that the students appropriately asked for classroom and testing accommodations, and the students reported that the seminar increased their independence and self-confidence. These two measures suggest that the intervention gains (assuming gains were made) were meaningful and relevant to important aspects of the participants' lives.

The social relevance of the second group of intervention results also was frequently unclear. Whether skill enhancement, increases in protected sex, and decreases in unwanted or unsafe sexual practices actually enhanced the participants' lives in some way was not measured. Other socially relevant results, such as whether the participants' assertion of their right to refuse unwanted or unprotected sexual activity was actually honored by their partner, was not evaluated. The evaluations also did not determine the relation between changes in behavior and skill development and important social outcomes such as lower rates of STDs and unwanted pregnancies. Few evaluations reported whether the intervention results were meaningful from the perspective of the participants. An example of an exception is the participants' rating the degree to which the program helped them to reduce AIDS risk (Kelly et al., 1989). The rating was high.

Only one evaluation of the previously discussed interventions reported unpredictable or unsatisfactory results (Durlak et al., 1994). Some of the students participating in this program experienced embarrassment and uncomfortable feelings when they acknowledged and discussed their LD with teachers. This failure to evaluate unexpected or negative results of the interventions is surprising, given the number of possible, or even likely, negative consequences that can result from asserting one's legal and personal rights. Asserting one's right to work accommodations might result in negative interactions between the employee and employer or co-workers, or the employer might view the employee as a trouble maker and retaliate. For students, disclosing a disability to instructors might result in embarrassment or might alter instructors' expectations for or perceptions of the students. Refusing sexual activity, or making it contingent on the use of protection, might result in pleas, threats, actual physical harm, unwanted sexual behavior despite the assertion, and loss of the relationship. Finally, as Gambrill (1995a) cautioned, clients might experience negative consequences if practitioners communicate unrealistic expectations of what clients can accomplish by themselves or without changes in broader social, economic, and political environments (e.g., social attitudes, economic resources, and additional disability and civil rights legislation). Practitioners, as well as researchers, need to assess and assist clients in coping with possible negative outcomes of the interventions and work toward changing broader environmental factors.

Socially relevant intervention procedures. A few of the programs in the first group of CB interventions included only participants who were referred because they lacked legal knowledge or assertive behavior. Several of the interventions in the second group conducted some type of individual assessment, such as determining whether potential participants engaged in certain high-risk behaviors, before they were selected for participation. Other interventions involved group members assessing their own antecedent conditions (e.g., drug use and mood) that triggered unsafe or unwanted sexual behavior. However, none of the interventions conducted a comprehensive, functional assessment to determine whether the participants already had the required assertive, self-advocacy, or other skills or whether other maintaining conditions were impeding the clients from exhibiting already acquired skills. Such maintaining conditions might include negative reactions from others (e.g., employers, instructors, sexual partners), fear or expectation of negative reactions, value or cultural conflicts, failure of relevant agencies to enforce rights policies, and lack of relevant resources (e.g., contraceptives or the money to purchase them).

Comprehensive assessments completed before participation in the previously discussed CB programs might have suggested more appropriate interventions. Even so, practitioners and researchers might learn from the methods that were used to enhance the appropriateness, acceptability, and applicability of their interventions to participants and their life circumstances. For example, intervention materials designed to teach clients with disabilities their legal rights and self-advocacy skills can be based on a review of the disabilities civil rights literature and the consumer complaint process. Individuals knowledgeable in the legal, advocacy, and relevant service fields can evaluate the content of intervention materials.

Given the cultural and developmental nature of sexual behavior and interactions, practitioners and developers of CB interventions must pay particular attention to the relevancy and acceptability of their interventions designed to change these types of behaviors. Obtaining information on sexual behavior and interactions from research, related literature, surveys, and focus groups and pretesting the materials with individuals with similar characteristics (e.g., age, gender, and race/ethnicity) as the target participants are examples of strategies used to inform the previously described interventions. Other techniques that might enhance the relevance and acceptability of group interventions are group members coaching one another, serving as coping models, and sharing personal situations and strategies. Group facilitators can build social support and consensus among women about safe-sex norms; identify benefits related directly to the women's children, family, and ethnic group; emphasize the importance of power relationships between men and women, particularly in the context of economic insecurity, cultural sexual norms, and male-female relationships. Using culturally relevant and age-appropriate activities and reinforcing and discussing African American gay men's self-identity as members of both a sexual and racial minority group are also ways to address the particular characteristics of the clients and the contexts of their lives.

In the context of the standardized programs, CB interventions can be individualized to enhance their appropriateness, acceptability, and feasibility. For example, in Rumrill's intervention, clients establish individual areas for work accommodations and practitioners revise role plays based on clients' unique situations. Practitioners also assist clients in developing a personal list of accommodation needs and the skills and strategies needed to attain the accommodations. In one of the two programs that assist college students with LD in requesting academic accommodations, students meet with college instructors to request accomodations and discuss their individual accommodation needs.

The second group of interventions provides additional methods to focus on clients' unique situations. For example, group members identify personal cues that trigger high-risk sexual behavior, apply CB strategies to their personal situations in the group and in natural settings, and choose risk-reduction behaviors consistent with their own values and relationships. Several of the other interventions are particularly empowering. For example, group facilitators reinforce positive behavior and past successes. They communicate the expectation that clients will be successful in asserting their right to refuse unwanted or unprotected sexual activity and to engage in safer sexual behaviors.

If interventions are to be appropriate, acceptable, and feasible, they must address the special needs of vulnerable clients. Several examples of special accommodations for clients with disabilities are incorporated into the first group of interventions. Clients are provided with a telephone directory containing phone numbers of relevant agencies for persons with disabilities interested in securing their legal rights, a checklist for redressing rights violations, and a handout providing provisions of ADA's title 1. For clients with visual impairments, information is offered in various forms, including large print, Braille, and audiotape. Finally, the personal list developed in the intervention assisting employees with disabilities in requesting work accommodations prompts clients to use their newly acquired skills to attain their goals. Practitioners are likely to find that many of these materials and strategies are relevant to any client but may be particularly relevant to some vulnerable groups because of their special learning, cognitive, and other special needs.

As the second group of programs demonstrates, other accommodations can enhance the acceptability of CB interventions that assist low-income women in asserting their right to refuse unwanted or unsafe sexual activity. Acknowledging and addressing the women's lack of economic resources and the multiple stressors that can prevent them from attending group sessions and engaging in assertive and healthy sexual behaviors are among the interventions. Specific examples include providing assistance with transportation and babysitting, scheduling meetings that do not conflict with work or educational responsibilities, and incorporating strategies into the group sessions for achieving education and employment goals. Regardless of the sensitivity to client characteristics and life circumstances, cultural norms for some populations might prevent participation in activities related to sexual behavior, whether conducted in groups or individually.

Finally, several of the evaluations of the second group of interventions solicited qualitative judgments of the interventions from participants, teachers, and parents. Ratings were related to satisfaction, enjoyment, interest, and value of the interventions. The ratings generally were very positive, but some female participants were embarrassed by some of the HIV-prevention interventions. These social validity evaluations suggest that practitioners need not hesitate in offering such programs to clients. However, practitioners should describe the interventions, including realistic benefits and risks, in order for clients to make an informed decision whether to participate.

Maintenance and generalization. Evaluations of the first group of interventions either failed to measure whether the enhanced knowledge, skills, or self-advocacy behaviors were maintained after formal intervention or measured maintenance of the behaviors within a short period of time. Strategies that practitioners might adopt from these interventions to transfer clients' skills to natural settings and/or to maintain them include prompting clients to request an accommodations review from their employer and to use the acquired skills and conducting a follow-up session to monitor progress. The two programs that teach students to request academic accommodations ask students to practice the skills with relevant staff and faculty to assist them in transferring the skills to natural settings. In one of the programs, students hold meetings with instructors to describe their LD, to identify accommodations they might require in the class, and to request appropriate accommodations. As previously discussed, determining whether clients' enhanced self-advocacy skills generalize to natural settings and result in clients actually securing their rights can be difficult to evaluate, and only one study conducted such an evaluation (Rumrill, 1999). However, one evaluation measured whether the enhanced self-advocacy skills transferred to relevant role plays in community settings. None of the studies determined whether the acquired skills or other intervention gains generalized to other individuals, such as other employers or instructors, or to multiple settings.

The majority, but not all, of the second group of interventions evaluated whether the assertiveness and other acquired skills, as well as some of the other intervention gains (e.g., increases in the percentage of protected sex), were maintained after formal intervention. The follow-up period ranged from one to eighteen months. Whether the skills or other intervention gains were maintained varied across the evaluations and depended on the outcome being examined. All of the evaluations measured in some way whether the behaviors generalized to natural settings, primarily through self-reports of assertive and various sexual and related behavior. The interventions also suggest strategies that practitioners can use to maintain clients' acquired skills and/or transfer them to real-life situations. Examples include assigning homework to be carried out in natural settings, teaching clients strategies to maintain safer sexual behaviors (e.g., developing social supports and maintaining a balanced lifestyle), and implementing relapse prevention (e.g., assisting clients in identifying and planning for obstacles that might prevent them from continuing and increasing safer sexual behavior). Group facilitators also can assist group members in making a contract or commitment to safer sexual activity and can stress the importance of ongoing vigilance and peer support for maintaining safer sexual practices.

As previously discussed, only a few of the interventions prepare clients for coping with situations in which their behavior does not accomplish the intended result or is met with negative or harmful consequences. Researchers also did not examine whether clients had other necessary resources or information (e.g., names of organizations to obtain free contraceptive devices or available funds to purchase them) to maintain the intervention gains after intervention. Given the potential adversarial nature of self-advocacy and assertive behavior and the limited resources of many vulnerable clients, practitioners and researchers should address both of these omissions. Otherwise, intervention gains might be short lived.

Kelly and Murphy (1992) caution against being overly optimistic about the long-term maintenance of increases in protected and low-risk sexual behavior. They provide evidence, for example, that gay men initially make behavioral changes but frequently do not maintain the changes over time, in all contexts, or with all partners. Their other observation that the men most likely to maintain behavioral change are well educated and white also is relevant here. This suggests that many individuals who are the focus of this book are at risk of failing to assert their sexual rights and of exhibiting high-risk sexual behavior before intervention, as well as failing to maintain enhanced skills or safer sexual behaviors after intervention.

Kelly and Murphy's (1992) summary and the analysis here suggest several strategies that practitioners and researchers might use to enhance the effectiveness of interventions designed to assist vulnerable clients in asserting their legal and personal rights, as well as to generalize and maintain intervention gains. First, conduct individualized assessments before intervention and design interventions consistent with the assessments. Second, provide multiple opportunities, including multiple role-play partners and different contexts, for clients to practice the relevant skills. Third, assign homework for clients to practice the skills in the context of their own lives. Fourth, increase clients' awareness of and identify strategies for coping with possible refusals or other aversive responses from partners, employers, instructors, and other relevant individuals when clients assert their rights. Finally, practitioners should assess and, if possible, intervene to change other maintaining conditions, such as school policies, peers, family, economic circumstances, and broader social policies. In the future, researchers also can develop and evaluate strategies to change those conditions.

As discussed in this chapter, as well as in the previous two chapters, an individual's goals, options, and choices are frequently defined and limited by social policy and organizational and community practices. Unless these broader policies and practices are changed, choices and opportunities of vulnerable populations can be unnecessarily limited. The first chapter in part V examines CB interventions that empower vulnerable populations by assisting them in changing limiting social policies and organizational and community practices.

ADDITIONAL READINGS AND RESOURCES

Baptiste, D. R., Paikoff, R. L., McKay, M. M., Madison-Boyd, S., Coleman, D., & Bell, C. (2005). Collaborating with an urban community to develop an HIV and AIDS prevention program for black youth and families. *Behavior Modification, 29,* 370–416.

Barth, R. P. (1996). *Reducing the risk: Building skills to prevent pregnancy, STD and HIV* (3rd ed.). Santa Cruz, CA: ETR Associates.

Freedom Self-Advocacy Curriculum. National Mental Health Consumers' Self-Help Clearinghouse, 1211 Chestnut Street, Suite 1207. Philadelphia, PA 19107. Curriculum for conducting three workshops (attitudes, skills, and knowledge) to teach self-advocacy skills to mental health consumers can be downloaded at http://www.mhselfhelp.org/training/view.php?training_id=7.

Hovell, M., Blumberg, E., Sipan, C., Hofstetter, C. R., Burkham, S., Atkins, C., et al. (1998). Skills training for pregnancy and AIDS prevention in Anglo and Latino youth. *Journal of Adolescent Health, 23,* 139–149.

Kalichman, S. C. (1998). *Preventing AIDS: A sourcebook for behavioral interventions.* Mahwah, NJ: Erlbaum.

Lock, R., & Layton, C. (2001). Succeeding in postsecondary ed through self-advocacy. *Teaching Exceptional Children, 34,* 66–71.

Pedlow, C. T., & Carey, M. P. (2003). HIV sexual risk-reduction interventions for youth: A review and methodological critique of randomized controlled trials. *Behavior Modification, 27,* 135–190.

Roessler, R., & Rumrill, P. (1994). Strategies for enhancing career maintenance self-efficacy of people with multiple sclerosis. *Journal of Rehabilitation, 60,* 54–59.

Roessler, R., Rumrill, P., Battersby, J., & Garnette, M. (1996). *Employee's guide to the Americans with Disabilities Act: The "win-win" approach to reasonable accommodations.* Hot Springs, AR: Arkansas Research and Training Center in Vocational Rehabilitation.

Rumrill, P., Roessler, R., & Brown, P. (1997). *Self-advocacy training: Preparing students with disabilities to request classroom accommodations.* University of Arkansas: Arkansas Research and Training Center in Vocational Rehabilitation.

Thomason, B. T., Bachanas, P. J., & Compos, P. E. (1996). Cognitive behavioral interventions with persons affected by HIV/AIDS. *Cognitive and Behavioral Practice, 3,* 417–442.

PART

FIVE

Increasing Involvement in Macro Decision Making and Summary

13 Changing Social Policies and Community and Organizational Practices

Policy decisions in this country are made primarily through political processes. Understanding political processes and structures and using effective political and advocacy skills increase the probability that groups will influence social policy consistent with their goals (Baker, Leitner, & McAuley, 2001). The importance of social workers assisting all individuals in becoming meaningfully involved in the decisions that influence their lives is reflected in the NASW (1999) Code of Ethics. Unfortunately, vulnerable populations frequently have little input into the macro decisions that affect their education, rehabilitation, health care, and mental health services and other services, and other important areas of their lives. This lack of involvement, in turn, can result in a variety of negative outcomes.

This chapter first discusses reasons for the limited involvement of vulnerable populations in macro decision making. It then considers beneficial outcomes that can result from vulnerable groups participating in the social policy and organizational and community practice decisions that affect their lives. CB interventions that assist vulnerable populations, including individuals with low income, mental retardation, physical disabilities, and severe mental illness, women, and the elderly, in influencing macro policies and practices are described next. Finally, a more critical evaluation of the interventions is presented and implications for practice and future research are discussed.

Several of the CB interventions and programs discussed in this chapter teach participants self-advocacy skills, as did some of the interventions described in the previous chapters on enhancing self-determination. Here, however, the goal of teaching self-advocacy skills is to assist vulnerable individuals not only in accessing resources and services and making changes that benefit themselves, but in making organizational, community, and social policy changes that enhance the lives of individuals with shared problems. The interventions discussed here also differ from those in the three previous parts of this book in three ways. First, in addition to CB methods, the more complex multicomponent government and privately sponsored programs include other instructional techniques to a greater extent than previously discussed CB interventions. Second, because relatively few CB interventions that assist vulnerable populations in influencing macro-level practices and decision making have been evaluated, programs that were not rigorously evaluated or only provided evidence that the interventions enhanced skill development are included to a greater extent than in previous chapters. Whether actual changes were made in organizations, communities, or social policy as a result of the interventions was less frequently evaluated. Third, in addition to vulnerable populations, many of the programs discussed in this chapter increase the advocacy and political skills and activity of other interested individuals, such as family members.

Although the ultimate goal of the CB interventions described in this chapter is to change macro policies and practices, these interventions do not require practitioners to mobilize vulnerable groups or to advocate for social change. Instead, practitioners use the strategies to assist vulnerable populations and interested others in acquiring the knowledge and skills to advocate macro changes. Advocating macro practices and policies that affect one's own life and the lives of others with similar problems, instead of depending on others, can be particularly empowering.

MACRO DECISION MAKING AMONG VULNERABLE POPULATIONS

Constrained Involvement

As discussed in the introduction to chapter 10, many factors can constrain the self-determined behavior of vulnerable populations. Similar factors can prevent vulnerable groups from influencing the social policies and organizational and community practices that affect their lives. For some vulnerable groups, problems such as cognitive limitations and symptoms of severe mental illness can impair their ability to learn or use already acquired skills to influence the macro decisions that affect the services they receive and other areas of their lives. Other factors, such as discrimination, stigma, and paternalism, can lead policy makers and service providers to develop negative assumptions about the capability of vulnerable groups to make sound choices for themselves. As a result, the input of vulnerable populations is frequently discounted and undervalued. In addition, policy makers and service providers make available few or no opportunities for consumers of health, mental health, geriatric, disability, and other social services to participate in the policy, organizational, and community decisions that influence their lives. Instead, policy makers, interested others, and professional staff inappropriately make many of these decisions for them (Sabin & Daniels, 2002; Stringfellow & Muscari, 2003).

Vulnerable populations frequently have few opportunities to acquire the knowledge and skills needed to become effective advocates for macro practices and policies. These skills include understanding and analyzing power relationships and the issues involved in social policies and practices, identifying and reporting issues, making informed choices, engaging in strategic planning, and advocating for change. Economic resources, such as funds to pay for transportation, child care, and time off work, and negotiating the demands and additional burdens associated with various disabilities, old age, and poverty also can constrain involvement in influencing macro decision making and practices (Baker et al., 2001; Fawcett et al., 1984; Hess, Clapper, Hoekstra, & Gibison, 2001; Stringfellow & Muscari, 2003).

The previously discussed constraints are particularly relevant for many racial/ethnic minority groups. Compared with their white peers, racial/ethnic minorities are disproportionately disabled and poor and less likely to participate in the political activity that can influence the social polices and macro practices that affect their lives (Marschall, 2001; Putnam, 2000). Reasons for these disparities include language and communication problems, particularly for Latinos, which result in increased difficulty in obtaining relevant information and assistance from local service agencies. A distrust of government policies and programs and a lack of awareness of their legal rights also might constrain involvement of minorities with disabilities in advocacy and political activity (Balcazar, Keys, & Suarez-Balcazar, 2001).

Individuals with low income who are involved in community self-help, one approach to addressing community problems related to poverty, can lack skills for conducting effective meetings and for group problem solving and have few opportunities to learn the skills. Disorganized and ineffective meetings, in turn, can result in low levels of member participation, poorly planned strategies, unresolved issues, and unclear direction for advocacy activity (Seekins, Mathews, & Fawcett, 1984). And for a self-help group to successfully influence social policy and macro practices, it must be able to maintain member participation. Long-range and often indirect benefits resulting from activities of self-help groups, such as cleaner neighborhoods and educational improvement, likely are not sufficiently strong reinforcers to maintain participation of low-income group members (Miller & Miller, 1970).

Women traditionally have been underrepresented in the political and organizational decision making that affect their lives, including decisions made about medical and health research. Women frequently lack the knowledge and skills required to influence decisions made on biomedical research, treatment options, and the availability of treatment for health problems, such as breast cancer, that are experienced disproportionately by women (Dickersin et al., 2001; Low et al., 1994).

Finally, as Aspis (1997) argues, other types of knowledge and motivation are necessary if vulnerable groups, such as those with disabilities, are to engage in activities that can influence macro practices and social policy. Vulnerable populations must recognize and understand the importance of making personal decisions that immediately affect their own lives, as well as engaging in longer-term activities that change social policies and organizational and community practices. Vulnerable populations also must be willing and able to clearly identify alternatives to choices offered to them, recognize the importance of supporting one another to achieve common goals, and challenge the political system to be responsive to their needs.

Beneficial Outcomes from Macro Involvement

Involving vulnerable groups in the macro decisions made about the services they receive and other aspects of their lives can have important implications both at the individual and group level. For example, participating in service decisions and experiencing changes in environmental conditions as a result of their own efforts can empower individuals with severe mental illness. Some evidence also suggests that personal empowerment gained from such experiences can enhance the well-being of individuals with severe mental illness (Stringfellow & Muscari, 2003). In addition, clients who personally experience the problems and services are usually best positioned to evaluate the usefulness and appropriateness of the policies and services and to suggest improvements and better alternatives (Hess et al., 2001).

Influencing social policy and community and organizational practices can have other positive outcomes for individuals, as well as for groups of individuals experiencing similar problems. As Aspis (1997) pointed out, instituting policy change is necessary if the change is to become a protected right, and not solely dependent on the goodwill of others, such as service providers. For example, an individual with a disability might self-advocate and obtain a wage for his or her work activity in a particular work program. However, without legislation that guarantees a right to a wage, organizations or staff will arbitrarily decide whether other workers with disabilities receive a wage in similar programs.

The importance of vulnerable populations' involvement in macro decision making has been demonstrated historically. Individuals with disabilities, as well as family members, have played important roles in passing legislation protecting their rights, such as the IDEA of 1990 and the ADA of 1990. Individuals with physical disabilities also have influenced community practices and social policies through advocacy groups formed as part of the Independent Living and People First movements (Cunconan-Lahr & Brotherson, 1996). Independent living groups are based on the philosophy that the environment, not the disabling condition, produces the obstacle (Seekins, Fawcett, & Mathews, 1987). The People First movement challenges the stereotyped view that individuals with disabilities necessarily need others to speak on their behalf. After acquiring relevant skills, individuals with disabilities, sometimes with the assistance of family members, can represent themselves on issues that affect their own lives (Zirpoli, Hancox, Wieck, & Skarnulis, 1989).

As a result of these movements and related legislation, individuals with disabilities have become empowered to safeguard their own rights, assume greater control over their lives, and provide others with education on disability-related issues, activities that have resulted in a more inclusive society (Cunconan-Lahr & Brotherson, 1996). Enacting legislation, however, does not guarantee that organizations and communities will protect the rights and respond to the needs of vulnerable populations. Vulnerable groups frequently must advocate on their own behalf to ensure that their rights are protected and communities respond to their needs, such as ensuring that communities are accessible and supportive of independent living for individuals with disabilities (Balcazar, Seekins, Fawcett, & Hopkins, 1990).

Community self-help involves the organized efforts of low-income community members affected by problems related to poverty, such as inadequate housing, substandard education, crime, and unemployment, to help themselves. Self-help group meetings provide opportunities for members to share information, identify problems, propose solutions, make decisions, and work toward resolution of identified problems. In effective self-help groups, members access locally available resources and identify and implement solutions to shared problems (Seekins et al., 1984).

A final advantage of vulnerable groups participating in policy-related activity is their ability to correct myths and misinformation. For example, in the area of aging, policy makers might lack knowledge or accurate knowledge about the older population, the effectiveness of aging programs, and the characteristics and needs of older people (Baker et al., 2001). In addition, Baker et al. argue that elderly advocates and others who advocate on behalf of the elderly can provide appropriate responses to public campaigns that create intergenerational conflict over resources and offer negative views of public programs for the elderly. Advocates also can influence macro decision makers to provide responsive and innovative programs.

INCREASING INVOLVEMENT IN MACRO DECISION MAKING

The CB interventions described here address many of the factors that prevent vulnerable populations from participating in the macro decisions that influence the services they receive and other areas of their lives. For example, the interventions teach vulnerable groups, and sometimes family members and interested others, the necessary knowledge and skills to advocate for changes in social policies and organizational and community practices. Vulnerable populations include individuals with a variety of disabilities (e.g., physical disabilities, mental retardation, LD, and severe mental illness), women with a serious health problem (e.g., breast cancer), the elderly, and individuals with low income.

CB interventions that assist vulnerable groups in learning relevant knowledge and skills and in increasing attendance at self-help meetings to change community and organizational practices and social policies are presented first. This is followed by descriptions of more complex multicomponent government and privately sponsored programs. The programs teach political and advocacy knowledge and skills and provide resources and opportunities for vulnerable groups to become active in political processes at community, state, and national levels.

Skills Training and Increasing Group Attendance

CB interventions that assist vulnerable groups in learning relevant knowledge and skills to make changes in social policies and community and organizational practices are discussed here. The skills are related to writing letters to public officials and newspaper editors, preparing and presenting testimonies in public forums, chairing and leading advocacy groups, identifying and reporting relevant issues, problem solving, and public speaking. Finally, reinforcement is used to increase attendance at self-help group meetings where members strive to resolve shared community problems. Unless otherwise stated, the interventions were evaluated using single-system and multiple-baseline designs.

Adults with disabilities. The goal of this behavioral program is to increase the involvement of members attending disability advocacy groups in three types of advocacy activities (Seekins et al., 1987). The activities include preparing and presenting personal testimonies at city commission meetings and state legislative hearings, writing letters to public officials, and writing letters to newspaper editors. In this intervention, no direct skills training is provided. Instead, group members use prepared guides as a "behavioral prosthetic" to assist them in preparing effective letters and testimony. To ensure the social relevance of the content of the guides, Seekins et al. conducted a task analysis of the three advocacy skill areas. Potential relevant skills for presenting personal testimonies were identified through observations of testimony presented at city commission meetings and state legislative hearings. Effective skills for letter writing to public officials were determined through the examination of letters in several newspapers for common response components. Advocacy group members then determined which response components constituted an effective letter to a public official. The identified responses for effective testimony, letter writing to public officials, and letter writing to an editor are presented in table 13.1.

Consistent with skills training, the self-help guides provide instruction for

Table 13.1. Responses for Effective Personal Testimony and Letter Writing

Personal Testimony Responses
1. Go to podium.
2. Stop at podium and pause.
3. Briefly look a each member of panel.
4. Look directly at chairperson.
5. State your name.
6. Make a statement about yourself.
7. Describe your circumstances.
8. Tell how this happened.
9. Tell what this means to you in your everyday life.
10. Pause.
11. Tell how the decision the panel makes will affect you personally.
12. Tell how the decision will affect others.
13. Ask a value question.
14. Pause, and look at members of the panel.
15. Leave the podium.

Letter to Public Official Responses
1. Open the letter
2. Write something about yourself
3. Tell why you are writing the letter.
4. Summarize your understanding of the issue (decision) being considered.
5. Tell why you think a decision should be made.
6. Tell what changes mean to you personally.
7. If you think others will also be affected, identify them.
8. Acknowledge past support.
9. Describe the action you hope the official will take.
10. If you have written a letter that opposed some action, offer an alternative.
11. If you have time and you are committed, ask how you can help.
12. Close the letter.
13. Sign the letter.

Letter to the Editor Responses
1. Open the letter.
2. Tell why you are writing.
3. Tell why it is important.
4. Praise or criticize something someone has said or done.
5. Tell why this is good or bad.
6. State your opinion about what should be done.
7. Make a general recommendation.
8. Sign the letter.

Note. From "Effects of Self-Help Guides on Three Consumer Advocacy Skills: Using Personal Experiences to Influence Public Policy," by T. Seekins, S. B. Fawcett, & R. M. Mathews, 1987, *Rehabilitation Psychology, 36*, p. 30. Copyright 1987 by the Division of Rehabilitation Psychology of the American Psychological Association. Reprinted with permission.

effective responses for each skill area, including a rationale for learning the skills, examples of supportive or opposing statements for a particular issue, behavioral definitions of effective skill performance, and space to prepare personal letters or testimony (see Seekins & Fawcett in "Additional Readings and Resources" at the end of this chapter for information on obtaining the guides).

Members of an independent living advocacy organization who had multiple types of disabilities (i.e., multiple sclerosis, epilepsy, quadriplegia, and a variety of chronic health problems) participated in the evaluations of the intervention. The evaluations were conducted using a single-system design with one female member, then through the random assignment of ten members either to a treatment group receiving the self-help guides or to a comparison group receiving an introduction to the guides and a model letter prepared in response to another local issue. The participant in the first evaluation prepared letters to a newspaper editor and a public official on eleven different issues related to local independent living and disability rights (e.g., modifying a city antidiscrimination ordinance, cuts in state-supported medical services, a tax to fund independent living services, obstacles to voting, and disabled parking problems) and prepared public testimony when relevant. In the second evaluation, all of the members wrote letters to newspaper editors and to public officials to persuade them to allocate funds from a community development block grant to remove architectural barriers and to purchase a lift van.

In the first evaluation, the woman's percentage of target testimony and letter writing responses increased after she used the self-help guides. Expert ratings (e.g., by a public administrator, former mayor, community organizers, and an independent living center board president) of the overall quality of the woman's testimony and letters, the likelihood of editors publishing the letters, and the likely influence of the testimony and letters on the decisions of public officials all increased after intervention. In the second evaluation, the percentages of identified responses used in writing letters to public officials and newspaper editors were higher in the experimental group, compared with the comparison group. Expert ratings similar to those used in the first evaluation demonstrated better performance by the experimental group in writing effective letters to public officials and newspaper editors. Finally, the researchers found a statistically significant correlation between the percentages of the members' targeted responses and the expert ratings.

This second behavioral intervention focuses specifically on advocacy letter writing skills (White, Thompson, & Nary, 1997). The intervention was developed in response to a rural independent living center's request to assist members of their community advocacy group in writing effective advocacy letters to resolve disability-related community problems affecting their members. The intervention involves self-paced lessons contained in an Action Letter Portfolio training manual. The manual was developed with assistance and feedback on the readability and usefulness of the content from individuals with disabilities. Two readability scoring programs also ensured that the manual's content was at the appropriate high school reading level (see White, Thomson, & Nary, 1998, in "Additional Readings and Resources" at the end of this chapter for information on obtaining the manual).

The manual, which the group members use independently, contains the following five main sections.

1 Key components of a quality advocacy letter and rationales for the components
2 Strategies for analyzing and breaking down larger problems into smaller ones (the goal is to win small victories)
3 Strategies to follow up on the letter if no response or an unacceptable response is received
4 Examples of advocacy letters written by members of other independent living centers
5 Relevant facts, figures, and information on disability policy

To guide future revisions of the manual, the authors collected feedback from the participants on the clarity and usability of the manual. After intervention, the four participating members with physical, psychiatric, or learning disabilities demonstrated small to large increases in advocacy letter writing skills. Maintenance of the skills was not evaluated, but two of the four participants received responses from their personal letters. Unfortunately, at a six-month follow-up none of the participants had written additional letters.

Balcazar and his colleagues (1990) developed an additional behavioral intervention to assist individuals with disabilities involved in an advocacy organization in achieving three goals related to advocacy activities. The goals of the intervention are to (1) enhance a chairperson's ability to conduct action-oriented advocacy group meetings, (2) increase group members' skills for identifying and reporting relevant advocacy issues during the meetings, and (3) increase group members' advocacy actions and related achievements as a result of the actions. The goals were chosen based on previous observations, interviews, and reviews of audiotapes of the group's meetings. The assessment determined several factors impeding effective advocacy meetings. They included being disorganized, reaching few decisions, implementing few proposed actions, and focusing on internal organizational issues versus issues directly relevant to members with disabilities. During the process of developing the intervention, members assisted the researchers in identifying relevant skills and provided feedback on the materials and procedures.

The first of the two main identified skills—reporting disability-related issues—is defined in two ways. First, a group member reports on a community event that affects the ability of individuals with physical disabilities to live independently. Examples of issues include the need for curb cuts in downtown streets, violations of the disability parking ordinance, and failure to enforce fire safety codes in a local residential care facility. Second, a group member provides an update on a previously identified issue; for example, he or she might read a report on an ongoing project. The second main skill involves closing discussion of a new disability-related issue. This skill is defined as the chairperson directing group members to decide on an action for the reported issue. Closure can be attained in three ways: (1) members vote on a motion, (2) a committee is formed to plan or implement the actions, or (3) the item is tabled until the next meeting. No specific interventions are used to teach implementation of the agreed on action, but several methods (e.g., interviewing group members, reviewing relevant records, and reading meeting minutes) are used to identify the advocacy actions and the outcomes of the actions.

The group facilitator uses two training manuals providing about twelve hours of instruction to teach group members to effectively identify and report disability-related issues. The first manual defines the skills for identifying the issues and provides steps for writing related reports, examples of disability-related issues and completed reports, and exercises for selecting relevant issues and preparing reports. The second manual contains thirty-five possible actions requiring different degrees of complexity and effort, ranging from postponing action to organizing a boycott. For each action, the manual provides descriptions of the activities involved, necessary resources, and possible positive and negative consequences of the actions.

A manual with an instructional format similar to the training manuals for group members is used to enhance the chairperson's skills to lead action-oriented meetings. During the first of the four sessions, the practitioner provides the chairperson with a summary of managing action-oriented meetings and steps for agenda preparation, opening the meeting, and initiating group discussion of issues. In the second session, the chairperson is taught skills for handling votes, closing discussion of issues, planning action steps, and closing the meetings. In the final two sessions, the chairperson practices the skills in role plays (see Seekins, Balcazar, & Fawcett, 1986, in "Additional Readings and Resources" for information on obtaining the training manuals).

During twenty-one monthly meetings of the advocacy organization involved in the intervention evaluation, the trained members (six of the fourteen members; two consecutive chairpersons) demonstrated a statistically significant increased trend in reporting disability-related issues, while the untrained members showed no significant trend. The performance of both chairpersons in closing discussion of new issues and the number of advocacy actions taken by group members, as well as the positive outcomes of those actions, all increased after intervention. For example, for the issue of increasing curb cuts for wheelchairs in a downtown area, actions included writing a letter to the city manager and meeting with the city manager and city planner. The actions resulted in the installation of curb cuts at four downtown street corners. Other examples of successfully resolved issues for which multiple actions were taken include the installation of an emergency alarm safety system for disabled persons living in their homes and the enhancement of fire safety procedures for disabled and elderly residents of local nursing homes. Finally, participants' ratings of their overall satisfaction with the interventions averaged 6.5 (1 = very dissatisfied; 7 = very satisfied), and their average rating of the importance of the training was 7.0.

Adults with low income. In an older study, Briscoe, Hoffman, and Bailey (1975) used PST to teach socioeconomically disadvantaged policy board members of a self-help rural black community project to increase their problem-solving skills. The board meetings focused on identifying and solving community problems, such as repairing a community center, organizing educational and social events, and identifying community resources and distributing them to residents. A preliminary analysis of the board meetings over a one-year period determined that the board members were unable to clearly define a problem, agree on specific actions to take, and identify a responsible person to carry out the actions. The observations suggested teaching the three basic skills necessary for effective problem solving: (1) identifying the problem, (2) stating and evaluating alternative solutions, and (3) agreeing on a specific action to resolve the problem and the method for implementing the action (i.e., what would be done, by whom, when, and how?).

The intervention uses SST techniques to teach board members the problem-solving process, which includes key statements to facilitate learning. Examples of key statements for the three steps are: "The problem is _____"; "One solution is _____"; "What actions are we going to take?" In the first step, the practitioner describes the skill and shows the board member a card with the respective key phrase printed on it (e.g., "The problem is _____"). The practitioner and board member read the phrase together; the board member reads it alone; then the board member repeats the phrase after the card is removed. In step 2, the board member learns to apply the skills to a simple problematic situation depicted pictorially on a card, then to gradually more complex situations described verbally. For example, the practitioner shows the board member a picture of a problematic situation (e.g., a dentist examining a girl's teeth), after which various problematic situations (e.g., in an adult education class, fifteen students are required to use a book to practice reading, but only seven books are available) are read. In both types of situations, the practitioner asks the board member to identify the problem, using the key phrase "The problem is _____." The practitioner then prompts the board members during subsequent board meetings to use the key statement to state the problem. The remaining two problem-solving skills are taught in a similar manner. After intervention, as demonstrated by different raters, including community leaders active in local policy boards, the group members involved in the program evaluation (N = 9; median education was eighth grade) increased their problem-solving skills during actual board meetings. Not all participants, however, maintained their skills at high levels at the six-week follow-up.

This second behavioral intervention discussed here was developed by Fawcett and Miller (1975) to enhance public-speaking skills of paraprofessional staff members employed by a neighborhood service center serving low-income community members. The staff were members of the speaker's bureau of the center, which responds to requests from community organizations and groups (e.g., churches, businesses, and civic and social organizations) to present and promote the activities and services of the center. Based on the literature identifying effective speaking behaviors, the intervention focuses on speaking skills in three main categories: eye contact, gestures, and speaking behaviors. Speaking skills are further defined as the following five initial and four closing skills.

Initial Skills

1 Assume appropriate position on stage
2 Scan the audience
3 Acknowledge the introduction
4 Preliminary greeting
5 Introduce the topic

Closing Skills

1 Final scan of the audience
2 Final greeting
3 Request for questions
4 Introduction of the next speaker, if applicable

The researchers prepared a *Public Speaking Manual* (available from Fawcett) containing behavioral definitions of the skills, written instructions, examples, and quizzes. For participants who have difficulty with written instruction, the content of the manual can be administered orally. After the instructional material is mastered, behavioral rehearsal is used to teach participants each public-speaking skill. After acquiring the skills, the participants speak before several live audiences composed of friends or other individuals familiar with the speaker training program, who provide feedback on the participants' performance. After intervention, the percentage of the identified skills increased for all three of the staff members involved in the evaluation (African American, Latina, and white females). Audience ratings of the staff members' overall performance in speaking publicly at a variety of community engagements also demonstrated marked improvement after intervention. In addition, the confidence of two of the three staff members' in their ability to speak in public increased after intervention. All participants rated their satisfaction with the training as a 7 (very happy) on a scale of 1 to 7.

This behavioral program was designed to enhance the leadership skills of chairpersons of the executive board of low-income neighborhood centers (Seekins et al., 1984). The intervention was developed in response to the request of members of a low-income neighborhood service center for assistance in making group decisions. The main responsibilities of the board included establishing organizational policy and advising staff on the agency's daily operations. Examples of agenda items of the executive board meetings included reports and announcements (e.g., date of a government food distribution), proposals (e.g., development of a community canning kitchen), and community problems (e.g., complaints that the emergency distribution food policy was unfair). Based on a review of the literature on effective chairpersons' skills, the following three main categories of skills are targeted by the intervention.

1. Opening and closing meetings (i.e., ending discussion of an item by communicating the result of a vote, forming a committee, tabling discussion, announcing member agreement, or accepting a report)
2. Initiating discussions and handling motions
3. Brainstorming and selecting solutions

A task analysis of the relevant skills and observations of effective leaders of group meetings suggested forty-two responses were involved in the three skill areas. Examples include calling the meeting to order, encouraging questions and comments, calling on quiet members, asking for the advantages of various suggestions, and asking the secretary to summarize the board's decisions. Based on the analysis, a manual was developed (*Chairing Meetings: Building Leadership in Community Organizations*, available from Seekins or Fawcett) to teach the identified responses. The manual, which is divided into chapters corresponding to the identified skill areas, includes behavioral definitions of the skills, study guides, examples, and rehearsal scripts.

The practitioner begins the intervention by asking the chairperson to read the instructional material and complete the study guide and examples, for which he or she receives praise for appropriate responses and corrective feedback for inappropriate responses. The chairperson then practices the relevant skills using the scripted role-play situations. Finally, the chairperson practices the identified skills with additional persons in the room where board meetings are conducted, which is followed by appropriate feedback.

Evaluation of the intervention indicated that it was successful in improving the skills of both participating chairwomen. For example, before intervention, an average of 30% of the agenda items were closed, compared with 85% after intervention. Assessment also indicated that after intervention the board made more decisions. Both findings were consistent with ratings of a panel of experts, including an organizational development consultant and an urban planner. Finally, both women were highly pleased with the training, as indicated by their rating of 7 (very happy) on a scale of 1 to 7.

This final reinforcement intervention, which was designed to increase the attendance of low-income women in two self-help groups (Miller & Miller, 1970), was discussed in both chapters 6 and 9. The intervention is briefly discussed again, because in addition to enhancing social support and addressing economic problems, one of the main objectives of these self-help groups is to discuss and take action on community issues affecting group members. Community issues include urban renewal, school board policies, police problems, and city government. During the group meetings, members agree to focus on a problem, and they devise strategies for resolving it. Presidents of the self-help groups also meet on a quarterly basis to discuss strategies, organizational responses, and members' reactions, and to coordinate their groups' activities. The counselor for the self-help groups uses one intervention—reinforcement of group member attendance.

Evaluation of the intervention demonstrated that providing reinforcers, such as donated items (e.g., clothing, toys, household goods), relevant information (e.g., on welfare services, birth control), and services (e.g., assistance in negotiating a welfare payment grievance, negotiating house improvements with a landlord, clearing up a police/court problem), significantly increased attendance at the meetings ($N = 52$; average of three participants before intervention, and fifteen after intervention). Increased participation in the self-help groups also generalized to other self-help activities, as indicated by the two presidents' increased attendance at other community groups (e.g., a citizen's advisory board and a school integration committee). Casual observations also indicated increases in the community involvement of group members as well.

Government- and Foundation-Sponsored Programs

The interventions described here all incorporate CB strategies into complex, multicomponent programs. The programs include the government-sponsored PPM, which assists individuals with disabilities and their family members in learning the necessary knowledge and skills to advocate for themselves and/or their children and to influence policy at the local, state, and federal levels. Government-sponsored leadership academies also assist adults with severe mental illness, the elderly, and interested others (primarily family members) in acquiring relevant knowledge and skills to influence social policy and community and organizational practices. The final program, Project LEAD (Leadership, Education, and Advocacy Development), assists breast cancer activists (primarily women with a history of breast cancer) in learning the relevant scientific knowledge and skills needed to participate in and influence policy decisions related to breast cancer research.

The most common CB methods incorporated into these programs are identification of specific skills, provision of standardized information and instruction, use of SST to teach advocacy and related skills (e.g., securing services, contacting elected officials, public speaking, and legislative testimony), social reinforcement, role modeling, homework assignments, and a variety of strategies to prompt and maintain involvement after formal training ends. Evaluations of these programs were minimal, and frequently simply descriptive. Only one of the four PPM programs compared preintervention and postintervention outcomes, as did only one of the three evaluations of the leadership academies. Both evaluations of the LEAD program used preintervention and postintervention measures to assess the program's effectiveness.

PPM: Individuals with disabilities. Partners in Policymaking (PPM) is a federally funded empowerment and self-advocacy training program based in St. Paul, Minnesota (Zirpoli et al., 1989). A description of the program is presented first, followed by a discussion of four evaluations of the program. The goals of the PPM are to provide information, training, and the necessary skills for parents with young children and for adults with developmental disabilities to obtain appropriate services, enhance their leadership potential, and influence policies at the local, state, and national levels. Special efforts are made to select program participants from different backgrounds (e.g., racial/ethnic minorities and individuals with low income, developmental disabilities, and residence in different areas of the state). The one-year program covers travel, meals, lodging, and respite and child care expenses.

The PPM program consists of three main training components. The first component provides sixteen days of training focusing on specific service topics and different levels of government. The topics are presented by a variety of experts, including legislators and representatives from advocacy organizations. During the second component of the program, participants complete homework assignments. The assignments include making personal contacts with policy makers at the local, state, and national levels; reading (e.g., a summary of existing legislation affecting people with disabilities); attending community meetings (e.g., a city council or school board meeting); and making presentations on the concerns of individuals with disabilities (e.g., to PTA groups or conferences). The third training component requires participants to complete a major project, such as serving an internship or organizing a meeting with public officials. During the sessions, trainers provide handouts, reference material, and formal presentations on a variety of topics. Topics include relevant issues at different levels of government, advocacy organizations and skills, behavior management, and educational issues applicable to students with disabilities, such as IEPs and classroom integration.

Six months after attending the program, the participants (N = 35) rated the degree to which the program improved their self-advocacy skills (95% responded positively) and enabled them to receive more appropriate services for themselves or for a family member (89% responded positively). The participants also reported on the degree to which the PPM program prepared them to be an effective advocate (82% responded, "I was very prepared"). All but two of the participants reported making contact with a public official in some way, such as through letters, phone calls, office visits, and testifying, or by serving on a committee or commission. Additional advocacy efforts included publishing newspaper articles or letters, presenting at conferences and to parent groups, and making media appearances. Participants reported other program benefits. They included developing a strong support network, acquiring a better understanding of various systems and ways to access them, and obtaining more appropriate services for themselves or someone else, as well as increased self-confidence, especially when interacting with public officials and educators.

After five years of operation, Zirpoli and his colleagues (Zirpoli, Wieck, Hancox, & Skarnulis, 1994) conducted a similar evaluation of Minnesota's PPM program. At the time, the program had 163 graduates and was being offered in several other states. Participants were primarily females, educated (73% had more than a high school education), and parents of children with a developmental disability. However, 22% of the participants had a disability. When evaluating the overall program, 93% of the participants rated it excellent or very good, and 88% rated the program's effectiveness in teaching them to become a better advocate as excellent or very good. Feedback was similar to the first evaluation in terms of the high percentage of participants who reported contacting public officials, advocating in other ways for themselves or others with disabilities, and educating the public on the rights and needs of individuals with disabilities.

The impact of Iowa's PPM program on the advocacy activities of participants with developmental disabilities and their family members also was evaluated through a survey, telephone interviews, and focus groups (Cunconan-Lahr & Brotherson, 1996). Similar methods were used to evaluate barriers to advocacy. Consistent with the results of the two previously discussed evaluations of Minnesota's PPM program, Iowa participants reported that the program had an important impact on enhancing their self-advocacy skills, on their advocacy concerning disability-related issues, and on other areas of their lives. Examples of advocacy activities also were very similar. The reported barriers to advocacy included time, expense (e.g., transportation, costs for personal supports, attendant care, child care, missed work), and negative emotions, such as embarrassment resulting from telling one's story.

Balcazar, Keys, Bertram, and Rizzo (1996) conducted a more rigorous evaluation of the Illinois PPM program. The researchers examined self-reports of advocacy actions and advocacy outcomes of three participants with disabilities (two with mental retardation and one with multiple sclerosis) and twenty-one parents of children with disabilities before, during, and five months after completion of the program. The PPM program provided support services to two of the individuals with disabilities, which included reviewing and discussing the agenda for the training sessions and the content of the presentations, answering questions during the presentations, and providing assistance with homework assignments. Because one goal of the evaluation was to determine whether posttraining differences in engaging in advocacy actions were related to participants' previous level of advocacy experience, participants were classified into three groups—beginner, involved, and activist—based on their advocacy experience prior to their participation in the PPM program.

Actions reported by the participants included phone calls, meetings or office visits, letter writing and organization of mass mailings, media activities (e.g., participating in radio interviews), and a variety of other actions (e.g., school presentations, speaking at public hearings, and fund-raising). Advocacy issues were defined as any disability-related event or situation requiring action and affecting individuals with disabilities and/or their families. Examples were unmet needs for information, services, or support; negative or positive changes in services and supports; and budget allocations or policies. Outcomes referred to changes in the community and/or in relevant processes related to disability issues and resulting at least in part from participants' actions. Outcomes were categorized into school inclusion (e.g., getting a son/daughter enrolled in a neighborhood school), advocacy supports (e.g., forming a new local advocacy group), legislative changes (e.g., assisting with passage of a bill), community education activities (e.g., making a presentation), appointment to a decision-making board, and fund raising.

All three groups—beginner, involved, and activist—significantly increased the number of their advocacy-related actions and outcomes compared with their respective baseline levels. The mean of the activist group, however, was significantly higher than the other two groups. Further analysis suggested that participants in the activist group gained greater benefit from the PPM program, compared with the other groups, because of their increased involvement in local or state networks, supports, and knowledge about activist strategies. After intervention, participants in the beginner group significantly increased their membership in relevant organizations and in the number of services they received. Participants in the activist group also reported significant improvement in their satisfaction with services.

Leadership academies: Severe mental illness. The information on the Idaho Leadership Academy (ILA) provided here is summarized from Hess and colleagues (2001). Mental health consultants, in conjunction with human service personnel (including a Native American health and human services agency), advocacy groups, and researchers developed the ILA. The ILA has three main goals: first, to teach participants the skills necessary to assume a leadership position in enhancing supports for mental health consumers and in the state's system of mental health services; second, to teach participants the skills needed to collect information to assess the impact of their mental health leadership activities on the local, state, and national levels; and third, to provide Academy graduates with an ongoing support system and opportunities to use their acquired skills in their local communities.

Each of the five ILA sessions is conducted for two- and a-half days. During the sessions, instructors teach leadership and advocacy skills using four workbooks, discussion, small group exercises, and role-play activities. The workbooks are based on those designed to teach advocacy skills to individuals with physical disabilities discussed in the previous sections of this chapter (e.g., Balcazar et al., 1990; Seekins et al., 1987). The advocacy skills include identifying and reporting relevant issues, conducting effective meetings, planning action steps to address identified issues, writing effective letters, and giving testimony to public officials. A team consisting of mental health professionals, a consumer, a family member, and a Native American modified the workbooks to enhance the content's relevance for the Idaho participants. Participants practice the skills by leading simulated meetings, writing action plans and letters, and making group presentations.

The ILA also uses the "concerns report method" to teach mental health consumers and family members to identify relevant local and state issues. The method has been previously used to identify community problems and possible solutions from the perspective of individuals with disabilities (Fawcett et al., 1988) and from economically disadvantaged backgrounds (Seekins & Fawcett, 1987). When using the concerns report method, the academy participants ask community groups to rate the importance of a variety of issues and their level of satisfaction with the community's efforts to address each issue. They determine a score for each issue by multiplying the level of importance by the level of satisfaction. Issues with the lowest level of satisfaction and highest level of importance are identified as high priority issues (see Consumer Concerns Report Method in "Additional Readings and Resources" at the end of this chapter to obtain a report of a Native American center using this method).

To identify high-priority issues for adults with severe mental illness and their families, a representative group of mental health consumers and family members is given a list of more than 100 possible issues for revision. The revised list is further reduced by mental health consumers and family members at the first ILA session. The issues can include employment, housing, health care, and stigma. The process results in two twenty-item concerns report surveys, one containing consumer concerns for use in surveys of consumers and the other concerns for use in surveys of families. The two concerns report surveys are then distributed to mental health consumers and family members in different regions of the state, including regions represented by minority populations, such as Native American reservations. After the top four issues and the top four strengths are determined, town meetings attended by mental health consumers and their families, the media, governmental staff, and members of the general public are held in the various regions. During the meetings, issues, as well as strengths, obstacles, and resources, are discussed and clarified. Participants brainstorm various methods to address concerns and develop action plans, and they form a number of teams to begin work on identified issues.

The ILA incorporates a number of strategies to achieve the third goal of providing Academy graduates with an ongoing support system and opportunities to use their acquired skills in their local communities. Graduates are invited to attend subsequent sessions of the Academy, where they serve as role models for new participants. The graduates provide an orientation, report on their recent advocacy actions, and discuss concerns and activities of local advocacy groups. Graduates also are given opportunities to participate in advanced training, in which they practice giving legislative testimony and learn skills for interacting with the media, public speaking, developing local advocacy groups, fund-raising, and computer networking. To provide further opportunities for support and networking, telephone conference calls are held approximately every six to eight weeks. During the conference calls, the graduates discuss their accomplishments, exchange advocacy information, engage in problem solving, and provide one another with support.

Evaluations of the ILA included assessments of both action and outcomes. Action is defined as "the working steps one takes on an issue, such as planning an event, researching a funding source, making significant telephone calls, putting together mailings, attending meetings, or preparing testimony." Outcomes are defined as "a tangible product of one or more advocacy actions, such as a group presentation, a response from a legislator, a consumer receiving a new service, an event held, an article printed in the newspaper, or a grant received" (Hess et al., 2001, p. 260). Data were gathered from 160 Academy graduates (only 1% of Idaho's population is Native American, but 20% of graduates were Native American) over a twenty-seven-month period. During this time, graduates participated in 1,345 advocacy actions and achieved 400 advocacy outcomes as a result of those actions.

Examples of specific outcomes at the local level include opening a facility that provided respite care and room and board for individuals with severe mental illness and reducing stigma in the community by developing a speaker's bureau and distributing educational brochures. At the state level, mental health consumers and their families increased the availability of information on consumer rights by participating in a task force that assisted in the adoption of a family involvement and consumer rights policy in mental health services. The task force also wrote an informational booklet on the topic, which was distributed throughout the state. Advocates in the Shoshone-Bannock tribe formed a suicide prevention task force.

Another evaluation determined that 68% of the 130 participants attending the first four ILA sessions continued involvement in mental health advocacy activities six months after attending the Academy; 43% of those attending one of the first three sessions continued their advocacy activities after one year. Illness or personal/family crisis, entering school or employment, and residential relocation were among the reasons for discontinuing advocacy activities. Opportunities to network with other consumers and family members, the increased support and confidence gained from the process, and learning advocacy skills were the three most helpful aspects of the program reported by the graduates. Participants ranked advocacy training the highest among additional types of assistance they would like to receive. Difficulties in choosing issues, deciding on the level of government on which to focus advocacy efforts, and finding and balancing time and energy between personal lives and advocacy activities were among the challenges the participants reported facing.

In 1995, in cooperation with existing advocacy organizations for the mentally ill and their families, Robert Hess established the West Virginia Leadership Academy (WVLA) for Consumers and Families (Sabin & Daniels, 2002). The remainder of the description of the WVLA is summarized from Stringfellow and Muscari (2003). The goals and training of the WVLA are similar to those of the ILA, and the training consists of two main components: (1) three to four days of structured training and (2) subsequent networking activities designed to reinforce and support application of the acquired skills. Most of the training is provided by volunteer Leadership Academy graduates using a standardized manual. The class content is structured around acquiring knowledge and skills in the six critical advocacy areas identified by Fawcett et al. (1984). The areas include the following.

1. Knowledge of relevant problems
2. Skills for reporting issues
3. Skills for group formation and leadership
4. Strategic planning
5. Controlling positive and negative consequences for decision makers (e.g., votes for elected officials and unfavorable media attention)
6. Structural variables (accessing critical information from various sources, such as from meeting agendas of elected officials)

In addition to developing skills and attitudes, the WVLA reinforces behaviors in groups and classes that are consistent with collective advocacy. For example, instructors assist academy participants in making the transition from the role of patient or client to the role of student and advocate by refocusing discussions and reinforcing advocacy behaviors.

The WVLA accomplishes the objective of its second component—maintaining the acquired knowledge and skills—by providing a network of advocacy activities through cooperation with the Academy, the West Virginia Bureau for Behavioral Health and Health Facilities, and the state's mental health advocacy community. An example of an activity is arranging conference calls, which provide opportunities for graduates to report on and discuss advocacy issues. Graduates are invited to attend an annual Leadership Academy conference, which provides additional training and opportunities to make presentations, and the biannual meetings of the West Virginia Mental Health Planning Council, which advocates, plans, and monitors the state's mental health system.

The graduates also are encouraged to participate in consumer organizations throughout the state and are active in a variety of other networking activities initiated by the Academy or by the graduates themselves. Examples of networking activities include sending out issue alerts, networking with one another, and attending a variety of other conferences (for additional information, see Consumer Organization and Networking Technical Assistance Center [CONTAC] in "Additional Readings and Resources" at the end of the chapter). More than 375 individuals have graduated from the WVLA. As a service of CONTAC, it assists in the organization and training of mental health consumers throughout the nation. However, no formal evaluation of the WVLA was provided.

Leadership academies: Elderly individuals. The Oklahoma Aging Advocacy Leadership Academy (OAALA) is a statewide training program providing skills and knowledge to assist elderly and other interested individuals in advocating aging services and programs (Baker et al., 2001; information that follows is summarized from this reference). The program consists of ten weekend sessions, which provide content on issues relevant to the elderly and advocacy and leadership skills training in the area of aging. To ensure the relevance of the curriculum, program developers conducted focus groups with senior advocates and members and leaders from relevant organizations (e.g., the AARP and the State Council on Aging). The groups assisted in identifying program topics and evaluating the developing curriculum. The OAALA recruits participants from both retired and baby boomer populations. The latter are recruited because they frequently cope with issues of the elderly, particularly in the caregiver role. Participants are selected based on their application, narrative statements, and letters of recommendation. However, efforts are made to select representative participants with regard to gender, age, geographic region, and type of employment.

The instructional approach of the academy considers the needs and interests of elderly learners. Didactic instruction is brief and limited. Instead, instructors emphasize discussions, experiential and small group activities, and homework assignments designed to apply the acquired skills and knowledge. For example, homework includes developing a personal resource file on an age-related topic, gathering information on age-related resources, researching an issue that participants would like to become social policy, and writing a letter to a legislator on a relevant issue. During the sessions, participants present their projects, complete exercises in critical thinking, and participate in role-play exercises. Elements of the two curricula tracks—age-related content and advocacy skills training—are blended throughout the ten sessions. Basic content of the ten sessions is related to the following topics: purpose of training; social issues related to aging; the state legislature; organizing for social change; older people's health and wellness; long-term care; caregiving, decision making, and ethics; diversity and aging and influencing the media; home care services; and putting it all together. Advocacy skills training teaches skills in communication, lobbying, strategies for change, media engagement, and negotiations for a home care services agreement.

Pretraining and posttraining assessments of participants' ratings of their familiarity with the sixty-five advocacy and volunteer leadership areas taught in the OAALA demonstrated a significant increase in scores across all items after training. Participants also rated the quality of eighteen aspects of the Academy (e.g., the presentations and appropriateness of the topics and exercises) very high (a mean of 5.7 on a scale of 1 to 6; 6 = excellent). While the participants were enrolled in the Academy during the eleven months, they were involved in multiple advocacy and volunteer activities. For example, the participants established a local voluntary organization for elders requiring assistance with dental and visual services; produced a video program on rural transportation problems faced by the elderly and individuals with disabilities and presented it to the state transportation department and other government officials; assisted older individuals and local service groups in obtaining free computers, installation, and software; and organized to save a local hospital by increasing the sales tax.

Women's health issues: Breast cancer. Staff at the National Breast Cancer Coalition (NBCC) developed Project LEAD, which teaches breast cancer activists relevant scientific knowledge and skills to assist them in participating in decision making related to breast cancer medical research and policy (Dickersin et al., 2001). The five-day course is offered four times a year in various cities across the United States, and NBCC provides the classes, course materials, and meals without charge. The organization also provides travel scholarships for eligible participants. Participants are selected based on a personal experience with breast cancer. In addition, they must demonstrate a desire to learn scientific concepts, a willingness to actively participate in the course, and a commitment to engaging in the process of breast cancer research and policy.

The main course topics of the LEAD program include (1) an introduction to basic science and epidemiology concepts, (2) a critical appraisal of the scientific literature and grant proposals, (3) the clinical features of breast cancer and the research process, (4) advocacy training for participating in research decisions, and (5) formulating an individual action plan for research involvement. Participants are given standardized material for each session, including lecture outlines, homework assignments, study group questions, and reference materials. A range of teaching methods is used. For example, college-level lectures are presented by distinguished scientists on topics focused primarily on science education, and instructors use interactive discussions of case scenarios. Lecture topics also include behavioral strategies for serving as members of research and related groups, and relevant advocacy opportunities are provided. Each evening, participants complete individual or group homework assignments (e.g., discussing lecture material). In order to prepare for participation in an Institutional Review Board or grant review study process, groups review a successful grant proposal and role-play their discussion points. Instructors and other participants provide feedback to group members on their scientific approach, problem-solving skills, and interactions (Dickersin et al., 2001).

After four years, 460 participants (81.7% white; 11.6% African American; 6.7% other racial/ethnic groups; all but one were female) attended Project LEAD. The precourse and postcourse measures demonstrated improvement in the participants' understanding of basic scientific concepts, enhanced critical appraisal skills, and increased reliance on academic sources versus advice of others (e.g., friends) to answer questions related to breast cancer. Participants also gained confidence in their ability to explain basic science and epidemiology concepts to others. Although Project LEAD provides some advocacy training to assist activists in fulfilling their commitment to advocate in science settings, NBCC's Annual Advocacy Conference specifically focuses on training activists (Dickersin et al., 2001; see National Breast Cancer Coalition in "Additional Readings and Resources" for information on the conference).

Training programs for breast cancer advocates similar to Project LEAD have been developed in Canada, some European countries, and Australia. Researchers evaluated the effectiveness of such a program in Australia (Davis, Salo, & Redman, 2001). The primary goal of the Australian program is to empower women to participate in various forums in which decisions concerning breast cancer are made. The program involves three days of science and advocacy training, using teaching techniques such as role playing, critically reviewing research, and interviewing a local politician. The women are taught skills for engaging in activities such as research, decision making (within the government, scientific community, and industry), increasing breast cancer awareness, serving on relevant committees, lobbying for policy changes, engaging in public speaking, writing for the media, and networking.

The evaluation involved fifty-one women (84.3% were breast cancer survivors; the majority had a college education) participating in the program in three different Australian states. A pretraining and posttraining assessment demonstrated that participants' involvement in breast cancer advocacy activities and organizations significantly increased after program participation. The activities included serving as a board or committee member, working on recruitment issues for clinical trials, enhancing patient resources (e.g., establishing support groups or patient advocacy programs), and participating in breast cancer advocacy groups. After training, participants also reported significant increases in feeling qualified to engage in advocacy-related breast cancer issues. However, the researchers found no changes in other advocacy areas, such as lobbying for change, circulating petitions, reviewing research protocols, writing letters to the editor, or involvement in key breast cancer organizations.

ANALYSIS AND CRITIQUE FOR PRACTICE AND RESEARCH

The CB interventions described in this chapter, which frequently are combined with other instructional techniques into multicomponent programs, empower vulnerable populations by assisting them in advocating their individual and collective rights, improving community and organizational practices, and actively participating in macro decision making that affects important areas of their lives. The CB strategies include PST and reinforcement but primarily involve SST, including specification of the skills, instruction, examples and exercises, rehearsal, reinforcement, feedback, and homework assignments. Strategies to prompt and sustain program gains also are used. Evaluations of the interventions and multicomponent programs suggest that they can increase the knowledge and enhance the advocacy and political skills of individuals with physical and developmental disabilities, severe mental illness, and low income; the elderly; and women with a history of breast cancer, as well as interested others.

Many of these interventions can be used by social workers, community organizers, educators, or other helping professionals working in any setting in which vulnerable groups (and significant others) desire to acquire the knowledge and skills to influence macro decision making, to advocate their rights, and to challenge organizational and community services or practices to be more responsive to their needs. Settings might include rehabilitation, health, mental health, education, and child welfare settings; community action agencies; and services for the elderly. Of course, government- and foundation-sponsored programs, including PPM, leadership academies, and Project LEAD, require significant financial resources to develop and to implement. However, social workers might make appropriate referrals when such programs are available. Social workers holding social policy–related or administrative positions also might find the content of this chapter relevant. These social workers are in a unique position to influence state and federal governments to support programs that develop the leadership and political skills of vulnerable populations and/or to foster similar programs in their own organizations and agencies.

Effectiveness and Additional Applications

Evaluations of the previously discussed CB interventions and programs were not rigorous. Only one study randomly assigned participants to an intervention or control group. More commonly, researchers used multiple-baseline and pretest-posttest designs. Researchers evaluated several of the multicomponent programs solely by asking participants to rate the effectiveness of the programs (e.g., the degree to which the program improved their advocacy skills) and to report on their advocacy and political activity after completing training. No baseline measures or comparison groups were used. In the more complex multicomponent programs, CB strategies were used in conjunction with other instructional approaches. Given these research design limitations, the extent to which the programs or specific CB interventions can enhance participants' knowledge and skills and increase their attempts to influence macro decision making and practices has not yet been determined. Whether involvement in advocacy and political activity actually results in macro-level change is even more difficult to establish.

Even if the interventions and programs are effective in achieving their stated goals, which vulnerable groups and individuals are able to benefit from them is unclear. This is particularly the case because of the self-selection and/or screening that occurred before participation. Even though efforts sometimes were made to recruit diverse participants (e.g., of different socioeconomic status and race/ethnicity), participants frequently varied little on background measures. The participants in many of the interventions were active in advocacy and other community and policy-related issues before training. In the case of the more comprehensive programs (e.g., Project LEAD, state PPMs, and OAALA), individuals were screened based on multiple criteria, such as commitment to advocacy, motivation, and possession of other personal resources needed to acquire and apply the knowledge and skills taught in the programs. Even when less cognitively demanding training materials, such as manuals that teach skills to effectively write letters and give personal testimony, were used, some ability to read, write, and/or speak cogently would be required. Many vulnerable groups, such as those with severe physical and cognitive disabilities, severe mental illness that is not in remission, and non-English speakers, would probably not benefit from such interventions, or additional types of assistance would need to be provided.

Despite these limitations, the interventions and programs suggest unique opportunities for practitioners to assist clients in becoming more active in influencing macro decision making. Practitioners can teach clients relevant knowledge and skills to enhance their ability to become actively involved in the type of services they receive, as well as in other community and social policy decisions that affect their lives. The quality of the research evaluating the CB interventions and programs also suggests opportunities for researchers to more rigorously evaluate them.

Practitioners also might use the interventions described in this chapter to assist the same vulnerable groups in influencing macro decision making in other areas, or to assist other vulnerable groups in identifying issues and advocating macro changes in areas that affect their lives. Researchers also have many opportunities to design and evaluate additional CB interventions and programs. Other areas might include welfare reform and other government programs for individuals with low income, and equal pay, hiring and promotion discrimination, maternity leave, and workplace harassment for women. Researchers might develop and evaluate CB programs for other vulnerable groups, such as racial/ethnic minorities, LGBT individuals, and recent immigrants, to assist them in advocating their group rights and influencing the macro decisions and practices that have an impact on their lives. Group rights and macro policies and practices might be related to immigration, and employment and housing discrimination, and other types of discrimination, involvement in the child welfare system, access to quality education and health care, safe and humane working conditions, and health issues, such as those related to AIDS care.

Freedom, Control, and Social Justice

The ultimate goals of the CB interventions and multicomponent programs discussed in this chapter—influencing organizational and community practices and social policies that affect the lives of vulnerable populations—are directly related to enhancing individual freedom and control. The goals also are consistent with social justice and the social work profession's commitment to ensuring that all individuals have access to relevant information and actively participate in making the decisions that influence their lives.

While the interventions discussed in this chapter are standardized to varying degrees, practitioners and researchers can use strategies incorporated into the interventions to enhance individual input and control over the standardized procedures. For example, self-paced self-help guides can be used as a "behavioral prosthetic" for writing advocacy letters and making personal testimony. In developing the guides, the researchers refrained from teaching specific content and choosing a particular issue of concern (i.e., telling individuals what to say) but used strategies to prompt effective style and organization. Other interventions and programs discussed in this chapter also enhance individual freedom and control by providing opportunities for participants to make choices and to establish their own goals both during and after intervention. For example, after advocacy groups learn particular skills, such as problem solving, leadership, decision making, letter writing, and public speaking, the skills can be applied to issues selected by the group and individual members. Finally, the more comprehensive programs discussed in this chapter used strategies to prompt participants to choose homework assignments and projects consistent with their own interests and goals.

Social Validity

Socially relevant goals and results. The developers of the CB interventions and multicomponent programs established the social validity of their outcome measures in a variety of ways. The ultimate goals of advocating individual and group rights and participating in macro decision making are consistent with societal and community group (e.g., the Independent Living movement) values. The ultimate goals of the interventions and programs should be important, desirable, and acceptable from the participants' perspective because the participants choose which issues and level of involvement (e.g., local, state, or national) their advocacy actions target. Steps also were taken to ensure the social relevance of the advocacy and political skills and knowledge that are the instrumental outcomes identified for change. They were selected through the use of methods such as surveying existing research, experts in the area, and advocacy groups, and observing actual testimony in public forums.

A number of the evaluations only determined whether the interventions resulted in participants achieving instrumental-type goals. These include increasing knowledge and skills such as problem solving, group decision making, public speaking, testimony, letter writing, and other advocacy behaviors, and group attendance. The social validity of these results is limited when it is not determined whether increasing knowledge, skills, and group attendance and improving group process translate into meaningful involvement in macro decision making or in influencing macro practices.

Other evaluations demonstrated that activities related to influencing macro decision making (e.g., contacting public officials and making media presentations) and involvement in organizations, committees, and groups consistent with the goals of the interventions increased after participation. The evaluations, however, only rarely measured whether increases in advocacy activity resulted in advocacy groups or participants successfully accomplishing their objectives. An example of more socially relevant results is that obtained by Balcazar and his colleagues (1990). The researchers determined that advocacy actions and favorable outcomes of those actions (e.g., increased curb cuts in a downtown area for wheelchairs) increased after intervention enhanced the group process of a disabilities advocacy group.

Evaluations of the CB interventions and multicomponent programs also varied in the methods and the degree to which they measured whether intervention gains were meaningful and relevant to the participants or to the contexts in which the skills were to be used. Some evaluations used participants' self-reports or paper-and-pencil assessments of changes in knowledge (e.g., basic scientific concepts and advocacy issues) yet provided no criteria to judge whether the changes were meaningful. Other evaluations suggest methods that practitioners and researchers might use to determine the social validity of intervention gains. Expert raters, such as a public administrator, a former mayor, and an independent living center board president, can judge the overall quality and likely influence of advocacy behaviors, such as public testimony and letters to public officials. Establishing a correlation between expert ratings and the percentage of targeted responses exhibited by participants (e.g., for making public testimonies) is another indicator of socially valid intervention gains. Performance of target skills can be observed in natural settings, such as evaluating problem-solving skills in the context of a policy board meeting for low-income members. Researchers can also evaluate whether intervention gains are meaningful, relevant, and important from the participants' perspective by asking participants to rate their attitudes (e.g., self-confidence in applying specific knowledge and skills), the effectiveness of the program (e.g., improved self-advocacy skills), and the importance of the training.

An example of informing participants of possible positive and negative consequences as a result of engaging in different advocacy actions is provided in the manuals prepared to assist individuals with disabilities in achieving goals related to advocacy activities. Few evaluations of the interventions and programs described in this chapter, however, reported investigating whether unfavorable outcomes occurred as a result of engaging in the advocacy and political behaviors. An example is experiencing embarrassment as a result of discussing one's life circumstances. Assessing unfavorable and unexpected results of an intervention is an important aspect of evaluating the social validity of an intervention, and such an assessment also has other important implications. Practitioners and researchers can use this information to assist clients and participants in anticipating and planning for such outcomes, which also should assist in maintaining intervention gains.

Socially relevant intervention procedures. Efforts to establish the social validity of the interventions and content of the multicomponent programs described in this chapter varied. Some of the programs screened individuals based on certain criteria, such as motivation and commitment to advocacy, but none of the interventions were preceded by individual functional assessments. A functional assessment could have determined other maintaining antecedents (e.g., time, transportation, limitations of various disabilities, and cultural values) or consequences (e.g., aversive reactions from others) that were deterring participants from performing the skills they already possessed. The results of such assessments could indicate the need for additional relevant interventions. However, before researchers developed the interventions for assisting the self-help and advocacy groups to function more effectively, they assessed the groups' processes. Problems such as a lack of problem-solving skills, disorganization, inability to reach decisions, implementation of few actions, and a focus on internal organizational issues were assessed and relevant skills were identified to change these maintaining conditions.

In addition to completing functional assessments, practitioners and researchers might adopt other methods identified in this chapter to enhance the social validity of their interventions. For example, experts on particular topics (e.g., science education) can teach program content. Current literature can be surveyed to determine appropriate responses, exercises, and examples. Socially relevant content for effective advocacy letters can be identified through an examination of examples of advocacy letters written by other individuals with similar problems (e.g., a disability). Advocates and leaders in relevant areas (e.g., aging) can be involved in curriculum design and evaluation. A team composed of multiple shareholders (e.g., mental health professionals, consumers, family members, and Native Americans) can assist in evaluating and modifying content of workbooks to ensure their relevance to participants interested in advocating for particular issues (e.g., mental health). Finally, researchers and practitioners can evaluate the acceptability and feasibility of training procedures after intervention by asking participants to rate the overall quality of the program, as well as their satisfaction and happiness with the content.

Many of the CB interventions used to teach advocacy knowledge and skills, such as problem solving, public speaking, testimony, letter writing, and group decision making, and to increase group attendance can be carried out in many different types of settings by practitioners trained in CB methods. This is particularly the case with the assistance of the intervention manuals. Although adopting some of the interventions from the multicomponent programs might be practical and feasible in some settings, administering the overall programs requires time, effort, specialized resources (e.g., scientific knowledge), and government or another type of financial support that might not always be available.

Practitioners and researchers also can learn from the special accommodations and adaptations used in the interventions and multicomponent programs discussed in this chapter. They include using oral instead of written instruction to teach public speaking skills and ensuring written materials are at a high school reading level to accommodate the participants' educational backgrounds. Programs such as Project LEAD provide the training free of charge and travel scholarships for eligible participants, and the Illinois PPM program provides support services to individuals with developmental disabilities. The services include reviews and discussions of the agendas and content of the training sessions, answering questions, and providing assistance with homework assignments. For older learners, adaptations include focusing on brief and limited didactic instruction and on learning activities that are experiential and active.

Maintenance and generalization. Several evaluations of the interventions and multicomponent programs described in this chapter failed to determine whether intervention gains, such as in specific skills, knowledge, or advocacy activity, were maintained after formal intervention. One of the evaluations assessed gains in group problem-solving skills six weeks after training and found that only some of the participants' skills were maintained at high levels. Other evaluations assessed both maintenance and transfer of the skills to natural settings (e.g., involvement in advocacy and related activities to influence organizational and community practices and social policy) five to six months after intervention. One study (White et al., 1997) determined that the participants wrote no advocacy letters during the six-month follow-up but failed to determine possible reasons for this outcome.

Practitioners and researchers might learn from the reasons provided by participants in the PPM programs and leadership academies for failing to transfer the acquired skills to their own lives or to continue their advocacy activities. Barriers to engaging in or continuing advocacy activities included time, expense, negative emotions resulting from disclosing personal stories, illness, personal or family crisis, enrolling in school, starting a new job, and residential relocation. These responses suggest that practitioners teaching advocacy interventions and researchers developing related programs might assist participants in transferring advocacy activities to natural settings and continuing them by identifying and addressing such conditions.

The multicomponent programs discussed in this chapter recognize that graduates require ongoing reinforcement, prompting, opportunities to practice the advocacy skills, and additional training to maintain and build on their skills. Practitioners and future advocacy program designers might adopt some of these strategies. For example, program graduates are invited to attend subsequent sessions where they provide orientation to new participants, report on their advocacy actions, and discuss concerns and activities of their local advocacy groups. Graduates are provided with opportunities to participate in advanced training. Establishing supportive advocacy networks that prompt and reinforce use of the acquired knowledge and skills also might maintain training gains. Examples include conference calls, annual conferences, ongoing encouragement from other graduates, and mailings of issue alerts and legislative updates. The evaluation conducted by Balcazar and his colleagues (1996) with former participants of the Illinois PPM also illustrates the importance of social supports and social change knowledge if engaging in advocacy-related actions and achieving relevant outcomes are to continue.

This and the previous nine chapters described and evaluated CB interventions that empower vulnerable populations by assisting them in achieving four main types of goals: increasing and accessing social resources, securing economic resources, enhancing self-determination, and influencing organizations, communities, and social policy. The next and final chapter provides a brief summary of the effectiveness of the interventions discussed in the intervention chapters, discusses the consistency between empowerment and the CB interventions, and provides directions for practice and future research.

ADDITIONAL READINGS AND RESOURCES

Balcazar, F. E., Keys, C. B., Bertram, J. F., & Rizzo, T. (1996). Advocate development in the field of developmental disabilities: A data-based conceptual model. *Mental Retardation, 6,* 341–351.

Consumer Concerns Report Method. Lawrence, KS: Research and Training Center on Independent Living, University of Kansas. A report on using this method by the American Indian Disability Technical Assistance Center is available at http://rtcil.org/concerns.htm

Consumer Organization and Networking Technical Assistance Center, P. O. Box 11000, Charleston, WV 25339. Additional information is available at http://www.contac.org

National Breast Cancer Coalition, 1101 17th St., NW, Suite 1300, Washington, DC 20036. Additional information on the NBCC is available at http://www.natlbcc.org/, on Project LEAD at http://www.natlbcc.org/bin/index.asp?strideq552&depid=18&btnid=7, and on the Annual Advocacy Conference at http://www.natlbcc.org/bin/index.asp?strid=713&depid=7&btnid=2

Oklahoma Aging Advocacy Leadership Academy (OAALA). Additional information is available at http://www.workworld.org/wwwebhelp/aging_services_overview_oklahoma.htm

Partners in Policymaking. Further information on state programs and online courses are available at http://www.partnersinpolicymaking.com/

Seekins, T., Balcazar, F., & Fawcett, S. B. (1986). *Consumer involvement in advocacy organizations. Vol I: Monitoring and reporting events. Vol II: Conducting effective meetings. Vol III: Project planning guide. Vol IV: Teaching advocacy skills.* Lawrence, KS: Research and Training Center on Independent Living, University of Kansas.

Seekins, T., & Fawcett, S. B. (n.d.). *A guide to writing letters to public officials: Contributing to important decisions affecting you and others; A guide to writing letters to the editor: Expressing your opinion to the public effectively; a guide for personal testimony: The art of using your personal experiences to influence policy decisions.* Lawrence, KS: Research and Training Center on Independent Living, University of Kansas. Available at http://www.rtcil.org/products/index.shtml

West Virginia Leadership Academy, Technical Assistance Center, P. O. Box 11000, Charleston, WV 25339. Additional information is available at http://wvla.wvmhca.org/

White, G. W., Thomson, R., & Nary, D. E. (1998). *The action letter portfolio.* Lawrence, KS: Research and Training Center on Independent Living, University of Kansas. Available at http://www.rtcil.org/products/index.shtml

14 Summary, Practice Implications, and Future Research

As the previous ten chapters suggest, CB interventions can be used to assist vulnerable populations in attaining four broad goals consistent with an empowerment perspective. In this final chapter, a summary of the effectiveness of the previously discussed interventions is provided and additional applications are suggested. The consistency between CB methods and empowerment is considered again, including issues of personal freedom and control, social justice, and social validity. In each section, suggestions are provided for practice and future research on CB interventions to assist vulnerable populations in attaining empowerment-related goals. The chapter ends with a few concluding comments.

EFFECTIVENESS AND ADDITIONAL APPLICATIONS

Evaluations of the CB interventions described in the previous chapters provide varying degrees of evidence that the interventions can assist vulnerable populations, including racial/ethnic and sexual minorities, the poor and elderly, females, and individuals with mental health, developmental, learning, physical, and sensory disabilities, in achieving empowerment goals. The goals are (1) accessing and increasing social resources, such as social interactions and friendships, leisure/recreational activity, and assistance to enhance well-being; (2) acquiring, maintaining, and increasing economic resources through employment and public and private sources; (3) enhancing self-determination by increasing control and input into personal decision making, increasing choice making in routine and more long-term decisions, and securing legal and personal rights; and (4) influencing the social policies and organizational and community practices that affect the lives of vulnerable groups.

A variety of CB interventions are used, including skills training, SST, prompting, reinforcement, enriching and changing the physical and social environments, cognitive restructuring, problem solving, and several other self-managed strategies, such as self-recording, self-instruction, self-monitoring, and self-reinforcement. Some CB applications involve a few simple procedures, while others combine a variety of interventions into multicomponent programs that are implemented with standardized manuals or training modules. Although the majority of the interventions and programs involve only CB strategies, some multicomponent programs (e.g., in chapter 13) integrate these methods with other education techniques.

As I have noted, the quality of the research that evaluated the CB interventions varies but relied heavily on single-system, multiple-baseline, and pretest-posttest designs. Relatively few of the interventions were evaluated using experimental methods in which participants were randomly assigned to a CB intervention or to a control or other intervention group. Even when research indicated a change in an ultimate outcome, such as in loneliness or employment, whether those changes were a result of attaining instrumental goals, such as enhanced social or job interview skills, was infrequently formally examined. In addition, participants rarely benefitted equally from the interventions, and outcome measures for a few of the participants even deteriorated. Finally, which CB interventions are the most effective to achieve particular outcomes for particular clients is far from determined. Given the research design limitations of the majority of the evaluations of the interventions presented in this book, firm conclusions on their effectiveness to achieve particular outcomes, and whether the interventions are more effective than alternative methods, cannot be established without further research.

The interventions described in the previous chapters were chosen because they were designed to achieve particular goals for individuals who share common characteristics, such as gender, low income, race/ethnicity, or a disability. Whether the study findings are applicable to others with similar characteristics is uncertain, because none of the evaluations randomly selected participants from a population of individuals who met the inclusion criteria. Participants were self-referred or referred by agency staff, educators, or significant others. In studies that included participants who had some similar characteristics (e.g., a psychiatric or physical disability) but varied in other characteristics (e.g., race/ethnicity), researchers rarely determined whether the interventions were equally effective for all participants. Other screening procedures, such as including only participants with a particular level of communicative ability or excellent school attendance, further complicate determining the applicability of the interventions to clients who share a common vulnerability.

Determining whether the interventions are applicable to individuals with different vulnerabilities, but striving to achieve similar goals, also requires further research. Some interventions, such as those used to teach knowledge and self-advocacy skills to achieve individual, community, and social policy goals, obviously are not applicable to certain groups (e.g., those with severe cognitive disabilities). The interventions presented here also are not a panacea for the complex and multiple problems that confront vulnerable clients. Many of these clients require additional assistance, such as pharmacological intervention for clients with severe mental illness.

Although the effectiveness of the interventions is inconclusive, social workers and other professionals might find them useful for assisting vulnerable clients in achieving the empowerment goals identified in this book. Further suggestions for applications to other vulnerable clients in a variety of settings are provided in the end-of-chapter summaries. Practitioners can offer the interventions as options to achieve a mutually established individual or group goal, accompanied with an explanation of the evidence supporting the effectiveness of the interventions, along with any evidence supporting alternative interventions, and potential benefits and risks. That participants did not respond equally to the previously described interventions suggests two important practice implications. First, practitioners should conduct individual functional assessments before intervention to determine whether the planned interventions are appropriate. Second, ongoing assessments should be conducted to determine whether client goals are being met. Offering informed choices to clients, conducting individual assessments, and assessing goal attainment all are consistent with an empowerment perspective.

The quality of the research that evaluated the interventions described in this book suggests opportunities for researchers to conduct more rigorous evaluations. Opportunities also exist for developing and evaluating CB methods to achieve similar goals for vulnerable populations for whom current interventions have not yet been developed and evaluated. The end-of-chapter summaries provide suggestions for such applications. Other areas of research also can enhance the effectiveness of CB interventions for vulnerable clients. Among these are identifying the reasons for participants' failure to achieve their goals or deterioration on outcome measures, and using that information to develop more effective interventions. Within samples sharing common characteristics, such as a physical disability, evaluating the effect of other characteristics, such as gender, sexual identity, and race/ethnicity, on goal achievement also can inform the development of more effective interventions. Determining whether acquiring particular skills (e.g., social or advocacy skills) is related to attaining ultimate goals (e.g., forming friendships or securing one's legal rights) is another important line of research. Finally, examining the ideal intensity and length of sessions, developing valid and reliable assessment instruments, and identifying the necessary components in multi-intervention programs and special accommodations for specific vulnerable groups can make important contributions to developing CB interventions that empower vulnerable populations.

The breadth and depth of the interventions within the chapters of this book also highlight areas for future design and evaluation of CB interventions to empower vulnerable groups. For example, the interventions described in part II, which assist vulnerable populations in accessing and increasing social resources, are relatively numerous. The relatively few interventions in chapter 13, which discusses CB methods that assist vulnerable groups in influencing organizations, communities, and social policy, reflect the scarcity of applications in these contexts. Compared with researchers in other fields (e.g., education, psychology, community psychology, psychiatry), social work researchers are absent or underrepresented in many of the intervention chapters. This is particularly the case in the chapters discussing CB interventions that assist vulnerable populations in enhancing personal control, advocating their legal rights, and participating in the macro decisions that affect their lives. The lack of social work research on CB applications that achieve these types of outcomes might be the reason some social work scholars have concluded that CB interventions are politically conservative. That is, the interventions only assist individuals and groups in adapting to unresponsive or unjust environments rather than effecting change of the social context. Interventions described in this book demonstrate that researchers can develop and practitioners can use CB methods to assist vulnerable groups not only in accessing available social and economic resources, but in attaining their own goals, securing their personal and legal rights, and changing environments when they are unjust or unresponsive to their needs.

Some of the interventions described in the previous chapters are relatively old, particularly those provided in part III, which focuses on acquiring, maintaining, and increasing economic resources. The final chapter in part III, which discusses CB interventions that assist vulnerable groups in accessing economic resources from their social support networks and other community sources, is comparatively small. These interventions are particularly relevant to social work, a field that has been traditionally concerned about the welfare of the economically disadvantaged. As social work scholars have argued, the profession is in a unique position to develop and evaluate interventions to assist the working poor, the underemployed, recent immigrants, older workers, and clients in Welfare-to-Work programs in enhancing their economic well-being (Iversen, 1998; Mor-Barak & Tynan, 1993). Social work researchers can develop and evaluate CB methods that can be used alone or in conjunction with the multiple other interventions frequently needed to assist individuals who are economically disadvantaged in acquiring, maintaining, and increasing their economic resources.

EMPOWERMENT AND COGNITIVE-BEHAVIORAL INTERVENTIONS
Individual Freedom and Control

Labeling CB interventions designed to achieve certain goals as "empowering" is not meant to imply that social workers and other professionals who use them are not "experts" or do not serve social control functions, thus constraining clients' personal freedom in different ways. Selection of treatment goals and interventions is limited by many factors, including the characteristics, capabilities, and skills of the clients themselves; societal standards and laws; and organizational or agency norms, goals, and funding sources. Regardless of practitioners' values or theoretical approach to practice, they assume primary responsibility for making final decisions on client goals, interventions, and the degree to which clients are involved in the decision-making process (Rothman, 1989). Practitioners need to acknowledge to clients, as appropriate, the social control function of their position and involve clients as far as possible, and significant others when applicable, in establishing treatment goals and in choosing interventions.

As Gambrill (1985) noted, the greater the power differential between individuals, the more caution practitioners, supervisors, and others must take to ensure that clients play a significant role in selecting goals and interventions. Clearly, the application of many interventions described in this book highlights power imbalances between the participants and the researchers, practitioners, educators, and staff who played significant roles in defining the goals and in selecting and administering the interventions. This power differential is heightened by participants' characteristics, including cognitive, mental, and physical disabilities, and the constraints inherent in many of the settings (e.g., schools, residential facilities, group homes, and employment sites) in which the interventions were administered. In many of these settings, as Bannerman, Sheldon, Sherman, and Harchik (1990) observe, a conflict exists between an individual's right to choose, and refuse, service goals and interventions, and the individual's "right to habilitation." The latter they define as learning the skills "needed to live as independently as possible" (p. 79).

Unfortunately, practitioners, educators, agency staff, family members, and guardians unnecessarily compromise personal freedom to achieve habilitation. For example, clients with disabilities too frequently are given little or no input into setting their own goals, establishing preferences to reach their goals, or choosing among procedures to attain their goals. As Bannerman and her colleagues (1990) recommend, and as this book demonstrates, practitioners can use methods to identify the preferences of vulnerable clients when they have difficulty in clearly communicating them. Methods include observation, interviewing significant others, and teaching clients to select among paired alternatives. Practitioners then can teach clients choice-making skills, offer relevant choices, and also train staff and significant others to offer client choices and teach clients to make their own choices. In addition, clients can be taught to use communication-enhancing devices and strategies (e.g., communication books, choice charts, and augmented communication systems) to communicate their choices.

CB interventions and technology, however, cannot resolve other issues related to the degree of choice clients are given and to clients' choices that conflict with habilitation or educational and other goals or place their safety and well-being at risk. These issues of choice and freedom can only be informed by societal and professional values and ethics, agency and organizational mandates, funding sources, and the skills and capacities of clients. However, practitioners and administrators are obligated to evaluate whether the freedom of vulnerable clients in organizational, educational, residential, work, and institutionalized settings is being unnecessarily constrained. For example, staff might be untrained and offer few or no choices to clients, and clients might lack the necessary technology to communicate their choices. Those constraints frequently are built into institutional and organizational practices, which practitioners can advocate to change, or they can teach advocacy skills to clients and/or significant others to advocate the changes themselves. Providing opportunities for client input into administrative decisions also can provide other advantages. For example, the evaluation of design changes in a psychiatric facility for elderly patients described in chapter 4 (Bakos et al., 1980) determined that residents who participated in making the changes improved their social interactions more than other residents.

Using any of the standardized CB interventions or multicomponent programs described in the previous chapters certainly can restrict clients' freedom to some degree, which can be inconsistent with an empowerment perspective. The use of standardized or manual-based interventions, which have been routinely used with clients sharing the same diagnosed disorder or problem, has both supporters and challengers (Eifert, Schulte, Zvolensky, Lejuez, & Lau, 1997). Challengers argue that even if clients share the same disorder or problem, the maintaining conditions are not necessarily the same. In such cases, standardized interventions might lead to inappropriate or insufficient intervention. In addition, some clients might not require all of the many components of standardized or manual-based interventions, and rigid application of such interventions might be counterproductive. For example, clients might drop out of treatment after being asked to engage in irrelevant or unnecessary activities. Consistent with these arguments is anecdotal case information suggesting that when practitioners use structured, directive interventions, they might send the message that clients *need* directing, thereby causing resistance and undermining self-efficacy (Goldfried & Castonguay, 1993).

On the other hand, Eifert and colleagues (1997) argue that standardized intervention manuals have made important contributions to developing, evaluating, and disseminating evidence-based therapies. Applying standardized interventions can be time efficient and cost effective, which has obvious benefits for clients, agencies, funding sources, and society. These researchers also present evidence that for many common problems individualizing treatment beyond a clinical diagnosis does not improve intervention outcomes, thus questioning the assumption that intervention always must be narrowly tailored to an individual behavior and its maintaining conditions. A consensus appears to be forming that not enough evidence is available to determine under which conditions matching interventions to the maintaining conditions of an identified behavior is more effective than using standardized interventions for particular disorders or problems (e.g., Eifert et al., 1997; Gresham, 2003; Heckaman, Conroy, Fox, & Chait, 2000; Van Acker et al., 2005).

The extent to which individuals and groups value structured, directive, or didactic instruction and the extent to which negative consequences (e.g., noncompliance, resistance, or dropping out of treatment) result from using such interventions are unclear. These are topics of future research. Despite this ongoing debate, strategies that practitioners can use to enhance client freedom and control of the CB interventions exist. Practitioners can adopt a more collaborative, nonjudgmental, and empathic interaction style, such as that used by the group facilitators described in one of the HIV-risk reduction interventions (Carey et al., 2000). This is consistent with Gutiérrez's (1990) belief that adopting a teaching style similar to a consultant or facilitator, not an instructor or a trainer, is central to empowerment. Practitioners can take advantage of treatment manuals that are designed to be flexible by including assessment procedures, guidance on the use of relevant modules for particular situations, and optional sections, and applying validated principles of behavior rather than fixed strategies (Eifert et al., 1997; Henin, Otto, & Reilly-Harrington, 2001). The interventions in the previous chapter provide many examples of adapting commonly accepted interventions to the specific circumstances of clients. Some of these are discussed in the social validity section of this chapter.

Clients' freedom and control of the intervention process also can be enhanced by instruction in a variety of self-management strategies, including self-recording, self-instruction, self-prompting, self-evaluation, self-reinforcement, and problem solving. Practitioners can provide an opportunity for clients to exhibit an identified behavior (e.g., social, work, leisure, and advocacy skills) before using techniques such as direct instruction and modeling. Graduated prompting strategies, which use the least intrusive intervention necessary to assist clients in performing the target skill (e.g., ranging from visual prompts to physical guidance), also can enhance client control over the intervention process while recognizing clients' strengths and capabilities.

Finally, any contradiction between the use of CB procedures and empowerment was addressed in chapter 3, where it was argued that there is no inconsistency between the use of standardized interventions and empowerment if clients are knowledgeable about and choose the intervention. In addition, if the intervention results in a client or group acquiring the desired knowledge and skills, the intervention gains can enhance freedom of choice and control. For example, individuals can choose to establish social relationships; to engage in a particular recreational, work, or routine activity; to establish and achieve their employment, educational, and personal goals; to advocate their legal and personal rights; and to participate in the macro decisions that affect the services they receive and other areas of their lives. Many of the standardized CB interventions discussed in this book were designed with the specific goal of enhancing those aspects of individual freedom and control.

This discussion, as well as the end-of-chapter summaries, suggests a number of methods for practitioners, administrators, and those involved more directly in social policy decisions to enhance vulnerable clients' freedom, control, and input into the intervention process, as well as into other decisions that affect their lives. Researchers also can design and evaluate additional CB interventions that enhance clients' freedom and control in a variety of areas, including mental health, child welfare, education, employment, health and rehabilitation, and social action. The interventions can (1) provide guidelines for individual functional assessments; (2) incorporate CB principles and research-based interventions, while maximizing flexibility and opportunities for clients to make choices, including goal and intervention selection; (3) assist clients with communicative difficulties in choosing and communicating their preferences and goals and in carrying out the interventions; and (4) enhance the self-determination, self-advocacy, and political action skills of vulnerable groups to achieve more control over the macro decisions that affect their treatment and other areas of their lives.

The Social Justice Perspective

Margolin (1997) admonished the social work profession for deceiving itself and others by invoking the word *empowerment*. She argues the use of the word *empowerment* promotes the view that the profession is changing the structural, institutional, and attitudinal causes of social problems, such as poverty and racism. In reality, Margolin says, social workers primarily use individual-level interventions that only perpetuate inequalities. As discussed in chapter 3, scholars from social justice and strengths-based perspectives also have criticized interventions focusing on individual deficits for similar reasons.

This book also uses the word *empowerment* and focuses on individual- and group-level interventions to assist vulnerable populations in acquiring knowledge and skills that are assumed to be lacking. The direct targets of the interventions are not social attitudes, institutions, or political structures. For example, teaching social or choice-making skills to children with disabilities does not necessarily change the negative attitudes about disabilities held by others, affect political processes that provide insufficient resources, or alter organizational practices that offer few choices. Acquiring employment, job hunting, and job-related social skills does not guarantee that even when individuals secure or maintain employment they will command a living wage, obtain reasonable benefits, become socially integrated into the workplace, or work in environments that are free from discrimination. Even when the ultimate goals are more consistent with traditional social justice issues, such as securing legal rights and changing attitudes, social policy, and community and organizational practices, vulnerable groups and significant others are taught the identified knowledge and skills to achieve the goals.

On the other hand, assisting vulnerable groups in acquiring knowledge and skills that enhance their ability to access existing social and economic resources, when they are adequate, to become more integrated into work, educational, and community settings, to choose a desired option, and to secure their personal and legal rights is consistent with social justice and an empowerment perspective. In addition, social change can be effected only through individual behavior. Offering opportunities to vulnerable groups and significant others to learn and use political and self-advocacy knowledge and skills is not inconsistent with social justice and humanistic values. On the contrary, vulnerable groups have demanded to participate in such activities. Evaluations of the CB interventions described in part IV and chapter 13 of part V provide evidence that vulnerable groups can use their acquired knowledge and skills to advocate for themselves, to secure their own rights, and to influence structural and attitudinal constraints at the local, state, and national levels. However, a note of caution is necessary here. In many circumstances simply teaching relevant knowledge and skills to vulnerable groups and/or interested others is insufficient to make many of the necessary policy and structural changes that are required to gain access to decision-making processes, social and economic resources, and equal opportunity. Communicating such an expectation can be unrealistic without the use of other strategies and assistance of other groups.

Practitioners desiring to increase the consistency of their interventions with a social justice and empowerment perspective also might learn from the end-of-chapter summaries. For example, although maintaining conditions can involve individual limitations, such as a lack of knowledge or skills, they also can include other conditions. Negative reactions from others in residential, organizational, education, and other community settings; insufficient opportunities; inadequate existing social and economic resources; and constraining organizational, community, or social policies might be among those conditions. By conducting an individualized assessment, practitioners can identify such maintaining conditions and design strategies to change them.

Although this book has focused on using CB interventions to assist vulnerable individuals and groups in resolving community and social problems, other scholars have used CB theories and frameworks to analyze social and community problems and to suggest relevant interventions, programs, and social policies. The problems include substance abuse, world conflict, welfare reform, environmental community design, and discrimination in schools (e.g., Biglan, Glasgow, & Singer, 1990; Ellis, 1992; Fawcett, Mathews, & Fletcher, 1980; Mattaini, 1993; Mattaini & Thyer, 1996; Opulente & Mattaini, 1997; Thyer et al., 1986). The extent to which CB principles and methods can be used to analyze, inform, and change macro practices and policies, either by enhancing the ability of individuals and groups to advocate policy change or by informing policy makers directly, is yet to be determined. Nonetheless, those scholars and the content of this book suggest such opportunities.

Social Validity

Feminist and other scholars have criticized CB assessment, intervention, and evaluation procedures for a variety of reasons (see chapter 3), many of which CB scholars have referred to as issues of social validity or relevance. Social validity concerns the establishment of socially relevant goals; demonstration of meaningful change; use of acceptable, appropriate, and feasible interventions; and maintenance and generalization of intervention gains. Wolf's (1978) seminal article arguing that behavioral therapy researchers must measure the social validity of their goals, interventions, and results and the historic importance placed on the related problems of maintaining and transferring treatment gains might lead one to expect more recent evaluation studies to report on these issues. But, as the evaluations of the CB interventions discussed in this book, as well as reviews elsewhere (Carr, Austin, Britton, Kellum, & Bailey, 1999; Clarke et al., 2002) demonstrate, this is far from the case. In spite of the insufficient attention given to social validity, a number of practice and research implications related to this area can be drawn from the interventions described in this book, as well as from other sources. These implications are discussed in the following four sections.

Establishing socially relevant goals. Treatment goals that are socially relevant are important, acceptable, desirable, and achievable from the perspective of the client and others involved in the interventions. In addition to conducting individualized assessments and actively involving clients and relevant others in goal selection, the previous chapters of this book suggest several other methods that practitioners and researchers can use to enhance the social validity of instrumental and ultimate intervention goals. Five of those methods are discussed now.

First, establish intervention goals that are consistent with important social values, such as forming social relationships, engaging in recreational/leisure activity, increasing economic resources, enhancing self-determination (e.g., securing legal and personal rights), and participating in the macro decision making that influences individuals' lives. Of course, practitioners and researchers must use caution, because some intervention goals, such as teaching children choice-making and self-advocacy skills, might conflict with parental, cultural, or other organizational values.

Second, examine the research literature that establishes relations between an identified goal (e.g., obtaining necessary accommodations for individuals with disabilities) and other relevant outcomes (e.g., satisfactory job and educational performance).

Third, survey individuals with similar characteristics, significant others (e.g., parents, teachers, residential staff, job coaches, and work supervisors), and individuals with expertise or experience in the relevant area (e.g., consult members of a disabilities advocacy group to identify goals for an advocacy program) to assist in establishing important, acceptable, desirable, and achievable intervention goals.

Fourth, observe interactions in natural environments to identify relevant behaviors for which intervention goals are established (e.g., observing children interacting in a school setting to identify socially relevant social skills).

Fifth, facilitate individual goal setting within the broader goals of a standardized program (e.g., individuals and groups establish their own political advocacy goals within a program's broader goal of increasing involvement in decisions made at the local, state, and national levels of government).

Despite these suggestions, the previous chapters of this book indicate some problems in establishing socially valid intervention goals that practitioners and researchers should consider. Special care must be taken in identifying and establishing achievable goals for many vulnerable clients, particularly for those with multiple and/or severe physical, developmental, or psychiatric disabilities. For example, full-time independent employment might not be a feasible goal for some clients with severe mental illness, such as schizophrenia. Instead, working part time while receiving the lowest level of support necessary to maintain job performance might be a socially valid goal. For other clients, such as those with severe physical or developmental disabilities, a viable and important goal might be making very small changes in a specific behavior.

The example in chapter 11 of some students with severe disabilities being indifferent to or preferring other students to make choices regarding recreational activity, even though choice making is assumed to be a socially relevant goal, suggests three practice and research implications.

First, practitioners and researchers cannot assume that because a goal is consistent with societal, professional, or significant others' values it will be preferred by all clients or in all situations. Second, to determine whether the treatment goal is and continues to be acceptable, initial and ongoing client assessment is necessary. Finally, additional work is needed to identify methods to enhance the communicative capability of clients with limited ability to communicate their goals and desires.

A number of the intervention goals also appear to lack some dimension of social validity. For example, goals for increasing social relationships frequently measure the number, length, and quality of social interactions but neglect more meaningful goals, such as establishing relationships or becoming socially competent in a variety of contexts. Other interventions establish instrumental goals related to increasing knowledge of legal rights and enhancing advocacy skills but omit ultimate goals related to actually using the acquired skills to secure legal rights. Many clients probably would not consider goals such as increasing social interactions and legal rights knowledge and skills acceptable and desirable if goals related to establishing relationships and securing legal rights are not also set. These observations challenge practitioners and researchers to establish intervention goals that are viable and meaningful to those who participate in the interventions.

Socially relevant results. Practitioners and researchers also should determine whether their intervention results are socially valid. Socially valid results refer to the extent to which the intervention gains are meaningful, relevant, or sufficient for participants and/or relevant others to conclude that a difference has been made in an important aspect of the participants' lives. The CB interventions described in the previous chapters use a number of methods to assess and establish the social validity of the changes observed on both instrumental and ultimate outcomes. Six of those strategies follow.

First, use standardized scales (e.g., survival skills knowledge, self-determination, social support, self-efficacy, and social competence), particularly those with established validity and reliability, to measure the degree of intervention change. Second, observe the skills performed in natural settings, such as social interactions in a recreational setting or problem-solving skills in the context of a policy board meeting. However, practitioners and researchers cannot assume that group or individual increases on a behavioral scale or observations of improvements in identified behaviors necessarily indicate that the changes are relevant or meaningful to the clients and relevant others.

Third, conduct interviews and administer questionnaires requiring qualitative judgments of clients and relevant others (e.g., parents, teachers, residential staff, caretakers, job coaches, friends, and experts). For example, clients can rate their attitudes (e.g., self-confidence in applying the acquired knowledge and skills), their perceptions of program effectiveness (e.g., improved self-advocacy skills), and the importance of the training to some aspect of their lives. Experts, such as an independent living center's board president, can judge the overall quality and likely influence of changes in behaviors, such as in public testimony and writing letters to public officials.

Fourth, measure increases in other relevant behaviors after intervention. For example, practitioners and researchers can evaluate the social relevance of enhancing choice-making skills by determining whether clients are more likely to make choices when they are available and, after a choice is made, by observing whether clients are more likely to sustain the chosen activity, compared with baseline measures. Increases in workers' attention to job tasks, job independence, and self-confidence can suggest that enhanced choice making in employment settings is socially relevant. Another example is determining an increase in completed and correct class assignments after students with LD learn help-recruiting skills.

Fifth, compare intervention gains, such as increases in productivity and social interactions, with performance of normative or "normal" samples. Some, however, have questioned the social relevance of using the behavior of "normal" individuals as a standard for many vulnerable clients, such as those with physical and cognitive disabilities and visual impairments (Erin et al., 1991; Foster & Mash, 1999). Problems include the availability of appropriate normative data and the difficulties involved in setting cutoff points indicating the "normal" range for acceptable behavior or performance. In addition, for clients with multiple and/or severe disabilities, women, clients with low income, and sexual and racial/ethnic minorities, defining meaningful change must be placed in the context of their disability, capabilities, culture, and the persons with whom and contexts in which they interact or perform the acquired behaviors.

Erin et al. (1991), for example, argued that practitioners cannot assume that what might be considered acceptable and desirable social skills for sighted clients will ensure access to the experiences of the sighted world for clients with visual impairments. Furthermore, the identified social skills for sighted individuals will not include all of the skills that individuals with visual impairments require to engage in satisfying social interactions. In evaluating, intervening in, and measuring socially relevant change for clients with other types of disabilities, special considerations and training are necessary. For clients with hearing impairments, communication concerns and understanding deaf culture, such as their language and feelings of pride in being deaf, are examples (Myers & Thyer, 1997).

Sixth, assess negative outcomes, another indicator of whether intervention results are socially valid. Unfortunately, few evaluations of the interventions discussed in the previous chapters formally assessed or reported on unexpected or negative outcomes. Researchers who did provide the results of such assessments indicate their importance. For example, students with disabilities experienced embarrassment when discussing their disabilities with teachers, and the psychotic symptoms of some clients diagnosed with schizophrenia increased after participation in SST.

This lack of attention to negative outcomes is surprising, given the high probability that participation in many of the discussed interventions could lead to negative consequences. For example, conflicts could arise between children and teachers, parents, and others when children are taught to set their own goals and make their own choices. Disappointment and other negative reactions might result from not achieving personally set goals. Other adverse consequences can occur after social interactions are initiated or one's legal rights are asserted. For example, advocating one's work accommodation rights might result in conflict with the employer, impaired relationships with co-workers, and anger, disappointment, or demoralization if the request is denied.

Assessing, identifying, and assisting clients in coping with negative consequences that might result from using acquired skills is particularly important for vulnerable clients, who frequently have a history of experiencing unfavorable consequences (e.g., failure, rejection, ridicule). Assisting clients in coping with such consequences is also important for two other reasons. First, if clients anticipate and learn to effectively cope with possible negative consequences, they will be more likely to maintain and transfer their treatment gains. Second, consistent with an empowerment perspective and social work values, clients and research participants should be informed of the risks of participating in the interventions.

Despite the techniques that can be used to measure the social relevance of treatment gains, the evaluations of the interventions discussed in this book highlight important limitations in this area. Some evaluations reported changes in outcome measures, such as loneliness, help-seeking behavior, participation in leisure/recreation activity, enhanced productivity, and securing employment. However, the evaluations failed to determine whether such changes enhanced the quality of participants' lives in some way, resulted in meaningful activity and relationships, or provided sufficient income and other benefits that adequately met the workers' and/or their families' needs. Even when interventions increased choice making, whether the choices offered to clients were desirable or meaningful (e.g., offering a choice of which clothing to wear to residents with severe mental retardation) was not always evaluated. As this example suggests, assessing whether intervention gains are meaningful to the lives of some vulnerable clients, such as those with severe, multiple disabilities or restricted ability to communicate, is extremely difficult. Developing special techniques to assess the social relevance of intervention gains for these clients is an area of current and future research. A recent example is the development of happiness indices (Yu et al., 2002). The indices assess the reactions of clients with severe and profound disabilities, such as smiling and laughing, as they are engaging in an identified behavior during naturally occurring work and leisure activities.

The described strategies also suggest that the use of multiple informants and integration of qualitative and quantitative methods may be required to determine whether intervention gains are socially valid (Gresham et al., 2001). However, as observed by other researchers (Foster & Mash, 1999; Schwartz & Baer, 1991; Wolf, 1978), subjective opinions of different respondents are frequently inconsistent. Further research is needed to design valid and reliable social validity assessments, as well as to identify methods to understand and assess different perceptions among respondents.

Socially relevant intervention procedures. Socially valid interventions are feasible, relevant, and acceptable to clients and others involved in the interventions. Socially valid procedures take into consideration the client's culture, values, and compliance, and costs, need for special resources and training, ease of administration, and transferability to other settings. Obviously, interventions that are unacceptable, impractical, or irrelevant to clients and others involved in implementing them are less likely to be adopted. Therefore, determining socially relevant interventions is critical. One of the best methods to identify relevant interventions is to conduct an individual functional assessment. Because such an assessment identifies the conditions maintaining a target behavior and considers the client's unique circumstances and characteristics, it can assist in the development of appropriate interventions. However, as scholars have observed (Clarke et al., 2002; Van Acker et al., 2005), and the interventions presented in this book demonstrate, despite the touted value of and commitment to individualized assessment and intervention, CB researchers and practitioners frequently fail to conduct functional assessments and to design interventions based on that assessment. Instead, maintaining conditions, such as a skill deficit, are frequently assumed and standardized interventions applied. The problems associated with the latter practices were previously discussed in this chapter, as well as in the end-of-chapter summaries.

The previous chapters of this book suggest that in addition to completing functional assessments, practitioners and researchers can use a number of other strategies to evaluate and enhance the social validity of their interventions. Ten types of methods are discussed. First, because CB interventions are transparent, practitioners and researchers can assess their acceptability and consistency with the values, culture, and resources of individuals involved in the interventions by describing the procedures and asking for feedback.

Second, task and contextual analyses of the specific behaviors required to perform the identified activity can be conducted in natural settings. Examples include selling ice cream in the playground and performing job activities at a work site. However, a task analysis may result in behaviors that are unnecessarily narrow and mechanistic, such as identifying forty-six separate tasks to teach coffee purchase skills to adults with mental retardation (Storey et al., 1984).

Third, obtaining information from a variety of other sources can identify relevant interventions and materials (e.g., knowledge of political structures, role-play scenarios, and appropriate responses), such as for teaching political, advocacy, social, and work skills. Information can be gathered from related literature, focus groups, surveys, and interviews, and intervention materials can be pretested with potential clients and other relevant individuals. Relevant individuals might include professionals, employers, experts, advocates, a team of multiple stakeholders, and persons with similar characteristics (e.g., a physical disability, race/ethnicity, culture, gender, age) as the clients or participants.

Fourth, naturally occurring situations and relevant contexts can be integrated into the interventions. Examples from the previous chapters include group facilitators assisting group members in identifying the social contexts in which certain behaviors are appropriate (e.g., sharing information related to type 1 diabetes). In other SST and problem-solving interventions, practitioners assist clients in identifying their own personal situations and selecting responses that best solve the problem for themselves. For example, clients identify members of their social support networks to assist them in achieving a personal goal. Clients identify personal cues that trigger high-risk behavior and choose risk-reduction behaviors consistent with their own values, culture, relationships, and the context of their own lives. Clients are assigned homework relevant to their unique problems and real-life situations.

Fifth, socially relevant individuals can be involved in the interventions. Previous examples include group members with similar characteristics and backgrounds coaching and serving as role models and role-play partners for one another and sharing personal situations, strategies, and results of homework assignments. Group facilitators with similar characteristics as group members also serve as role models. Teachers, staff in residential facilities, peers, co-workers, and caregivers teach, prompt, reinforce, and provide opportunities for clients with disabilities to perform the identified skills.

Sixth, methods that are sensitive to the unique characteristics of the clients can be implemented. This includes clients' culture, values, socioeconomic status, gender, disability, and age. In the group interventions designed to teach knowledge and skills for asserting one's right to refuse unwanted or unprotected sexual activity, group facilitators develop a shared sense of community, culture, and norms for sexual behavior, and they build social support and consensus among group members for safe-sex norms. Facilitators assist group members in identifying benefits related directly to their own children, family, and ethnic group and emphasize the importance of power relationships between men and women, especially in the context of economic insecurity, cultural sexual norms, and male-female relationships. In teaching students with disabilities self-determination skills, a family support component addresses possible conflicts between increasing youths' self-determination and family values.

Several of the group interventions discussed in this book also demonstrate sensitivity to clients' economic situations. Practitioners acknowledge and address the economic circumstances and the multiple stressors that might preclude clients from attending sessions and engaging in the identified behaviors, such as assertive and healthy sexual behaviors. Examples include providing assistance with transportation and child care, scheduling meetings that do not conflict with work/education responsibilities, and incorporating strategies into the group sessions for achieving education and employment goals. Finally, the political advocacy programs provide free training and travel scholarships for eligible participants.

If CB interventions are to be viable and acceptable to other vulnerable clients, such as those with physical, sensory, developmental, learning, and mental health disabilities, they must accommodate their unique characteristics as well. The end-of-chapter summaries provide many examples of such accommodations. The examples include posting target skills and self-management strategies on walls and floors for clients with hearing impairments, and providing publications in large print or Braille and on audiotapes for clients with visual impairments. Peers participating in SST programs are sensitized to the special communication behaviors of children with disabilities. For clients with communication problems, mechanical or electronic devices and specially designed communication, picture, and instruction books are developed and used. Practitioners teach clients with learning and cognitive disabilities to use their hands and fingers to determine whether they receive correct change when ordering at a fast-food restaurant; to use pictures, mounted items, and graphs to prompt and provide performance feedback; and to use abbreviated self-management statements or acronyms to assist in remembering problem-solving and other skill-building processes. Support services (e.g., reviewing training content and providing assistance with homework assignments) also are provided to individuals with cognitive disabilities participating in advocacy training programs.

Multiple other techniques accommodate the special needs of clients diagnosed with schizophrenia, such as reducing external distractions and teaching techniques to control psychotic symptoms, in teaching problem-solving and social skills. Other accommodations assist clients with severe mental illness in securing employment, such as coordinating job-seeking programs with mental health treatment staff, assisting with daily living problems, and providing additional resources (e.g., transportation, clothing, living allowances, a post office box).

For adolescents, the use of videos, games, and personal testimonies of relevant role models might be particularly relevant interventions. For older learners, practitioners and researchers might use brief and limited didactic instruction and focus on learning activities that are experiential and active (for practical guidelines for using homework assignments for older adults, see Kazantzis, Pachana, & Secker, 2003).

Seventh, if practitioners and researchers are to design and offer acceptable and relevant CB interventions, accommodations must be made for clients' individual interests and preferences. In addition to the techniques previously described in this chapter, other examples include parents and youths identifying their own reinforcers and prompts, individualizing topics of conversation in "communication books," and designing manuals for teaching advocacy letter writing and giving personal testimonials that accommodate personal writing and speaking styles and issues of concern. Clients select personal activities to enhance their well-being (e.g., to combat depression) and engage in unique self-talk to cope with stressful situations. Students with disabilities identify their own choice options, strengths, limitations, needed accommodations, and educational preferences. When teaching self-advocacy skills for academic and work accommodations, clients develop a personal list of work and academic accommodation needs and preferences for accommodating the needs.

Eighth, treatment compliance, which has important implications for both practice and research, also is a measure of the social relevance of interventions. If clients and others involved in the interventions decline to attend sessions, to actively participate during sessions, or to carry out homework assignments in natural settings, the interventions cannot be effective. In the evaluations of the interventions discussed in the previous chapters, few researchers assessed why clients and/or significant others dropped out of treatment or declined to carry out homework assignments. This was the case even when dropout rates (e.g., in Job Clubs) were shown to be high among some client groups (e.g., clients with severe mental illness). Lack of attention to evaluating treatment adherence is consistent with other analyses of evaluations of CB interventions (Hansen et al., 2000).

Hansen and his colleagues (2000) suggest that practitioners conduct a functional analysis of clients' noncompliance to identify appropriate strategies to resolve this problem. Possible maintaining conditions of noncompliance for vulnerable clients include ongoing stress and other competing demands related to poverty and adverse living conditions, such as lack of transportation, child care, or a telephone to call to reschedule an appointment, instead of discontinuing treatment. For clients with disabilities, communication problems and their multiple needs, chronic health problems, and limited endurance might be antecedent conditions. As previously discussed, unexpected negative consequences as a result of carrying out the interventions will likely result in subsequent noncompliance.

Hansen et al. (2000) identified strategies that practitioners might use to maintain or increase participation of vulnerable clients in the interventions. They include providing clear and detailed instructions, using prompts (e.g., reminder cards), and starting with small homework assignments and gradually increasing them. Teaching problem solving to identify and resolve barriers to adherence, identifying and changing cognitions that precede or accompany noncompliance, and providing frequent feedback and positive reinforcement for compliance are additional methods. Practitioners can make appropriate referrals, coordinate services, and advocate for clients in a variety of settings to ensure that opportunities and the support required to perform the identified skills are provided. Identifying reasons for treatment noncompliance and developing and evaluating strategies to increase treatment adherence for vulnerable clients are important areas for future qualitative and quantitative research.

Ninth, evaluations of the interventions described in the previous chapters suggest that the use of interviews and qualitative surveys after intervention are the most commonly used methods to assess intervention social validity. Methods include asking clients and others involved in the interventions (e.g., teachers, co-workers, supervisors, staff, and parents) to evaluate the interventions on various dimensions, including whether they were suitable, helpful, enjoyable, or preferred to other methods. Others involved in the intervention process (e.g., teachers) report on their observations of the participants' active engagement and enjoyment of the interventions (e.g., students with disabilities learning to set and attain their own goals). The results of the postintervention evaluations overall were very positive, which are consistent with conclusions of other research that has examined evaluations of the social validity of CB interventions (Heckaman, Conroy, Fox, & Chait, 2000).

These positive evaluations of CB interventions are relevant to both practitioners and researchers who might hesitate to offer clients or to develop and evaluate these types of interventions. The hesitation might result from a fear that the characteristics of the interventions (e.g., relative directiveness and focus on changing specific behavior) might be unacceptable to clients and significant others. The evaluations of the discussed CB interventions, as well as the Heckaman et al. (2000) review, suggest little reason for such hesitancy. Of course, CB interventions would not be acceptable to everyone or in all settings. This is indicated by individuals who declined to participate and some of the responses to the social validity measures reported by evaluations of the previously described interventions. For example, a structured play intervention designed to enhance social interactions between preschool children with hearing impairments and their peers might conflict with some teachers' philosophy of child-directed play; and some programs, such as those teaching self-determination skills in schools, may compete with other required education curricula. Whether clients and/or significant others find CB methods less acceptable, compared with other types of interventions, is an important research topic.

Tenth, continued use of the intervention in the same locale and adoption of the intervention in other settings are other social validity indicators. The Job Club method, for example, has been adopted for use with many different clients and in a variety of settings, suggesting that the procedures are acceptable and feasible to clients, agency personnel, and social policy makers in terms of costs, values, required resources, and ease of administration. However, if interventions are expected to be continued in the same setting or adopted in other settings, barriers to their use must be assessed. In employment settings, for example, training or continued use of strategies that interfere with ongoing work activities are likely to be rejected. If the interventions are to be acceptable and feasible in similar or other settings, practitioners need to determine whether the required resources (e.g., time, transportation, expertise, and money to purchase specialized materials and equipment) are available, and if necessary to assist in providing them. Even when CB interventions appear to be acceptable and feasible because they can be taught to staff in natural environments (e.g., in group homes), ongoing training, evaluation, and support, as well as updating of intervention materials, are likely to be necessary if the interventions are to continue to be relevant, viable, and acceptable to those involved with their use.

As many of the previously described CB interventions suggest, researchers frequently are sensitive to the characteristics of vulnerable populations, including their culture, age, socioeconomic status, race/ethnicity, sexual orientation, disability, and unique life situations. However, the interventions discussed in this book also have limitations related to their social relevance to vulnerable groups. For example, the larger sociocultural context is not always taken into account when interventions, are designed; for example, they may fail to identify in which circumstances particular social and advocacy skills might be most appropriate, to anticipate and plan for adverse outcomes, or to examine and incorporate ways in which other characteristics (e.g., socioeconomic status, race/ethnicity, culture, gender) might influence the relevance of SST programs. Instead of waiting until after intervention to evaluate the social relevance of CB interventions, a better approach would be to involve clients, potential participants, and significant others in the design of the interventions and provide ongoing opportunities for continued evaluation of the social validity of the interventions. Although many examples of methods adapting intervention procedures to accommodate the special needs of vulnerable groups are evident in the previously discussed interventions, practitioners and researchers are challenged to continue to identify, develop, and evaluate additional strategies.

Maintaining and generalizing intervention gains. As evaluations of the interventions described in the previous chapters demonstrate, researchers and practitioners cannot assume that gains observed immediately after formal intervention ends will transfer to other settings, situations, materials, and/or individuals or will be maintained. Generalization and maintenance of intervention gains must be planned for and assessed. Although maintenance and transfer of treatment gains are important issues in their own right, they also are interrelated with socially valid intervention goals, results, and procedures and treatment effectiveness. As Hansen et al. (2000) contend, the greater the extent to which the goals and interventions are socially valid, the more likely it is that clients will participate. If clients carry out the interventions, the interventions are more likely to be effective, and intervention gains are more likely to transfer to natural settings and contexts and to be maintained. Finally, the greater the extent to which treatment gains generalize and are maintained, the more socially valid the results are.

Although no consensus exists on the length of time that treatment gains should be maintained after formal intervention ends, some researchers suggest at least six months (Dobson & Khatri, 2000; Kennedy, 2002). The interventions examined in this book reveal a large variation in the degree to which maintenance and transfer of treatment gains were planned for and assessed. Methods that were used to assess transfer and maintenance of intervention gains include observations of role plays in natural settings, observations of naturally occurring behavior, use of standardized scales, and reports by participants and significant others. Evaluations of the interventions, however, suggest that measuring maintenance and generalization of intervention gains can be problematic.

Determining whether certain types of skills and outcomes generalize to and are maintained in natural environments is difficult if the target skills, such as securing one's legal rights or seeking emergency assistance, are used infrequently. Other problems include assessing whether gains in instrumental outcomes (e.g., choice making and social skills) are maintained, but failing to assess whether the skills continue to achieve the ultimate goals (e.g., actually making choices and initiating social interactions). Evaluations that did assess maintenance of intervention gains demonstrate that not all participants maintain their gains after formal intervention, and rarely were the reasons for this undesirable outcome examined. The evaluations also vary in the extent to which they determined whether the acquired skills (e.g., social, self-advocacy, recreational/leisure, employment, self-determination) transferred to multiple settings, individuals, and situations. Although some evaluations did determine transfer of the intervention gains to a variety of settings and to novel tasks, materials, and individuals, the individuals and settings were frequently within the same organization or institution in which intervention took place (e.g., in a school or group home). Other evaluations indicate the need for additional intervention before generalization occurs.

Although practitioners and researchers are expected to plan for and evaluate the maintenance and transfer of intervention gains to multiple settings and contexts, the previously described limitations are consistent with reviews of CB intervention research elsewhere (Brown & Odom, 1994; Gresham et al., 2001; Hansen et al., 2000; Harchik, Sherman, & Sheldon, 1992; Stokes & Osnes, 1989). These researchers also provide methods to assist clients in maintaining and generalizing the intervention gains. Stokes and Osnes's suggestions merit an extended discussion.

Stokes and Osnes (1989) identify three main types of methods that practitioners and researchers can use to actively plan for the generalization and maintenance of intervention gains. General methods include (1) taking advantage of current functional contingencies, especially natural communities of reinforcement, (2) teaching diversely, and (3) using functional mediators. Following a discussion of these methods, several additional strategies are briefly described.

Taking advantage of current functional contingencies. This first method, taking advantage of current functional contingencies, refers to using naturally occurring antecedents and consequences that can increase the likelihood that the identified behavior will be performed. Most of the examples in the literature and in the previously described CB interventions are consistent with this method, and they commonly focus on taking advantage of natural communities of reinforcement. If the identified behaviors are naturally reinforced in the home, school, work, and community environments in which they are to be performed, they are more likely to transfer to and be maintained in those settings.

Practitioners and researchers can take advantage of naturally occurring reinforcers by using three main strategies. First, teach behaviors that are likely to be followed by naturally reinforcing events. Second, teach clients to recruit others to provide reinforcing consequences. Third, recruit others in clients' natural environments who can provide reinforcing consequences. The content that follows also discusses the importance of ensuring that the required antecedent conditions (e.g., support and resources) are in place and provides examples of recruiting others to provide this assistance in order to maintain and transfer intervention gains to natural settings.

If the intervention goals, target skills, and intervention materials are socially valid, naturally reinforcing consequences are likely to follow. For example, if clients choose a preferred leisure/recreational activity, set their own goals, and learn responses and social interaction skills acceptable to their peers, then engaging in the chosen activity, attaining the goal, and using the social skills and responses are likely to be naturally reinforced. The naturally occurring reinforcers might be feelings of pleasure, satisfaction, and accomplishment, positive attention, and affiliation with others. As a result of these naturally occurring consequences, use of external prompts and reinforcers often can be discontinued. For example, a school social worker initially prompts and praises students with disabilities and their able-bodied peers to facilitate their social interactions. After the students experience positive social interactions, the practitioner fades the prompts and praise, and the natural positive reinforcement from the social interactions maintains the behaviors.

The use of acquired social, advocacy, problem-solving, and other skills, however, will not always result in naturally reinforcing consequences for clients and/or for others involved in the interactions. For example, a female refuses unwanted sex with her partner, and she loses the desired relationship; a student with LD fails to achieve an important personal goal, and he feels demoralized; an adolescent with a disability attempts to initiate a conversation with a nondisabled peer and is met with laughter, and he feels humiliated. As discussed in chapter 4, even establishing peer networks, which can change the perceptions and attitudes of able-bodied peers toward students with disabilities, might be insufficient to maintain and/or generalize the interactions between vulnerable students and their able-bodied peers. If the social interactions are to be maintained by naturally occurring consequences and to be transferred to multiple settings and peers, they must be reinforcing to everyone involved. Even after intervention, the physical, cognitive, or communicative abilities, or the selection of recreational or play activities of some students with disabilities, might not be reinforcing for their able-bodied peers.

In addition to negative consequences, a number of antecedent conditions can limit the use of acquired skills and goal attainment among vulnerable clients. Such factors include problems related to specific disabilities, such as a struggle to control psychiatric symptoms or the worsening of a chronic disease. The opportunities, support, and resources needed to use the skills, such as identifying and offering choices, transportation, and specialized equipment and materials, might be unavailable. The anticipation of negative consequences, such as embarrassment, fear, or adverse reactions from others, might preclude clients from maintaining and generalizing treatment gains. Other problems include changes in the wider social and economic environments, such as a company's closure for a past recipient of public benefits desiring to maintain employment.

The second type of strategies that take advantage of natural communities of reinforcement involves teaching clients to recruit others who can provide natural reinforcers. Several examples of this strategy are included in the interventions described in the previous chapters. Practitioners teach clients with disabilities to recruit play and recreational partners and teach students with disabilities to recruit teachers and peers to provide praise and feedback when completing class assignments. To increase productivity, workers with mental retardation are taught to recruit praise from their supervisors. Job Club counselors assist group members in recruiting others who reinforce their job search activities. Group facilitators assist clients in developing social supports who can reinforce performance of acquired behaviors, such as engaging in safer sexual activity.

A number of the previously described interventions also teach clients to obtain the needed information, resources, and social support to assist them in attaining their educational, employment, and other personal goals; in performing routine (e.g., opening doors, locating objects in stores, mounting curbs) and emergency help-seeking activities; and in caring for their medical and psychiatric needs. For example, minority youths and youths with disabilities are taught to recruit potential helpers to achieve their personal goals. Job Club counselors teach group members to recruit others to provide employment-related assistance, such as job leads and transportation. Pregnant and parenting adolescents and individuals with low income learn to recruit members of their social support networks to provide them with a variety of personal and economic assistance. Patients diagnosed with severe mental illness and the elderly are taught to obtain information on their medications from medical professionals and to recruit others to assist them in keeping their medical appointments. Teaching clients to recruit others in their natural environments who can provide reinforcing experiences and the necessary information, assistance, and support likely will result in transfer and maintenance of intervention gains.

Finally, taking advantage of current functional contingencies involves practitioners recruiting significant others to provide clients with reinforcing consequences, as well as the prerequisite resources and support. As the previous chapters demonstrate, practitioners can train teachers, peers, staff, and caregivers to teach a variety of skills (e.g., social, leisure, choice making) to children and youths, group home residents, and residents of residential treatment centers and to reinforce the performance of the skills and personal goal achievement in natural settings. Clients also are taught to praise each other, for example, during game playing.

After implementing many of the interventions described in the previous chapters, practitioners must recruit ongoing support before terminating services if clients are to continue performing the skills or other activities. Many interventions, such as those for clients with disabilities, involve specially designed materials and methods (e.g., communication books), which are necessary for clients to engage in the identified activities (e.g., social interactions, recreation/leisure, and choice making). The materials and methods likely would need to be adapted to settings and situations differing significantly from those in which the interventions were conducted. For the skills or activities to be maintained even in settings and situations identical or similar to those during intervention, some type of continued support would be necessary for many clients. For example, some elderly nursing home residents require assistance in writing letters to maintain their ongoing correspondence. Preferences also are likely to change over time, and clients are likely to become bored with the same food or recreational/leisure choices. If choice making is to be maintained by the natural reinforcer of the choice that is obtained, staff and significant others must be able to periodically assess and provide relevant choice options.

The CB interventions presented in this book provide few strategies to coordinate intervention with other relevant individuals in organizational, agency, community, and residential settings. Abery and his colleagues' (1995) multicomponent program designed to enhance the self-determination skills of students with mental retardation is an example of a school-based program involving the students' families. Using behaviorally trained case managers for clients diagnosed with schizophrenia is another example of coordinating efforts to maintain and transfer the social skills acquired in treatment settings to the daily lives of the clients. Case managers serve as the clients' liaison with other treatment staff, family members, and community agencies; they create opportunities and provide encouragement and reinforcement for the clients' use of the acquired skills. Finally, the leadership academies, which teach political advocacy skills to the elderly, individuals with developmental disabilities or severe mental illness, and interested others, use strategies to support, reinforce, and build on program gains. An example is telephone conferences, during which graduates can discuss their accomplishments and exchange advocacy ideas. Graduates also are encouraged to participate in consumer organizations and in a variety of other support activities, including networking with one another and attending conferences.

The previously discussed strategies for taking advantage of current functional contingencies provide a number of methods to assist clients in transferring and maintaining intervention gains. The discussion also suggests additional practice implications. First, practitioners must assess and teach clients strategies to cope with possible negative consequences of using the acquired skills, even when the skills are believed to be socially valid. In some circumstances continued support, external reinforcement, and/or adaptations to changing circumstances are necessary. Second, others involved in the interventions (e.g., staff, teachers, caregivers) must be adequately trained.

Third, when others are involved in the intervention process (e.g., teachers providing opportunities and reinforcement for students performing particular social skills), whether the clients can maintain the skills in absence of such intervention must be assessed before termination of services. If necessary, practitioners must ensure that the required supports, such as prompts, reinforcement, and resources, are in place. Finally, others involved in the intervention procedures might need incentives and support themselves, if they are to perform the necessary behaviors, provide reinforcement and support, and make any necessary modifications. In organizational settings, agency administrators may need to alter existing job descriptions and evaluation procedures to reflect the required behavior of staff (e.g., offering choices to residents with disabilities) and provide support, motivation, and booster sessions.

Teaching diversely. Teaching diversely is Stokes and Osnes's (1989) second set of methods that can enhance maintenance and generalization of intervention gains to multiple environments and contexts. That is, practitioners should vary the conditions of the interventions, including the antecedent stimuli, responses, and consequences, and the antecedents and consequences should be made less discriminable. The CB interventions described in this book provide a number of examples of teaching diversely.

First, the antecedent events are varied through the use of multiple instructors, practice partners, settings, and materials. For example, multiple instructors and peers are used in the interventions that teach play, leisure, self-advocacy, and interview skills, and other social interactions. Clients practice relevant skills in several classrooms within the schools and in other natural settings (e.g., restaurants, bars, group homes, and private homes). Psychiatric patients role-play and practice medication-related information-seeking and negotiation skills with a number of individuals, including a physician. Elderly clients call multiple pharmacies and physicians to learn skills for acquiring information about their medications. A variety of situations across many different settings are designed for individuals with disabilities to practice help-seeking skills. Many different materials and activities also are used in many of the skills-building interventions, including play materials and toys, leisure/recreational activities, and job applications. Finally, homework is assigned for clients to practice the identified skills in multiple natural settings.

Second, multiple examples of relevant social skills and related responses are incorporated into the interventions through written materials, modeling, and rehearsal. As described in the previous chapters, clients practice the social, self-advocacy, and political skills using different role-play situations requiring varied responses, and also practice the responses in natural settings. Different types of reinforcers, such as social, concrete, and edible reinforcers, can be used to vary consequences. The reinforcers also can be administered by different individuals (e.g., the practitioner, group members, teachers, parents, and other caretakers), as well as by clients themselves.

Third, antecedent events are made less discriminable, thereby making it less likely that only a narrow set of circumstances will prompt the client to perform the identified behavior. Stokes and Osnes refer to this as "loose training." Conducting interventions in natural settings has the advantage of the presence of multiple naturally occurring events and social responses, which can enhance maintenance of the identified behavior and generalization to other settings. Many of the interventions discussed in this book are designed to be taught in natural settings, including private residences, group homes, restaurants, schools, sheltered workshops, and competitive employment. A final strategy to make antecedents less discriminable is to fade artificial prompts, including monitoring devices, verbal statements, picture cues, and scripts.

Fourth, consequences should be made less discriminable. Gradually fading reinforcers and pairing artificial reinforcers (such as tokens and edibles) with naturally occurring reinforcers, then gradually fading the artificial reinforcers, are strategies to make consequences less discriminable. For example, peers are taught to praise the play behavior of students with mental retardation, as well as to provide prompts and feedback. As the students' skills improve, the practitioner teaches the peers to gradually withdraw their praise, as well as the prompts and feedback, and the natural reinforcer of the play interactions is expected to maintain the behavior. Additional techniques that make consequences less discriminable are using delayed reinforcement and reinforcing spontaneous performance of the behavior in natural settings.

Using functional mediators. The use of functional mediators is the last group of methods suggested by Stokes and Osnes to enhance the transfer and maintenance of intervention gains. A functional mediator is an event that is present in natural settings or can be carried by the client into those settings to facilitate generalization of the identified behaviors. Functional mediators also act as discriminative stimuli, which are present in the intervention and natural settings. Discriminative stimuli assist the client to determine the situations and contexts in which to perform the identified behavior.

Different types of functional mediators are used in the interventions examined in the previous chapters. For example, physical mediators, such as a picture of an emergency situation, can prompt help-seeking skills, and a photograph of an employee performing a work task can prompt work behaviors. Natural supports also can function as mediators. Peer tutors, peer networks, co-workers, and supervisors can be involved in the intervention and in natural settings to assist transfer and maintenance of a variety of social, play, and work skills. The use of specially designed materials and equipment, such as communication books and augmented communication systems, also might be considered functional mediators.

When interventions cannot be carried out in natural settings, either because of the type of behavior that is targeted (e.g., refusing unwanted sexual activity) or because of agency or organizational constraints, other functional mediators can be incorporated into the intervention. Involving others who are similar to individuals whom the clients are likely to encounter in their actual lives might facilitate transfer of the intervention gains. For example, when students with disabilities are taught to obtain academic accommodations, students practice with school staff and faculty. Using materials that are equivalent to or closely resemble those found in natural settings also can assist clients in transferring intervention gains. For example, the intervention that teaches adult clients with mental retardation to eat more independently in community fast-food restaurants is conducted in an artificial setting but incorporates materials similar to those found in the restaurants (e.g., counters and wall menus).

Finally, practitioners can teach clients a variety of self-mediated techniques, which also can serve as functional mediators. Previously described examples are using self-instruction to initiate and sustain clients' social interactions and job tasks. Clients self-monitor performance of their work and social skills using self-recording, timers, and a self-operated auditory prompting system. Checklists for homework assignments, determining housing preferences, and for redressing rights violations; forms to prompt clients to ask relevant questions about medications; and self-help guides to assist clients in writing advocacy letters are other examples. Clients self-reinforce, and they set and monitor their goals. Problem solving can enhance social interactions and can assist clients in developing strategies to cope with problematic situations with their physicians. All of these strategies can assist clients in maintaining intervention gains and generalizing them to the settings in which they live, play, work, learn, and engage in other activity.

Additional strategies. In addition to the three main methods advocated by Stokes and Osnes, the interventions described in previous chapters provide other maintenance and generalization strategies. These include relapse prevention, contracting, and follow-up and booster sessions. To prevent relapse, practitioners assist clients in identifying and planning for obstacles that might interfere with continuation or increases in the learned skills, such as asserting the right to decline unwanted sexual activity. Clients make a contract or commitment to engage in the identified behaviors, and practitioners stress the importance of ongoing vigilance and peer support to maintain behaviors, such as safer sexual practices.

Follow-up sessions are conducted to monitor progress in maintaining and transferring skills, such as requesting a work accommodation review from employers of clients with a disability. Practitioners hold booster sessions to refresh clients' skills and assist them in coping with unexpected situations and obstacles, which can increase the likelihood that the acquired skills and ultimate outcomes (e.g., an acquired personal relationship) will be maintained or continue to increase. Finally, clients are given opportunities to use and build on their skills. For example, the leadership academies provide conferences, networking opportunities, and training roles for their graduates.

Despite the availability of methods that can be used to increase the maintenance and transfer of intervention gains, the previous discussion suggests the need for additional research in these areas. First, researchers need to evaluate and report the degree to which treatment gains are transferred to other settings, individuals, materials, and contexts, and whether gains on both instrumental and ultimate goals are maintained for at least six months. Second, researchers need to develop valid and reliable methods to assess generalization and maintenance of treatment gains. Methods can be developed using both qualitative and more traditional objective measures, such as reliable and valid scales and direct observations of predefined skills.

Third, possible negative consequences of maintenance and generalization strategies need to be assessed. English et al. (1997), for example, believed that the main reason friendships did not develop between "peer buddies" and preschoolers with developmental disabilities was their decision to "teach diversely" by involving multiple peers. The peer rotation apparently did not allow sufficient time for friendships to develop. Fourth, further research is necessary to determine effective methods to integrate and coordinate treatment within and among various settings.

Finally, although self-management strategies might assist clients in learning, maintaining, and transferring skills to different settings and situations, further research must determine which self-mediated strategies are appropriate for which behavior, client, and situation. Additional areas for future research on self-management strategies that apply to many vulnerable clients are discussed by Harchick and his colleagues (1992). For example, researchers need to identify the prerequisite knowledge, abilities, or skills necessary for learning self-management strategies (e.g., language level, cognitive ability, ability to count, and skill at discriminating whether the behavior occurred). These researchers also advocate the inclusion of clients in designing and selecting specific procedures, as well as the development of methods for training others involved with the clients (e.g., parents, staff, teachers) to assist them in teaching clients to use the self-management procedures in natural settings.

As this discussion of social validity indicates, and as other scholars have observed (e.g., Foster & Mash, 1999), social validity is not a dichotomous construct (i.e., either it exists or it does not), but a multidimensional construct that can be assessed in multiple ways. Examples provided in this book suggest the need for researchers and practitioners to conduct individual functional assessments and to develop and use methods to establish socially relevant goals, interventions, and treatment outcomes, and to ensure that treatment gains are maintained and transfer to the environments in which vulnerable clients live, work, learn, and engage in other activity. Finally, even when goals, interventions, and results are shown to be socially valid, a conclusion cannot be drawn that the interventions are effective. Social validity might be necessary for effectiveness, but it does not demonstrate effectiveness. Researchers and practitioners need to supplement social validity measures with traditional research methods that assess changes in the behavior targeted by the intervention.

CONCLUDING COMMENTS

The CB interventions described in this book are not panaceas for the problems that vulnerable populations experience. Following assessment, however, the interventions can be used alone or with other types of interventions to assist vulnerable clients in achieving empowerment-related goals. These goals include accessing and increasing social resources; acquiring, maintaining, and increasing economic resources; enhancing self-determination, such as setting and attaining individual goals, making choices, and securing legal and personal rights; and influencing macro decisions that affect their lives, including organizational and community practices and social policies.

That some researchers or practitioners may have developed CB applications that lack social validity, or have applied the interventions unnecessarily to control vulnerable groups and force them to conform to societal norms, does not imply that such applications must be so directed. As many of the interventions described in this book demonstrate, CB interventions not only can offer hope but can increase opportunities, skills, resources, and power for some of society's most powerless individuals and groups, including those with multiple, severe disabilities. The interventions described here and elsewhere (e.g., Hurst & Genest, 1995; Lewis, 1994; Martell et al., 2004; McNair, 1996; Organista & Muñoz, 1996) also demonstrate that practitioners and researchers, including feminists and those providing services to sexual and ethnic/racial minorities, can develop and use CB applications that are consistent with feminist philosophy and responsive to the cultures and social-political environments of vulnerable populations.

Nearly two decades ago, Howard Goldstein (1990) observed what he called an historic paradox in the social work profession: while adopting a scientific perspective, it did not entirely abandon its humanistic and social ideals. He described a profession that has advanced on two distinct tracks—one adhering to humanistic traditions, and the other attempting to adopt the objectivity of scientific methods and social science theories, including those of behavioral psychology. This book has tried to demonstrate that there is no inherent contradiction between the profession's humanistic and social ideals and the application of social science theories and scientific methods. Traditional scientific methods can be used to evaluate effective interventions for vulnerable populations, and they can be combined with qualitative methods to develop socially valid goals, interventions, and results, and to maintain and transfer treatment gains. CB theories, and the interventions on which they are commonly based, also can be used to achieve individual and group goals consistent with the professional values of social work and its humanistic tradition. Social work researchers and practitioners must find effective ways to meet this challenge.

ADDITIONAL READINGS AND RESOURCES

Behavior and Social Issues. Edited by M. Mattaini. An online journal that advances the analysis of human social behavior, with an emphasis on issues of social justice and human rights. Available at http://www.bfsr.org/

Culturally sensitive CBT [Special issue]. (1996). *Cognitive and Behavioral Practice, 13*(4).

Ethnic and cultural diversity in cognitive and behavioral practice [Special issue]. (1996). *Cognitive and Behavioral Practice, 3*(2).

Finn, C. A., & Sladeczek, I. E. (2001). Assessing the social validity of behavioral interventions: A review of treatment acceptability measures. *School Psychology Quarterly, 16,* 176–206.

Galinsky, M. J., Terzian, M. A., & Fraser, M. W. (2006). The art of group work practice with manualized curricula. *Social Work with Groups, 29,* 11–26.

Gresham, F. M., McIntyre, L. L., Olson-Tinker, H., Dolstra, L., McLaughlin, V., & Van, M. (2004). Relevance of functional behavioral assessment research for school-based interventions and positive behavioral support. *Research in Developmental Disabilities, 25,* 19–37.

Hays, P. A., & Iwamasa, G. Y. (Eds.). (2006). *Culturally responsive cognitive-behavioral therapy: Assessment, practice, and supervision.* Washington, DC: American Psychological Association.

Henin, A., Otto, M. W., & Reilly-Harrington, R. (2001). Introducing flexibility in manualized treatments: Application of recommended strategies to the cognitive-behavioral treatment of bipolar disorder. *Cognitive and Behavioral Practice, 8,* 317–328.

Kendall, P. C., Chu, B., Gifford, A., Hayes, C., & Nauta, M. (1998). Breathing life into a manual: Flexibility and creativity with manual-based treatments. *Cognitive and Behavioral Practice, 5,* 177–198.

Lee, S., Simpson, R. L., & Shogren, K. A. (2007). Effects and implications of self-management for students with autism: A meta-analysis. *Focus on Autism and Other Developmental Disabilities, 22,* 2–13.

Lohrmann-O'Rourke, S., Browder, D. M., & Brown, F. (2000). Guidelines for conducting socially valid systematic preference assessments. *Journal of the Association for Persons with Severe Handicaps, 25,* 42–53.

Satterfield, J. M. (1998). Cognitive behavioral group therapy for depressed, low-income minority clients: Retention and treatment enhancement. *Cognitive and Behavioral Practice, 5,* 65–80.

Schwartz, I. S., & Baer, D. M. (1991). Social validity assessments: Is current practice state of the art?. *Journal of Applied Behavior Analysis, 24,* 189–204.

References

Abery, B., Rudrud, L., Arndt, K., Schauben, L., & Eggebeen, A. (1995). Evaluating a multicomponent program for enhancing the self-determination of youth with disabilities. *Intervention in School and Clinic, 30,* 170–179.

Agran, M., Blanchard, C., & Wehmeyer, M. L. (2000). Promoting transition goals and self-determination through student self-directed learning: The self-determined learning model of instruction. *Education and Training in Mental Retardation and Developmental Disabilities, 35,* 351–364.

Agran, M., Blanchard, C., Wehmeyer, M., & Hughes, C. (2002). Increasing the problem-solving skills of students with developmental disabilities participating in general education. *Remedial and Special Education, 23,* 279–288.

Agran, M., Fodor-Davis, J., & Moore, S. (1986). The effects of self-instructional training on job-task sequencing: Suggesting a problem-solving strategy. *Education and Training of the Mentally Retarded, 21,* 273–281.

Agran, M., & Moore, S. C. (1994). *How to teach self-instruction of job skills.* In D. Browder (Ed.), *Innovations* (series). Washington, DC: American Association on Mental Retardation.

Agran, M., Salzberg, C. L., & Stowitschek, J. J. (1987). An analysis of the effects of a social skills training program using self-instructions on the acquisition and generalization of two social behaviors in a work setting. *Journal of the Association for Persons with Severe Handicaps, 12,* 131–139.

Ahluwalia, I. B., Dodds, J. M., & Baligh, M. (1998). Social support and coping behaviors of low-income families experiencing food insufficiency in North Carolina. *Health Education & Behavior, 25,* 599–612.

Alberti, R. E., & Emmons, M. L. (2001). *Your perfect right: A guide to assertive living* (8th ed.). San Luis Obispo, CA: Impact.

Algozzine, B., Browder, D., Karvonen, M., Test, D. W., & Wood, W. M. (2001). Effects of interventions to promote self-determination for individuals with disabilities. *Review of Educational Research, 71,* 219–277.

Alinsky, S. D. (1971). *Rules for radicals: A practical primer for realistic radicals.* New York: Vintage.

Americans with Disabilities Act of 1990, Pub. L. No. 101-336, 104 Stat. 327 (1991).

Amrine, C., & Bullis, M. (1985). The Job Club approach to job placement: A viable tool? *Journal of Rehabilitation of the Deaf, 19,* 18–23.

Arnold, B. R., & Parrott, R. (1978). Job interviewing: Stress management and interpersonal-skills training for welfare-rehabilitation clients. *Rehabilitation Counseling Bulletin, 22,* 44–52.

Arns, P. G., Martin, D. J., & Chernoff, R. A. (2004). Psychosocial needs of HIV-positive individuals seeking workforce re-entry. *AIDS Care, 16,* 377–386.

Artz, L., Macaluso, M., Kelaghan, J., Austin, H., Fleenor, M., Robey, L., et al. (2005). An intervention to promote the female condom to sexually transmitted disease clinic patients. *Behavior Modification, 29,* 318–369.

Aspis, S. (1997). Self-advocacy for people with learning difficulties: Does it have a future? *Disability and Society, 12,* 647–654.

Austin, M. J., Coombs, M., & Barr, B. (2005). Community-centered clinical practice: Is the integration of micro and macro social work practice possible? *Journal of Community Practice, 13,* 9–30.

Azrin, N. H., & Besalel, V. A. (1980). *Job-Club counselor's manual: A behavioral approach to vocational counseling.* Baltimore: University Park Press.

Azrin, N. H., Flores, T., & Kaplan, S. J. (1975). Job-finding club: A group-assisted program for obtaining employment. *Behaviour Research and Therapy, 13,* 17–27.

Azrin, N. H., & Phillip, R. A. (1979). The Job Club method for the job handicapped: A comparative outcome study. *Rehabilitation Counseling Bulletin, 23,* 144–155.

Azrin, N. H., Philip. R. A., Thienes-Hontos, P., & Besalel, V. A. (1980). Comparative evaluation of the Job Club program with welfare recipients. *Journal of Vocational Behavior, 16,* 133–145.

Baer, D. M., Wolf, M. M., & Risley, T. R. (1987). Some still current dimensions of applied behavior analysis. *Journal of Applied Behavior Analysis, 20,* 313–327.

Baker, P., Leitner, J., & McAuley, W. J. (2001). Preparing future aging advocates: The Oklahoma aging advocacy leadership academy. *The Gerontologist, 41,* 394–400.

Bakos, M., Bozic, R., Chapin, D., & Neuman, S. (1980). Effects of environmental changes on elderly residents' behavior. *Hospital and Community Psychiatry, 31,* 677–682.

Balcazar, F. E. (1993). Intervention research and the empowerment of African-American men. *Journal of Men's Studies, 1,* 277–286.

Balcazar, F. E., Fawcett, S. B., & Seekins, T. (1991). Teaching people with disabilities to recruit help to attain personal goals. *Rehabilitation Psychology, 36,* 31–42.

Balcazar, F. E., Keys, C. B., Bertram, J. F., & Rizzo, T. (1996). Advocate development in the field of developmental disabilities: A data-based conceptual model. *Mental Retardation, 34,* 341–351.

Balcazar, F. E., Keys, C. B., & Garate-Serafini, L. (1995). Learning to recruit assistance to attain transition goals: A program for adjudicated youth with disabilities. *Remedial and Special Education, 16,* 237–246.

Balcazar, F. E., Keys, C. B., & Suarez-Balcazar, Y. (2001). Empowering Latinos with disabilities to address issues of independent living and disability rights: A capacity-building approach. *Journal of Prevention & Intervention in the Community, 21,* 53–70.

Balcazar, F. E., Majors, R., Blanchard, K. A., Paine, A., Suarez-Balcazar, Y., Fawcett, S. B., et al. (1991). Teaching minority high school students to recruit helpers to attain personal and educational goals. *Journal of Behavioral Education, 4,* 445–454.

Balcazar, F. E., Seekins, T., Fawcett, S. B., & Hopkins, B. L. (1990). Empowering people with physical disabilities through advocacy skills training. *American Journal of Community Psychology, 18,* 281–296.

Bambara, L. M., & Ager, C. (1992). Using self-scheduling to promote self-directed leisure activity in home and community settings. *Journal of the Association for Persons with Severe Handicaps, 17,* 67–76.

Bambara, L. M., Koger, F., Katzer, T., & Davenport, T. A. (1995). Embedding choice in the context of daily routines: A experimental case study. *Journal of the Association for Persons with Severe Handicaps, 20,* 185–195.

Bandura, A. (1969). *Principles of behavior modification.* New York: Holt, Rinehart & Winston.

Bandura, A. (1977). *Social learning theory.* Englewood Cliffs, NJ: Prentice-Hall.

Bannerman, D. J., Sheldon, J. B., Sherman, J. A., & Harchik, A. E. (1990). Balancing the right to habilitation with the right to personal liberties: The rights of people with developmental disabilities to eat too many doughnuts and take a nap. *Journal of Applied Behavior Analysis, 23,* 79–89.

Barbee, J. R., & Keil, E. C. (1973). Experimental techniques of job interview training for the disadvantaged: Videotape feedback, behavior modification and microcounseling. *Journal of Applied Psychology, 58,* 209–213.

Barth, R. P., & Maxwell, J. S. (1985). Preventing depression and dysfunction among adolescent mothers. In L. D. Gilchrist & S. P. Schinke (Eds.), *Preventing social and health problems through life skills training* (pp. 15–28). Seattle: Center for Social Welfare Research, University of Washington.

Barth, R. P., Middleton, K., & Wagman, E. (1989). A skill building approach to preventing teenage pregnancy. *Theory into Practice, 28,* 183–190.

Barth, R. P., & Schinke, S. P. (1984). Enhancing the social supports of teenage mothers. *Social Casework, 65,* 523–531.

Barth, R. P., Schinke, S. P., & Maxwell, J. S. (1985). Coping skills training for school-age mothers. *Journal of Social Service Research, 8,* 75–94.

Beaulaurier, R. L., & Taylor, S. H. (2001). Social work practice with people with disabilities in the era of disability rights. *Social Work in Health Care, 32,* 67–91.

Beck, A. T. (1976). *Cognitive therapy and the emotional disorders.* New York: International Universities Press.

Beck, J. S. (1995). *Cognitive therapy: Basics and beyond.* New York: Guilford.

Bell, M., Lysaker, P., & Bryson, G. (2003). A behavioral intervention to improve work performance in schizophrenia: Work behavior inventory feedback. *Journal of Vocational Rehabilitation, 18,* 43–50.

Belle, D. E. (1982). The impact of poverty on social networks and supports. *Marriage and Family Review, 5,* 89–103.

Berger, R. M. (1981). Social interactions in nursing homes. In S. P. Schinke (Ed.), *Behavioral methods in social welfare* (pp. 223–252). New York: Aldine de Gruyter.

Berlin, S. (1980). A cognitive-learning perspective for social work. *Social Service Review, 54,* 537–555.

Berlin, S. B. (2002). *Clinical social work practice: A cognitive-integrative perspective.* New York: Oxford University Press.

Biglan, A., Glasgow, R. E., & Singer, G. (1990). The need for a science of larger social units: A contextual approach. *Behavior Therapy, 21,* 195–215.

Blackman, D. K., Howe, M., & Pinkston, E. M. (1976). Increasing participation in social interaction of the institutionalized elderly. *The Gerontologist, 16,* 69–76.

Blandford, J. M. (2003). The nexus of sexual orientation and gender in the determination of earnings. *Industrial and Labor Relations Review, 56,* 622–642.

Blankstein, K. R., & Segal, Z. V. (2001). Cognitive assessment. In K. S. Dobson (Ed.), *Handbook of cognitive-behavioral therapies* (2nd ed., pp. 40–85). New York: Guilford.

Bloom, D., & Michalopoulos, C. (2001, May). How welfare and work policies affect employment and income: A synthesis of research. Retrieved November 23, 2004, from http://www.financeprojectinfo.org/win/workreq-evals.asp

Bond, G. R. (2004). Supported employment: Evidence for an evidence-based practice. *Psychiatric Rehabilitation Journal, 27,* 345–359.

Braddy, B. A., & Gray, D. O. (1987). Employment services for older job seekers: A comparison of two client-centered approaches. *The Gerontologist, 27,* 565–568.

Breen, C., Haring, T., Pitts-Conway, V., & Gaylord-Ross, R. (1989). The training and generalization of social interaction during breaktime at two job sites in the natural environment. *Journal of the Association for Persons with Severe Handicaps, 10,* 41–50.

Brey, P., Zadny, J. J., Gonzalez-Huss, M. J., & Ament, P. A. (1989). A Job Club at a state hospital. *Behavioral Residential Treatment, 4,* 15–22.

Brieland, D. (1995). Social work practice: History and evolution. In *Encyclopedia of social work* (19th ed., Vol. 3, pp. 2247–2257). New York: NASW Press.

Brinckerhoff, L. C. (1994). Developing effective self-advocacy skills in college-bound students with learning disabilities. *Intervention in School and Clinic, 29,* 229–237.

Briscoe, R. V., Hoffman, D. B., & Bailey, J. S. (1975). Behavioral community psychology: Training a community board to problem solve. *Journal of Applied Behavior Analysis, 8,* 157–168.

Brooks, F., Nackerud, L., & Risler, E. (2001). Evaluation of a job-finding club for TANF recipients: Psychosocial impacts. *Research on Social Work Practice, 11,* 79–92.

Browder, D. M., Cooper, K. J., & Lehigh, L. (1998). Teaching adults with severe disabilities to express their choice of settings for leisure activities. *Education and Training in Mental Retardation and Developmental Disabilities, 33,* 228–238.

Browder, D. M., & Minarovic, T. J. (2000). Utilizing sight words in self-instruction training for employees with moderate mental retardation in competitive jobs. *Education and Training in Mental Retardation and Developmental Disabilities, 35,* 78–89.

Browder, D. M., & Shapiro, E. S. (1985). Applications of self-management to individuals with severe handicaps: A review. *Journal of the Association for Persons with Severe Handicaps, 10,* 200–208.

Brown, F., Belz, P., Corsi, L., & Wenig, B. (1993). Choice diversity for people with severe disabilities. *Education and Training in Mental Retardation, 28,* 318–326.

Brown, M. A., & Munford, A. M. (1983). Life skills training for chronic schizophrenics. *Journal of Nervous and Mental Disease, 171,* 466–470.

Brown, W. H., & Odom, S. L. (1994). Strategies and tactics for promoting generalization and maintenance of young children's social behavior. *Research in Developmental Disabilities, 15,* 99–118.

Browne, C. V. (1995). Empowerment in social work practice with older women. *Social Work, 40,* 358–364.

Caplan, R. D., Vinokur, A. D., Price, R. H., & van Ryn, M. (1989). Job seeking, reemployment, and mental health: A randomized field experiment in coping with job loss. *Journal of Applied Psychology, 74,* 759–769.

Carey, M. P., Braaten, L. S., Maisto, S. A., Gleason, J. R., Forsyth, A. D., et al. (2000). Using information, motivation enhancement, and skills training to reduce the risk of HIV infection for low-income urban woman: A second randomized clinical trial. *Health Psychology, 19,* 3–11.

Carey, M. P., Maisto, S. A., Kalichman, S. C., Forsyth, A. D., Wright, E. M., & Johnson, B. T. (1997). Enhancing motivation to reduce the risk of HIV infection for economically disadvantaged urban women. *Journal of Consulting and Clinical Psychology, 65,* 531–541.

Carr, E. S. (2003). Rethinking empowerment theory using a feminist lens: The importance of process. *Affilia, 18,* 8–20.

Carr, J. E., Austin, J. L., Britton, L. N., Kellum, K. K., & Bailey, J. S. (1999). An assessment of social validity trends in applied behavior analysis. *Behavioral Interventions, 14,* 223–231.

Casas, J. M. (1988). Cognitive behavioral approaches: A minority perspective. *The Counseling Psychologist, 16,* 106–110.

Certo, N., Mezzullo, K., & Hunter, D. (1985). The effect of total task chain training on the acquisition of busperson job skills at a full service community restaurant. *Education and Training of the Mentally Retarded, 20,* 148–156.

Chadsey-Rusch, J., Drasgow, E., Reinoehl, B., Halle, J., & Collet-Klingenberg, L. (1993). Using general-case instruction to teach spontaneous and generalized requests for assistance to learners with severe disabilities. *Journal of the Association for Persons with Severe Handicaps, 18,* 177–187.

Charlop, M. H., & Milstein, J. P. (1989). Teaching autistic children conversational speech using video modeling. *Journal of Applied Behavior Analysis, 22,* 275–282.

Christian, L., & Poling, A. (1997). Using self-management procedures to improve the productivity of adults with developmental disabilities in a competitive employment setting. *Journal of Applied Behavioral Analysis, 30,* 169–172.

Clarke, S., Dunlap, G., & Stichter, J. P. (2002). A descriptive analysis of intervention research in emotional and behavioral disorders from 1980 through 1999. *Behavior Modification, 26,* 659–683.

Coates, T. J. (1990). Strategies for modifying sexual behavior for primary and secondary prevention of HIV disease. *Journal of Consulting and Clinical Psychology, 58,* 57–69.

Collet-Klingenberg, L., & Chadsey-Rusch, J. (1991). Using a cognitive-process approach to teach social skills. *Education and Training in Mental Retardation, 26,* 258–270.

Cooper, K. J., & Browder, D. M. (2001). Preparing staff to enhance active participation of adults with severe disabilities by offering choice and prompting performance during a community purchasing activity. *Research in Developmental Disabilities, 22*, 1–20.

Corrigan, P. W. (1997). Behavior therapy empowers persons with severe mental illness. *Behavior Modification, 21*, 45–61.

Corrigan, P. W., Reedy, P., Thadani, D., & Ganet, M. (1995). Correlates of participation and completion in a Job Club for clients with psychiatric disability. *Rehabilitation Counseling Bulletin, 39*, 42–53.

Council on Social Work Education. (2001). *Educational policy and accreditation standards*. Washington, DC: Author.

Cowger, C. D. (1994). Assessing client strengths: Clinical assessment for client empowerment. *Social Work, 39*, 262–268.

Craft, M. A., Alber, S. R., & Heward, W. L. (1998). Teaching elementary students with developmental disabilities to recruit teacher attention in a general educational classroom: Effects on teacher praise and academic productivity. *Journal of Applied Behavior Analysis, 31*, 399–415.

Crouch, K. P., Karlan, G. R., & Rusch, F. R. (1984). Competitive employment: Utilizing the correspondence training paradigm to enhance productivity. *Education and Training of the Mentally Retarded, 19*, 268–275.

Cunconan-Lahr, R., & Brotherson, M. J. (1996). Advocacy in disability policy: Parents and consumers as advocates. *Mental Retardation, 34*, 352–358.

Cuvo, A. J., Leaf, R. B., & Borakove, L. S. (1978). Teaching janitorial skills to the mentally retarded: Acquisition, generalization, and maintenance. *Journal of Applied Behavior Analysis, 11*, 345–355.

Danziger, S., Corcoran, M., Danziger, S., & Heflin, C. M. (2000). Work, income, and material hardship after welfare reform. *Journal of Consumer Affairs, 34*, 6–30.

Dattilo, J., & Camarata, S. (1991). Facilitating conversation through self-initiated augmentative communication treatment. *Journal of Applied Behavior Analysis, 24*, 369–378.

Davis, C., Brady, M. P., Hamilton R., McEvoy, M. A., & Williams, R. E. (1994). Effects of high-probability requests on the social interactions of young children with severe disabilities. *Journal of Applied Behavior Analysis, 27*, 619–637.

Davis, C., Salo, L., & Redman, S. (2001). Evaluating the effectiveness of advocacy training for breast cancer advocates in Australia. *European Journal of Cancer Care, 10*, 82–86.

Davis, P., Bates, P., & Cuvo, A. J. (1983). Training a mentally retarded woman to work competitively: Effect of graphic feedback and a changing criterion design. *Education and Training of the Mentally Retarded, 18*, 158–163.

Delamater, R. J., & McNamara, J. R. (1986). The social impact of assertiveness: Research findings and clinical implications. *Behavior Modification, 10*, 139–158.

Dibley, S., & Lim, L. (1999). Providing choice making opportunities within and between daily school routines. *Journal of Behavioral Education, 9*, 117–132.

Dickersin, K., Bruan, L., Mead, M., Millikan, R., Wu, A. M., Pietenpol, J., et al. (2001). Development and implementation of a science training course for breast cancer activists: Project LEAD (leadership, education and advocacy development). *Health Expectations, 4*, 213–220.

Dickson, M. B. (1979). Job seeking skills program for the blind. *Journal of Visual Impairment and Blindness, 73*, 20–25.

Dickson, M. B., & MacDonell, P. K. (1982). Career clubs for blind job seekers. *Journal of Visual Impairment and Blindness, 76,* 1–4.

Dilk, M. N., & Bond, G. R. (1996). Meta-analytic evaluation of skills training research for individuals with severe mental illness. *Journal of Consulting and Clinical Psychology, 64,* 1337–1346.

Diner, S. J. (1970). Chicago social workers and blacks in the Progressive Era. *Social Service Review, 44,* 393–410.

DiPipi-Hoy, C., & Jitendra, A. (2004). A parent-delivered intervention to teach purchasing skills to young adults with disabilities. *Journal of Special Education, 38,* 144–157.

Dobson, K. S., & Khatri, N. (2000). Cognitive therapy: Looking backward, looking forward. *Journal of Clinical Psychology, 56,* 907–923.

Donohue, B., Acierno, R., Hersen, M., & Van Hasselt, V. B. (1995). Social skills training for depressed, visually impaired older adults: A treatment manual. *Behavior Modification, 19,* 379–424.

Donohue, B. Acierno, R., Van Hasselt, V. B., & Hersen, M. (1995). Social skills training in a depressed, visually impaired older adult. *Journal of Behavior Therapy and Experimental Psychiatry, 26,* 67–75.

Dow, M. G., Verdi, M. B., & Sacco, W. P. (1991). Training psychiatric patients to discuss medication issues: Effects on patient communication and knowledge of medications. *Behavior Modification, 15,* 3–21.

Downing, J. (1987). Conversational skills training: Teaching adolescents with mental retardation to be verbally assertive. *Mental Retardation, 25,* 147–155.

Drake, R. E., McHugo, G. J., Becker, D. R., Anthony, W. A., & Clark, R. E. (1996). The New Hampshire study of supported employment for people with severe mental illness. *Journal of Consulting and Clinical Psychology, 64,* 391–399.

Ducharme, D. E., & Holborn, S. W. (1997). Programming generalization of social skills in preschool children with hearing impairments. *Journal of Applied Behavior Analysis, 30,* 639–651.

Duncan, G. J., & Brooks-Gunn, J. (1997). *Consequences of growing up poor.* New York: Russell Sage Foundation.

Durlak, C. M., Rose, E., & Bursuck, W. D. (1994). Preparing high school students with learning disabilities for the transition to postsecondary education: Teaching the skills of self-determination. *Journal of Learning Disabilities, 27,* 51–59.

D'Zurilla, T. J., & Nezu, A. M. (1999). *Problem-solving therapy: A social competence approach to clinical intervention.* New York: Springer.

Eamon, M. K. (2001). Antecedents and socioemotional consequences of physical punishment on children in two-parent families. *Child Abuse & Neglect, 6,* 787–802.

Eamon, M. K. (2005). Social-demographic, school, neighborhood, and parenting influences on the academic achievement of Latino young adolescents. *Journal of Youth and Adolescence, 34,* 163–174.

East, J. F. (2000). Empowerment through welfare-rights organizing: A feminist perspective. *Affilia, 15,* 311–328.

Eckert, S. P. (2000). Teaching the social skill of accepting criticism to adults with developmental disabilities. *Education and Training in Mental Retardation and Developmental Disabilities, 35,* 16–24.

Eifert, G. H., Schulte, D., Zvolensky, M. J., Lejuez, C. W., & Lau, A. W. (1997). Manualized behavior therapy: Merits and challenges. *Behavior Therapy, 28*, 499–509.

Elksnin, L. K., Elksnin, N., & Sabornie, E. (1994). Job-related skills instruction of adolescents with mild mental retardation. *Journal for Vocational Special Needs Education, 17*, 1–7.

Ellis, A. (1992). Rational-emotive approaches to peace. *Journal of Cognitive Psychotherapy: An International Quarterly, 6*, 79–104.

Ellis, A. (1998). *Better, deeper, and more enduring brief therapy.* New York: Brunner/Mazel.

Engelman, K. K., Altus, D. E., & Mathews, R. M. (1999). Increasing engagement in daily activities by older adults with dementia. *Journal of Applied Behavior Analysis, 32*, 107–110.

English, K., Goldstein, H., Shafer, K., & Kaczmarek, L. (1997). Promoting interactions among preschoolers with and without disabilities: Effects of a buddy skills-training program. *Exceptional Children, 63*, 229–243.

Erin, J. N., Dignan, K., & Brown, P. A. (1991). Are social skills teachable? A review of the literature. *Journal of Visual Impairment and Blindness, 85*, 58–61.

Evans, I. M. (1997). The effect of values on scientific and clinical judgment in behavior therapy. *Behavior Therapy, 28*, 483–493.

Everhart, G., Luzader, M., & Tullos, S. (1980). Assertive skills training for the blind. *Journal of Visual Impairment and Blindness, 74*, 62–65.

Farley, R. C. (1987). Rational behavior problem-solving as a career development intervention for persons with disabilities. *Journal of Rational-Emotive Therapy, 5*, 32–42.

Farley, R. C., & Akridge, R. L. (1987). Training in relationship skills and rehabilitation clients' behavior in career settings. *Rehabilitation Counseling Bulletin, 30*, 148–156.

Faw, G. D., Davis, P. K., & Peck, C. (1996). Increasing self-determination: Teaching people with mental retardation to evaluate residential options. *Journal of Applied Behavior Analysis, 29*, 173–188.

Fawcett, S. B., Mathews, M., & Fletcher, R. K. (1980). Some promising dimensions for behavioral community technology. *Journal of Applied Behavior Analysis, 13*, 505–518.

Fawcett, S. B., & Miller, L. K. (1975). Training public speaking behavior: An experimental analysis and social validation. *Journal of Applied Behavior Analysis, 8*, 125–135.

Fawcett, S. B., Seekins, T., Wang, P. L., Muiu, C., & Suarez de Balcazar, Y. (1984). Creating and using social technologies for community empowerment. *Prevention in Human Services, 3*, 145–171.

Fawcett, S. B., Suarez de Balcazar, Y., Whang-Ramos, P. L., Seekins, T., Bradford, B., & Mathews, R. M. (1988). The concerns report: Involving consumers in planning for rehabilitation and independent living services. *American Rehabilitation, 14*, 17–19.

Fawcett, S. B., White, G. W., Balcazar, F. E., Suarez-Balcazar, Y., Mathews, R. M., Paine-Adres, A., et al. (1994). A contextual-behavioral model of empowerment: Case studies involving people with physical disabilities. *American Journal of Community Psychology, 22*, 471–496.

Fernandez-Ballesteros, R., Izal, M., Diaz, P., Gonzalez, J. L., & Souto, E. (1988). Training of conversational skills with institutionalized elderly: A preliminary study. *Perceptual and Motor Skills, 66,* 923–926.

Field, S. (1996). Self-determination instruction strategies for youth with learning disabilities. *Journal of Learning Disabilities, 29,* 40–52.

Fodor, I. G. (1988). Cognitive behavior therapy: Evaluation of theory and practice for addressing women's issues. In M. A. Dutton-Douglas & L. E. Walker (Eds.), *Feminist psychotherapies: Integration of therapeutic and feminist systems* (pp. 91–117). Norwood, NJ: Ablex.

Foss, G., Autry, W. P., & Irvin, L. K. (1989). A comparative evaluation of modeling, problem-solving, and behavioral rehearsal for teaching employment-related interpersonal skills to secondary students with mental retardation. *Education and Training of the Mentally Retarded, 24,* 17–27.

Foster, S. L., & Mash, E. J. (1999). Assessing social validity in clinical treatment research: Issues and procedures. *Journal of Consulting and Clinical Psychology, 67,* 308–319.

Foxx, R. M., Faw, G. D., Taylor, S., Davis, P. K., & Fulia, R. (1993). "Would I be able to . . . "? Teaching clients to assess the availability of their community living preferences. *American Journal on Mental Retardation, 98,* 235–248.

Foxx, R. M., McMorrow, M. J., Storey, K., & Rogers, B. M. (1984). Teaching social/sexual skills to mentally retarded adults. *American Journal of Mental Deficiency, 89,* 9–15.

Freedberg, S. (1989). Self-determination: Historical perspectives and effects on current practice. *Social Work, 34,* 33–38.

Furman, W., Geller, M., Simon, S. J., & Kelly, J. A. (1979). The use of a behavior rehearsal procedure for teaching job-interviewing skills to psychiatric patients. *Behavior Therapy, 10,* 157–167.

Galinsky, M. J., Schopler, J. H., Safier, E. J., & Gambrill, E. D. (1978). Assertion training for public welfare clients. *Social Work with Groups, 1,* 365–379.

Gambrill, E. (1985). Social skills training with the elderly. In L. L'Abate & M. A. Milan (Eds.), *Handbook of social skills training and research* (pp. 326–357). New York: Wiley.

Gambrill, E. D. (1994). Concepts and methods of behavioral treatment. In D. K. Granvold (Ed.), *Cognitive and behavioral treatment* (pp. 32–62). Pacific Grove, CA: Brooks/Cole.

Gambrill, E. (1995a). Assertion skills training. In W. O'Donohue & L. Krasner (Eds.), *Handbook of psychological skills training: Clinical techniques and applications* (pp. 81–118). Needham Heights, MA: Allyn & Bacon.

Gambrill, E. (1995b). Behavioral social work: Past, present, and future. *Research on Social Work Practice, 5,* 460–484.

Gambrill, E. (1997). *Social work practice: A critical thinker's guide.* New York: Oxford University Press.

Gaylord-Ross, R., Park, H., Johnston, S., Lee, M., & Goetz, L. (1995). Individual social skills training and co-worker training for supported employees with dual sensory impairment. *Behavior Modification, 19,* 78–94.

Gee, K., Graham, N., Sailor, W., & Goetz, L. (1995). Use of integrated, general education, and community settings as primary contexts for skill instruction for students with severe, multiple disabilities. *Behavior Modification, 19,* 33–58.

German, S. L., Martin, J. E., Marshall, L. H., & Sale, R. P. (2000). Promoting self-determination: Using *Take Action* to teach goal attainment. *Career Development for Exceptional Individuals, 23,* 27–38.

Gilchrist, L. D., & Schinke, S. P. (1983). Coping with contraception: Cognitive and behavioral methods with adolescents. *Cognitive Therapy and Research, 7,* 379–388.

Gitterman, A. (Ed.). (1991). *Handbook of social work practice with vulnerable populations.* New York: Columbia University Press.

Glueckauf, R. L., & Quittner, A. L. (1992). Assertiveness training for disabled adults in wheelchairs: Self-report, role-play, and activity pattern outcomes. *Journal of Consulting and Clinical Psychology, 60,* 419–425.

Glynn, S. M., Marder, S. R., Liberman, R. P., Blair, K., Wirshing, W. C., Wirshing, D. A., et al. (2002). Supplementing clinic-based skills training with manual-based community support sessions: Effects on social adjustment of patients with schizophrenia. *American Journal of Psychiatry, 159,* 829–837.

Gold, J. A. (1981). Incorporating cognitive-behavioral techniques into a traditional group work model. *Social Work with Groups, 4,* 79–89.

Goldfried, M. R., & Castonguay, L. G. (1993). Behavior therapy: Redefining strengths and limitations. *Behavior Therapy, 24,* 505–526.

Goldfried, M. R., & D'Zurilla, T. J. (1969). A behavior analytic model for assessing competence. In C. D. Spielberger (Ed.), *Current topics in clinical and community psychology* (pp. 151–196). New York: Academic.

Goldstein, H. (1990). The knowledge base of social work practice: Theory, wisdom, analogue, or art? *Families in Society: The Journal of Contemporary Human Services, 71,* 32–43.

Goldstein, R. S., & Baer, D. M. (1976). R.S.V.P.: A procedure to increase the personal mail and number of correspondents for nursing home residents. *Behavior Therapy, 7,* 348–354.

Gorey, K. M., Thyer, B. A., & Pawluck, D. E. (1998). Differential effectiveness of prevalent social work practice models: A meta-analysis. *Social Work, 43,* 269–278.

Goroff, N. N. (1983). Social work within a political and social context: The triumph of the therapeutic. In S. Ables & P. Ables (Eds.), *Social work with groups: Proceedings of 1978 symposium* (pp. 133–145). Louisville, KY: Committee for the Advancement of Social Work with Groups.

Granvold, D. K. (1994). Concepts and methods of cognitive treatment. In D. K. Granvold (Ed.), *Cognitive and behavioral treatment: Methods and applications* (pp. 3–31). Pacific Grove, CA: Brooks/Cole.

Gray, D. (1983). A Job Club for older job seekers: An experimental evaluation. *Journal of Gerontology, 38,* 363–368.

Gray, D. O., & Braddy, B. A. (1988). Experimental social innovation and client-centered job-seeking programs. *American Journal of Community Psychology, 16,* 325–343.

Greenberg, D., Meyer, R., Michalopoulos, C., & Wiseman, M. (2003). Explaining variation in the effects of Welfare-to-Work programs. *Evaluation Review, 27,* 359–394.

Greenberg, M. H., Levin-Epstein, J., Hutson, R. Q., Ooms, T. J., Schumacher, R., Turetsky, V., et al. (2002). The 1996 welfare law: Key elements and reauthorization issues affecting children. *The Future of Children, 12,* 27–77.

Greif, G. L., & Ephross, P. H. (2005). *Group work with populations at risk* (2nd ed.). Oxford: Oxford University Press.

Gresham, F. M. (2003). Establishing the technical adequacy of functional behavioral assessment: Conceptual and measurement challenges. *Behavioral Disorders, 28,* 282–298.

Gresham, F. M., Sugai, G., Horner, R. H. (2001). Interpreting outcomes of social skills training for students with high-incidence disabilities. *Exceptional Children, 67,* 331–344.

Griffiths, D., Feldman, M. A., & Tough, S. (1997). Programming generalization of social skills in adults with developmental disabilities: Effects on generalization and social validity. *Behavior Therapy, 28,* 253–269.

Groden, G. (1989). A guide for conducting a comprehensive behavioral analysis of a target behavior. *Journal of Behavior Therapy and Experimental Psychiatry, 12,* 163–169.

Grossi, T. A. (1998). Using a self-operated auditory prompting system to improve the work performance of two employees with severe disabilities. *Journal of the Association for Persons with Severe Handicaps, 23,* 149–154.

Grossi, T. A., & Heward, W. L. (1998). Using self-evaluation to improve the work productivity of trainees in a community-based restaurant training program. *Education and Training in Mental Retardation and Developmental Disabilities, 33,* 248–263.

Gutiérrez, L. M. (1990). Working with women of color: An empowerment perspective. *Social Work, 35,* 149–153.

Gutiérrez, L. M., & Ortega, R. (1991). Developing methods to empower Latinos: The importance of groups. *Social Work with Groups, 14,* 23–43.

Hacker, J. S. (2004). Privatizing risk without privatizing the welfare state: The hidden politics of social policy retrenchment in the United States. *American Political Science Review, 98,* 243–260.

Halasz-Dees, M., & Cuvo, A. J. (1986). Teaching a functional leisure skill cluster to rehabilitation clients: The art of macrame. *Applied Research in Mental Retardation, 7,* 79–93.

Halford, W. K., & Hayes, R. (1991). Psychological rehabilitation of chronic schizophrenic patients: Recent findings on social skills training and family psychoeducation. *Clinical Psychology Review, 11,* 23–44.

Hall, C., Sheldon-Wildgen, J., & Sherman, J. (1980). Teaching job interview skills to retarded clients. *Journal of Applied Behavior Analysis, 13,* 433–442.

Hall, J. A., Dineen, J. P., Schlesinger, D. J., & Stanton, R. (2000). Advanced group treatment for developmentally disabled adults with social skill deficits. *Research on Social Work Practice, 10,* 301–326.

Hall, J. A., Schlesinger, D. J., & Dineen, J. P. (1997). Social skills training in groups with developmentally disabled adults. *Research on Social Work Practice, 7,* 187–201.

Hampton, B. A. M., James, J. E., Wrigley, J. D., & Fullwood, F. C. (1980). Brief social skills training and peer involvement with an isolated resident of a psychiatric rehabilitation center. *Journal of Behavior Therapy and Experimental Psychiatry, 11,* 321–325.

Hansen, D. J., Zamboanga, B. L., & Sedlar, G. (2000). Cognitive-behavior therapy for ethnic minority adolescents: Broadening our perspectives. *Cognitive and Behavioral Practice, 7,* 54–60.

Hanson, M., Cancel, J., & Rolon, A. (1994). Reducing AIDS risks among dually disordered adults. *Research on Social Work Practice, 4,* 14–27.

Harchik, A. E., Sherman, J. A., & Sheldon J. B. (1992). The use of self-management procedures by people with developmental disabilities: A brief review. *Research in Developmental Disabilities, 13,* 211–227.

Haring, T. G., & Breen, C. G. (1992). A peer-mediated social network intervention to enhance the social integration of persons with moderate and severe disabilities. *Journal of Applied Behavior Analysis, 25,* 319–333.

Harris, R. M., Bausell, R. B., Scott, D. E., Hetherington, S. E., & Kavanagh, K. H. (1998). An intervention for changing high-risk HIV behaviors of African American drug-dependent women. *Research in Nursing & Health, 21,* 239–250.

Hart, T. A., & Heimberg, R. G. (2001). Presenting problems among treatment-seeking gay, lesbian, and bisexual youth. *Psychotherapy in Practice, 57,* 615–627.

Hasenfeld, Y. (1987). Power in social work practice. *Social Service Review, 61,* 469–483.

Hayden, M. F., & Nelis, T. (2002). Self-advocacy. In R. L. Schalock, P. C. Baker, & M. D. Croser (Eds.), *Embarking on a new century: Mental retardation at the end of the 20th century* (pp. 221–233). Washington, DC: American Association on Mental Retardation.

Heckaman, K., Conroy, M., Fox, J., & Chait, A. (2000). Functional assessment-based intervention research on students with or at risk for emotional and behavioral disorders in school settings. *Behavioral Disorders, 25,* 196–210.

Heimberg, R. G., Cunningham, J., Stanley, J., & Blankenberg, R. (1982). Preparing unemployed youth for job interviews: A controlled evaluation of social skills training. *Behavior Modification, 6,* 299–322.

Henin, A., Otto, M. W., & Reilly-Harrington, R. (2001). Introducing flexibility in manualized treatments: Application of recommended strategies to the cognitive-behavioral treatment of bipolar disorder. *Cognitive and Behavioral Practice, 8,* 317–328.

Henly, J. R., & Lyons, S. (2000). The negotiation of child care and employment demands among low-income parents. *Journal of Social Issues, 56,* 683–706.

Hepler, J. B. (1997). Evaluating a social skills program for children with learning disabilities. *Social Work with Groups, 20,* 21–36.

Hess, R. E., Clapper, C. R., Hoekstra, K., & Gibison, F. P., Jr. (2001). Empowerment effects of teaching leadership skills to adults with a severe mental illness and their families. *Psychiatric Rehabilitation Journal, 24,* 257–265.

Hicks-Coolick, A., & Kurtz, P. D. (1997). Preparing students with learning disabilities for success in postsecondary education: Needs and services. *Social Work in Education, 19,* 31–43.

Hildebrand, R. G., Martin, G. L., Furer, P., & Hazen, A. (1990). A recruitment-of-praise package to increase productivity levels of developmentally handicapped workers. *Behavior Modification, 14,* 97–113.

Hobfoll, S. E., Jackson, A. P., Lavin, J., Britton, P. J., & Shepherd, J. B. (1994). Reducing inner-city women's AIDS risk activities: A study of single, pregnant women. *Health Psychology, 13,* 397–403.

Hollar, D. (2003). A holistic theoretical model for examining welfare reform: Quality of life. *Public Administration Review, 63,* 90–104.

Hovell, M., Blumberg, E., Sipan, C., Hofstetter, C. R., Burkham, S., Atkins, C., et al. (1998). Skills training for pregnancy and AIDS prevention in Anglo and Latino youth. *Journal of Adolescent Health, 23,* 139–149.

Hovell, M. F., Hillman, E. R., Blumberg, E., Sipan, C., Atkins, C., Hofstetter, C. R., et al. (1994). A behavioral-ecological model of adolescent sexual development: A template for AIDS prevention. *Journal of Sex Research, 31,* 267–281.

Huang, W., & Cuvo, A. J. (1997). Social skills training for adults with mental retardation in job-related settings. *Behavior Modification, 21,* 3–44.

Huber-Marshall, L., Martin, J. E., Maxson, L. L., Hughes, W., Miller, T. L., McGill, T., & Jerman, P. (1999). *Take action: Making goals happen.* Longmont, CO: Sopris West.

Hudson, B., & Macdonald, G. M. (1986). *Behavioral social work: An introduction.* London: Macmillan.

Hughes, C., Fowler, S. E., Copeland, S. R., Agran, M., Wehmeyer, M. L., & Church-Pupke, P. P. (2004). Supporting high school students to engage in recreational activities with peers. *Behavior Modification, 28,* 3–27.

Hughes, C., Harmer, M. L., Killian, D. J., & Niarhos, F. (1995). The effects of multiple-exemplar self-instructional training on high school students' generalized conversational interactions. *Journal of Applied Behavior Analysis, 28,* 201–218.

Hughes, C., & Petersen, D. L. (1989). Utilizing a self-instructional training package to increase on-task behavior and work performance. *Education and Training of the Mentally Retarded, 24,* 114–120.

Hughes, C., & Rusch, F. R. (1989). Teaching supported employees with severe mental retardation to solve problems. *Journal of Applied Behavior Analysis, 22,* 365–372.

Hunt, P., Alwell, M., Goetz, L., & Sailor W. (1990). Generalized effects of conversation skill training. *Journal of the Association for Persons with Severe Handicaps, 15,* 250–260.

Hunter, J., & Schaecher, R. (1994). AIDS prevention for lesbian, gay, and bisexual adolescents. *Families in Society: The Journal of Contemporary Human Services, 75,* 346–354.

Hunter, P., & Kelso, E. N. (1985). Feminist behavior therapy. *The Behavior Therapist, 10,* 201–204.

Hurst, S. A., & Genest, M. (1995). Cognitive-behavioural therapy with a feminist orientation: A perspective for therapy with depressed women. *Canadian Psychology, 36,* 236–257.

Individuals with Disabilities Education Act of 1990, Pub. L. No. 101-476, Title 20, U.S.C. 1400 et seq.

Iversen, R. R. (1998). Occupational social work for the 21th century. *Social Work, 43,* 551–566.

Iwamasa, G. Y. (1997). Behavior therapy and a culturally diverse society: Forging an alliance. *Behavior Therapy, 28,* 347–355.

Jacobs, H. E., Collier, R., & Wissusik, D. (1992). The job-finding module: Training skills for seeking competitive community employment. *New Directions for Mental Health Services, 53,* 105–115.

Jacobs, H. E., Kardashian, S., Kreinbring, R. K., Ponder, R., & Simpson, A. R. (1984). A skills-oriented model for facilitating employment among psychiatrically disabled persons. *Rehabilitation Counseling Bulletin, 28,* 87–96.

Johnson-Masotti, A. P., Pinkerton, S. D., Kelly, J. A., & Stevenson, L. Y. (2000). Cost-effectiveness of an HIV risk reduction intervention for adults with severe mental illness. *AIDS Care, 12,* 321–332.

Jolly, A. C., Test, D. W., & Spooner, F. (1993). Using badges to increase initiations of children with severe disabilities in a play setting. *Journal of the Association for Persons with Severe Handicaps, 18,* 46–51.

Jung, R. S., & Jason, L. A. (1998). Job interview social skills training for Asian-American immigrants. *Journal of Human Behavior in the Social Environment, 1,* 11–25.

Kahn, S. (1970). *How people get power: Organizing oppressed communities for action.* New York: McGraw-Hill.

Kalichman, S. C., Sikkema, K. J., Kelly, J. A., & Bulto, M. (1995). Use of a brief behavioral skills intervention to prevent HIV infection among chronic mentally ill adults. *Psychiatric Services, 46,* 275–280.

Kamps, D. M., Potucek, J., Lopez, A. G., Kravits, T., & Kemmerer, K. (1997). The use of peer networks across multiple settings to improve social interaction for students with autism. *Journal of Behavioral Education, 7,* 335–357.

Kantrowitz, R. E., & Ballou, M. (1992). A feminist critique of cognitive-behavioral therapy. In L. S. Brown & M. Ballou (Eds.), *Personality and psychopathology: Feminist reappraisals* (pp. 70–87). New York: Guilford.

Kaplan, H., Hemmes, N. S., Motz, P., & Rodriguez, H. (1996). Self-reinforcement and persons with developmental disabilities. *Psychological Record, 46,* 161–178.

Kazantzis, N., Pachana, N. A., & Secker, D. L. (2003). Cognitive-behavioral therapy for older adults: Practice guidelines for the use of homework assignments. *Cognitive and Behavioral Practice, 10,* 324–332.

Kazdin, A. E., & Weisz, J. R. (Ed.). (2003). *Evidence-based psychotherapies for children and adolescents.* New York: Guilford.

Kearney, C. A., Bergan, K. P., & McKnight, T. J. (1998). Choice availability and persons with mental retardation: A longitudinal and regression analysis. *Journal of Developmental and Physical Disabilities, 10,* 291–305.

Kelly, J. A., Laughlin, C., Claiborne, M., & Patterson, J. (1979). A group procedure for teaching job interviewing skills to formerly hospitalized psychiatric patients. *Behavior Therapy, 10,* 299–310.

Kelly, J. A., McAuliffe, T. L., Sikkema, K. J., Murphy, D. A., Somlai, A. M., Mulry, G., et al. (1997). Reduction in risk behavior among adults with severe mental illness who learned to advocate for HIV prevention. *Psychiatric Services, 48,* 1283–1288.

Kelly, J. A., & Murphy, D. A. (1992). Psychological interventions with AIDS and HIV: Prevention and treatment. *Journal of Consulting and Clinical Psychology, 60,* 576–585.

Kelly, J. A., Murphy, D. A., Washington, C. D., Wilson, T. S., Koob, J. J., Davis, D. R., et al. (1994). The effects of HIV/AIDS intervention groups for high-risk women in urban clinics. *American Journal of Public Health, 84,* 1918–1922.

Kelly, J. A., St. Lawrence, J. S., Hood, H. V., & Brasfield, T. L. (1989). Behavioral intervention to reduce AIDS risk activities. *Journal of Consulting and Clinical Psychology, 57,* 60–67.

Kelly, J. A., Urey, J. R., & Patterson, J. T. (1980). Improving heterosocial conversational skills of male psychiatric patients through a small group training procedure. *Behavior Therapy, 11,* 179–188.

Kelly, J. A., Wildman, B. G., & Berler, E. S. (1980). Small group behavioral training to improve the job interview skills repertoire of mildly retarded adolescents. *Journal of Applied Behavior Analysis, 13,* 461–471.

Kennedy, C. H. (2002). The maintenance of behavior change as an indicator of social validity. *Behavior Modification, 26,* 594–604.

Kennedy, C. H., & Haring, T. G. (1993). Teaching choice making during social interactions to students with profound multiple disabilities. *Journal of Applied Behavior Analysis, 26,* 63–76.

Keogh, D. A., Faw, G. D., Whitman, T. L., & Reid, D. H. (1984). Enhancing leisure skills in severely retarded adolescents through a self-instructional treatment package. *Analysis and Intervention in Developmental Disabilities, 4,* 333–351.

Kern, R. S., Liberman, R. P., Kopelowicz, A., Mintz, J., & Green, M. F. (2002). Applications of errorless learning for improving work performance in persons with schizophrenia. *American Journal of Psychiatry, 159,* 1921–1926.

Kim, R. Y. (2000). Factors associated with employment status of parents receiving Temporary Assistance for Needy Families. *Social Work Research, 24,* 211–222.

King, G. A., Specht, J. A., Schultz, I., Warr-Leeper, G., Redekop, W., & Risebrough, N. (1997). Social skills training for withdrawn unpopular children with physical disabilities: A preliminary evaluation. *Rehabilitation Psychology, 42,* 47–60.

Klebanov, P. K., Brooks-Gunn, J., & Duncan, G. J. (1994). Does neighborhood and family poverty affect mothers' parenting, mental health and social support? *Journal of Marriage and the Family, 56,* 441–455.

Koegel, L. K., Koegel, R. L., Hurley, C., & Frea, W. D. (1992). Improving social skills and disruptive behavior in children with autism through self-management. *Journal of Applied Behavior Analysis, 25,* 341–353.

Konarski, E. A., Jr., Johnson, M. R., & Whitman, T. L. (1980). A systematic investigation of resident participation in a nursing home activities program. *Journal of Behavior Therapy and Experimental Psychiatry, 11,* 249–257.

Kondrat, M. E. (1995). Concept, act, and interest in professional practice: Implications of an empowerment perspective. *Social Service Review, 69,* 405–428.

Kopels, S. (1995). The Americans with Disabilities Act: A tool to combat poverty. *Journal of Social Work Education, 31,* 337–346.

Krantz, P. J., & McClannahan, L. E. (1998). Social interaction skills for children with autism: A script-fading procedure for beginning readers. *Journal of Applied Behavior Analysis, 31,* 191–202.

Kregel, J., Wehman, P., & Banks, P. D. (1989). The effects of consumer characteristics and type of employment model on individual outcomes in supported employment. *Journal of Applied Behavior Analysis, 22,* 407–415.

Lagomarcino, T. R., Hughes, C., & Rusch, F. R. (1989). Utilizing self-management to teach independence on the job. *Education & Training in Mental Retardation and Developmental Disabilities, 24,* 139–148.

Lancaster, P. E., Schumaker, J. B., & Deshler, D. D. (2002). The development and validation of an interactive hypermedia program for teaching a self-advocacy strategy to students with disabilities. *Learning Disability Quarterly, 25,* 227–302.

Latimer, P. R., & Sweet, A. A. (1984). Cognitive versus behavioral procedures in cognitive-behavior therapy: A critical review of the evidence. *Journal of Behavior Therapy and Experimental Psychiatry, 15,* 9–22.

LeBlanc, L. A., & Matson, J. L. (1995). A social skills training program for preschoolers with developmental delays. *Behavior Modification, 19,* 234–246.

Lee, J. A. B. (1996). The empowerment approach to social work practice. In F. J. Turner (Ed.), *Social work treatment: Interlocking theoretical approaches* (4th ed., pp. 218–249). New York: Free Press.

Leslie, J. C. (1997). Ethical implications of behavior modification: Historical and current issues. *Psychological Record, 47,* 637–648.

Levine, O. H., Britton, P. J., James, T. C., Jackson, A. P., Hobfoll, S. E., & Lavin, J. P. (1993). The empowerment of women: A key to HIV prevention. *Journal of Community Psychology, 21,* 320–334.

Lewis, S. Y. (1994). Cognitive-behavioral therapy. In L. Comas-Díaz & B. Greene (Eds.), *Women of color: Integrating ethnic and gender identities in psychotherapy* (pp. 223–238). New York: Guilford.

Liberman, R. P., & Corrigan, P. W. (1993). Designing new psychosocial treatments for schizophrenia. *Psychiatry, 56,* 238–249.

Liberman, R. P., Eckman, T. A., & Marder, S. R. (2001). Training in social problem solving among persons with schizophrenia. *Psychiatric Services, 52,* 31–33.

Liberman, R. P., Glynn, S., Blair, K. E., Ross, D., & Marder, S. R. (2002). In vivo amplified skills training: Promoting generalization of independent living skills for clients with schizophrenia. *Psychiatry, 65,* 137–155.

Liberman, R. P., & Kopelowicz, A. (2002). Teaching persons with severe mental disabilities to be their own case managers. *Psychiatric Services, 53,* 1377–1379.

Liberman, R. P., Wallace, C. J., Blackwell, G., Eckman, T. A., Vaccaro, J. V., & Kuehnel, T. G. (1993). Innovations in skills training for the seriously mentally ill: The UCLA social and independent living skills modules. *Innovations and Research, 2,* 43–60.

Liberman, R. P., Wallace, C. J., Blackwell, G., Kopelowicz, A., Vaccaro, J. V., & Mintz, J. (1998). Skills training versus psychosocial occupational therapy for persons with persistent schizophrenia. *American Journal of Psychiatry, 155,* 1087–1091.

Likins, M., Salzerg, C. L., Stowitschek, J. J., Kraft, B. L., & Curl, R. (1989). Co-worker implemented job training: The use of coincidental training and quality-control checking on the food preparation skills of trainees with mental retardation. *Journal of Applied Behavior Analysis, 22,* 381–393.

Lindstrom, L. E., Benz, M. R., & Johnson, M. D. (1996). Developing Job Clubs for students in transition. *Teaching Exceptional Children, 29,* 18–21.

Linhorst, D. M., & Eckert, A. (2003). Conditions for empowering people with severe mental illness. *Social Service Review, 77,* 279–305.

Linsk, N., Howe, M. W., & Pinkston, E. M. (1975). Behavioral group work in a home for the aged. *Social Work, 20,* 454–463.

Long, D. A. (2001). From support to self-sufficiency: How successful are programs in advancing the financial independence and well-being of welfare recipients? *Evaluation and Program Planning, 24,* 389–408.

Lovett, D. L., & Harris, M. B. (1987). Important skills for adults with mental retardation: The client's point of view. *Mental Retardation, 25,* 351–356.

Low, K. G., Joliceour, M. R., Colman, R. A., Stone, L. E., Fleisher, C. L., et al. (1994). Women participants in research: Assessing progress. *Women & Health, 22,* 79–98.

Luthar, S. S. (1999). *Poverty and children's adjustment.* Thousand Oaks, CA: Sage.

Lynn, L. E. (2002). Social services and the state: The public appropriation of private charity. *Social Service Review, 76,* 58–82.

MacDonald, G., Sheldon, B., & Gillespie, J. (1992). Contemporary studies of the effectiveness of social work. *British Journal of Social Work, 22,* 615–643.

Marder, S. R., Wirshing, W. C., Mintz, J., McKenzie, J., Johnston, K., Eckman T. A., et al. (1996). Two-year outcome of social skills training and group psychotherapy for outpatients with schizophrenia. *American Journal of Psychiatry, 153,* 1585–1592.

Margolin, L. (1997). *Under the cover of kindness: The invention of social work.* Charlottesville, VA: University Press of Virginia.

Marschall, M. J. (2001). Does the shoe fit? Testing models of participation for African-American and Latino involvement in local politics. *Urban Affairs Review, 37,* 227–248.

Martell, C. R., Safren, S. A., & Prince, S. E. (2004). *Cognitive-behavioral therapies with lesbian, gay, and bisexual clients.* New York: Guilford.

Martin, G., & Hrydowy, E. R. (1989). Self-monitoring and self-managed reinforcement procedures for improving work productivity of developmentally disabled workers: A review. *Behavior Modification, 13,* 322–339.

Martin, G., Pallotta-Cornick, A., Johnstone, G., & Goyos, A. C. (1980). A supervisory strategy to improve work performance for lower functioning retarded clients in a sheltered workshop. *Journal of Applied Behavior Analysis, 13,* 183–190.

Martin, J. E., Marshal, L. H., Maxson, L. L., & Jerman, P. (1993a). *Student workbook: Self-directed IEP.* Colorado Springs: University of Colorado at Colorado Springs.

Martin, J. E., Marshal, L. H., Maxson, L. L., & Jerman, P. (1993b). *Teacher's manual for the self-directed IEP video and workbook.* Colorado Springs: University of Colorado at Colorado Springs.

Marwell, N. P. (2004). Privatizing the welfare state: Nonprofit community-based organizations as political actors. *American Sociological Review, 69,* 265–291.

Mathews, R. M. (1984). Teaching employment interview skills to unemployed adults. *Journal of Employment Counseling, 21,* 156–161.

Mathews, R. M., & Fawcett, S. B. (1984). Building the capacities of job candidates through behavioral instruction. *Journal of Community Psychology, 12,* 123–129.

Mathews, R. M., Whang, P. L., & Fawcett, S. B. (1984). *Occupational skills assessment instrument: Monograph 17.* Lawrence, KS: Research and Training Center on Independent Living, University of Kansas.

Mathur, S. R., & Rutherford, R. B., Jr. (1996). Is social skills training effective for students with emotional or behavioral disorders? Research issues and needs. *Behavioral Disorders, 22,* 21–28.

Matson, J. L., & Adkins, J. (1980). A self-instructional social skills training program for mentally retarded persons. *Mental Retardation, 18,* 245–248.

Matson, J. L., & Andrasik, F. (1982). Training leisure-time social-interaction skills to mentally retarded adults. *American Journal of Mental Deficiency, 86,* 533–542.

Mattaini, M. A. (1993). Behavior analysis and community practice: A review. *Research on Social Work Practice, 3,* 420–447.

Mattaini, M. A. (1997). *Clinical practice with individuals.* Washington, DC: NASW Press.

Mattaini, M. A., & Thyer, B. A. (Eds.). (1996). *Finding solutions to social problems: Behavioral strategies for change.* Washington, DC: American Psychological Association.

McClannahan, L. E., & Risley, T. R. (1975). Design of living environments for nursing home residents: Increasing participation in recreation activities. *Journal of Applied Behavior Analysis, 8,* 261–268.

McCuller, G. L., Salzberg, C. L., & Kraft, B. L. (1987). Producing generalized job initiative in severely mentally retarded sheltered workers. *Journal of Applied Behavior Analysis, 20,* 413–420.

McDonnell, J., Nofs, D., Hardman, M., & Chambless, C. (1989). An analysis of the procedural components of supported employment programs associated with employment outcomes. *Journal of Applied Behavior Analysis, 22,* 417–428.

McEvoy, M. A., Nordquist, V. M., Twardosz, S., Heckaman, K. A., Wehby, J. H., & Denny, R. K. (1988). Promoting autistic children's peer interaction in an integrated early childhood setting using affection activities. *Journal of Applied Behavior Analysis, 21,* 193–200.

McLeod, J. D., & Kessler, R. C. (1990). Socioeconomic status differences in vulnerability to undesirable life events. *Journal of Health and Social Behavior, 31,* 162–172.

McMahon, C. M., Wacker, D. P., Sasso, G. M., Berg, W. K., & Newton, S. M. (1996). Analysis of frequency and type of interactions in a peer-mediated social skills intervention: Instructional vs. social interactions. *Education and Training in Mental Retardation and Developmental Disabilities, 31,* 339–352.

McNair, L. D. (1996). African American women and behavior therapy: Integrating theory, culture, and clinical practice. *Cognitive and Behavioral Practice, 3,* 337–349.

McNally, R. J., Kompik, J. J., & Sherman, G. (1984). Increasing the productivity of mentally retarded workers through self-management. *Analysis and Intervention in Developmental Disabilities, 4,* 129–135.

Meichenbaum, D. (1993). Stress inoculation training: A twenty year update. In R. L. Woolfolk & P. M. Lehrer (Eds.), *Principles and practices of stress management* (2nd ed., pp. 373–406). New York: Guilford.

Meichenbaum, D. H., & Goodman, J. (1971). Training impulsive children to talk to themselves: A means of developing self control. *Journal of Abnormal Psychology, 77,* 115–126.

Melin, L., & Götestam, K. G. (1981). The effects of rearranging ward routines on communication and eating behaviors of psychogeriatric patients. *Journal of Applied Behavior Analysis, 14*, 47–51.

Meyer, L. H., & Evans, I. M. (1993). Science and practice in behavioral intervention: Meaningful outcomes, research validity, and usable knowledge. *Journal of the Association for Persons with Severe Handicaps, 18*, 224–234.

Michalopoulos, C., Schwartz, C., & Adams-Ciardullo, D. (2000, August). *National evaluation of Welfare-to-Work strategies. What works best for whom: Impacts of 20 Welfare-to-Work programs by subgroup.* New York: Manpower Demonstration Research Corporation.

Mickelson, K. D., & Kubzansky, L. D. (2003). Social distribution of social support: The mediating role of life events. *American Journal of Community Psychology, 32*, 265–281.

Miller, L. K., & Miller, O. L. (1970). Reinforcing self-help group activities of welfare recipients. *Journal of Applied Behavior Analysis, 3*, 57–64.

Miller, M. C., Cooke, N. L., Test, D. W., & White, R. (2003). Effects of friendship circles on the social interactions of elementary age students with mild disabilities. *Journal of Behavioral Education, 12*, 167–184.

Montague, M. (1988). Job-related social skills training for adolescents with handicaps. *Career Development for Exceptional Individuals, 11*, 26–41.

Moore, S. C., Agran, M., & Fodor-Davis, J. (1989). Using self-management strategies to increase the production rates of workers with severe handicaps. *Education and Training in Mental Retardation and Developmental Disabilities, 24*, 324–332.

Mor-Barak, M. E., & Tynan, M. (1993). Older workers and the workplace: A new challenge for occupational social work. *Social Work, 38*, 45–55.

Morgan, R. L., & Salzberg, C. L. (1992). Effects of video-assisted training on employment-related social skills of adults with severe mental retardation. *Journal of Applied Behavior Analysis, 25*, 365–383.

Mosley, J., & Tiehen, L. (2004). The food safety net after welfare reform: Use of private and public food assistance in the Kansas City metropolitan area. *Social Service Review, 78*, 267–283.

Msall, M. E., Avery, R. C., Tremont, M. R., Lima, J. C., Rogers, M. L., & Hogan, D. P. (2003). Functional disability and school activity limitations in 41300 school-age children: Relationship to medical impairments. *Pediatrics, 111*, 548–553.

Mueser, K. T., Foy, D. W., & Carter, M. J. (1986). Social skills training for job maintenance in a psychiatric patient. *Journal of Counseling Psychology, 33*, 360–362.

Myers, L. L., & Thyer, B. A. (1997). Social work practice with deaf clients: Issues in culturally competent assessment. *Social Work in Health Care, 26*, 61–76.

National Association of Social Workers. (1999). *Code of ethics of the National Association of Social Workers.* Washington, DC: Author.

National Association of Social Workers. (2000). *Social work speaks: National Association of Social Workers policy statements, 2000–2003* (5th ed.). Washington, DC: NASW Press.

Nietupski, J., Hamre-Nietupski, S., Green, K., Varnum-Teeter, K., Twedt, B., LePera, D., et al. (1986). Self-initiated and sustained leisure activity participation by students with moderate/severe handicaps. *Education and Training in Mental Retardation and Developmental Disabilities, 21*, 259–264.

Nietupski, J., & Svoboda, R. (1982). Teaching a cooperative leisure skill to severely handicapped adults. *Education and Training in Mental Retardation and Developmental Disabilities, 17,* 38–43.

Norman, J. L. (1996). Culturally sensitive implementation of cognitive therapy in treating depression. *Journal of Multicultural Social Work, 4,* 75–88.

Nyamathi, A., Flaskerud, J., Keenan, C., & Leake, B. (1998). Effectiveness of a specialized vs. traditional AIDS education program attended by homeless and drug-addicted women alone or with supportive persons. *AIDS Education and Prevention, 10,* 433–446.

O'Hare, T. (2005). *Evidence-based practices for social workers.* Chicago: Lyceum.

Olmeda, R. E., & Kauffman, J. M. (2003). Sociocultural considerations in social skills training research with African American students with emotional or behavioral disorders. *Journal of Developmental and Physical Disabilities, 15,* 101–121.

Opulente, M., & Mattaini, M. A. (1997). Toward welfare that works. *Research on Social Work Practice, 7,* 115–135.

O'Reilly, M. F., Lancioni, G. E., & Kierans, I. (2000). Teaching leisure social skills to adults with moderate mental retardation: An analysis of acquisition, generalization, and maintenance. *Education and Training in Mental Retardation and Developmental Disabilities, 35,* 250–258.

O'Reilly, M. F., Lancioni, G. E., & O'Kane, N. (2000). Using a problem-solving approach to teach social skills to workers with brain injuries in supported employment settings. *Journal of Vocational Rehabilitation, 14,* 187–194.

Organista, K. C., & Muňoz, R. F. (1996). Cognitive behavioral therapy with Latinos. *Cognitive and Behavioral Practice, 3,* 255–270.

Paine, A. L., Suarez-Balcazar, Y., Fawcett, S. B., & Borck-Jameson, L. (1992). Supportive transactions: Their measurement and enhancement in two mutual-aid groups. *Journal of Community Psychology, 20,* 163–180.

Palmer, C., & Roessler, R. T. (2000). Requesting classroom accommodations: Self-advocacy and conflict resolution training for college students with disabilities. *Journal of Rehabilitation, 66,* 38–43.

Palmer, S. B., & Wehmeyer, M. L. (2003). Promoting self-determination in early elementary school: Teaching self-regulated problem solving and goal-setting skills. *Remedial and Special Education, 24,* 115–126.

Palmer, S. B., Wehmeyer, M. L., Gipson, K., & Agran, M. (2004). Promoting access to the general curriculum by teaching self-determination skills. *Exceptional Children, 70,* 427–439.

Park, H., & Gaylord-Ross, R. (1989). A problem-solving approach to social skills training in employment settings with mentally retarded youth. *Journal of Applied Behavior Analysis, 22,* 373–380.

Parsons, M. B., Harper, V. H., Jensen, J. M., & Reid, D. H. (1997). Assisting older adults with severe disabilities in expressing leisure preferences: A protocol for determining choice-making skills. *Research in Developmental Disabilities, 18,* 113–126.

Parsons, M. B., & Reid, D. H. (1990). Assessing food preferences among persons with profound mental retardation: Providing opportunities to make choices. *Journal of Applied Behavior Analysis, 23,* 183–195.

Parsons, M. B., Reid, D. H., Reynolds, J., & Bumgarner, M. (1990). Effects of chosen versus assigned jobs on the work performance of persons with severe handicaps. *Journal of Applied Behavior Analysis, 23,* 253–258.

Perez-Johnson, I., Hershey, A., & Bellotti, J. (2000, June). *Further progress, persistent constraints: Findings from a second survey of the Welfare-to-Work Grants Program.* Princeton, NJ: Mathematica Policy Research Inc.

Peterson, J. L., Coates, T. J., Catania, J., Hauck, W. W., Acree, M., Daigle, D., et al. (1996). Evaluation of an HIV risk reduction intervention among African-American homosexual and bisexual men. *AIDS, 10,* 319–325.

Peterson, L. (1997). Commentary on "The Effect of Values on Scientific and Clinical Judgment in Behavior Therapy." *Behavior Therapy, 28,* 495–497.

Peterson, R. F., Knapp, T. J., Rosen, J. C., & Pither, B. F. (1977). The effects of furniture arrangement on the behavior of geriatric patients. *Behavior Therapy, 8,* 464–467.

Petrides, P., Petermann, F., Henrichs, H. R., Petzoldt, R., Rölver, K. M., Schidlmeier, A., et al. (1995). Coping with employment discrimination against diabetics: Trends in social medicine and social psychology. *Patient Education and Counseling, 26,* 203–208.

Plienis, A. J., Hansen, D. J., Ford, F., Smith, S., Jr., Stark, L. J., & Kelly, J. A. (1987). Behavioral small group training to improve the social skills of emotionally-disordered adolescents. *Behavior Therapy, 18,* 17–32.

Pollard, N. L. (1998). Development of social interaction skills in preschool children with autism: A review of the literature. *Child & Family Behavior Therapy, 20,* 1–16.

Purcell, D. W., Campos, P. E., & Perilla, J. L. (1996). Therapy with lesbians and gay men: A cognitive behavioral perspective. *Cognitive and Behavioral Practice, 3,* 391–415.

Putnam, R. (2000). *Bowling alone: The collapse and revival of American community.* New York: Simon & Schuster.

Quattrochi-Tubin, S., & Jason, L. A. (1980). Enhancing social interactions and activity among the elderly through stimulus control. *Journal of Applied Behavior Analysis, 13,* 159–163.

Rainwater, L., & Smeeding, T. M. (2003). *Poor kids in a rich country.* New York: Russell Sage Foundation.

Rappaport, J. (1981). In praise of paradox: A social policy of empowerment over prevention. *American Journal of Community Psychology, 9,* 1–25.

Rappaport, J. (1984). Studies in empowerment: Introduction to the issue. *Prevention in Human Services, 3,* 1–7.

Rasing, E. J., Coninx, F., Duker, P. C., & Van den Hurk, A. J. (1994). Acquisition and generalization of social behaviors in language-disabled deaf adolescents. *Behavior Modification, 18,* 411–442.

Reid, D. H., Parsons, M. B., & Green, C. W. (1991). *Providing choices and preferences for persons who have severe handicaps: Practical procedures for good times.* Morganton, NC: Habilitative Management Consultants.

Reid, D. H., Parsons, M. B., Green, C. W., & Browning, L. B. (2001). Increasing one aspect of self-determination among adults with severe multiple disabilities in supported work. *Journal of Applied Behavior Analysis, 34,* 341–344.

Reid, W. J. (2004). Contribution of operant theory to social work practice and research. In H. E. Briggs & T. L. Rzepnicki (Eds.), *Using evidence in social work practice: Behavioral perspectives* (pp. 36–54). Chicago: Lyceum.

Reid, W. J., Kenaley, B. D., & Colvin, J. (2004). Do some interventions work better than others? A review of comparative social work experiments. *Social Work Research, 28,* 71–81.

Reinhard, J. (2000). Limitations of mental health case management: A rational emotive and cognitive therapy perspective. *Journal of Rational-Emotive & Cognitive-Behavior Therapy, 18,* 103–117.

Remler, D. K., & Glied, S. A. (2003). What other programs can teach us: Increasing participation in health insurance programs. *American Journal of Public Health, 93,* 67–74.

Rife, J. C., & Belcher, J. R. (1994). Assisting unemployed older workers to become reemployed: An experimental evaluation. *Research on Social Work Practice, 4,* 3–13.

Risley, R. M., & Cuvo, A. J. (1980). Training mentally retarded adults to make emergency telephone calls. *Behavior Modification, 4,* 513–525.

Roffman, R. A., Downey, L., Beadnell, B., Gordon, J. R., Craver, J. N., & Stephens, R. S. (1997). Cognitive-behavioral group counseling to prevent HIV transmission in gay and bisexual men: Factors contributing to successful risk reduction. *Research on Social Work Practice, 7,* 165–186.

Rose, S. D. (1989). *Working with adults in groups.* San Francisco: Jossey-Bass.

Rose, S. D., & Edleson, J. L. (1987). *Working with children and adolescents in groups.* San Francisco: Jossey-Bass.

Rosen, A., & Proctor, E. K. (1981). Distinctions between treatment outcomes and their implications for treatment evaluation. *Journal of Consulting and Clinical Psychology, 49,* 418–425.

Rothman, J. (1989). Client self-determination: Untangling the knot. *Social Service Review, 64,* 589–612.

Ruben, D. H. (1987). Improving communication between the elderly and pharmacies: A self-initiative training program. *Journal of Alcohol and Drug Education, 32,* 7–12.

Rumrill, P. D., Jr. (1999). Effects of social competence training program on accommodation request activity, situational self-efficacy, and Americans with Disabilities Act knowledge among employed people with visual impairments and blindness. *Journal of Vocational Rehabilitation, 12,* 25–31.

Rusch, F. R., & Hughes, C. (1989). Overview of supported employment. *Journal of Applied Behavior Analysis, 22,* 351–363.

Rusch, F. R., McKee, M., Chadsey-Rusch, J., & Renzaglia, A. (1988). Teaching a student with severe handicaps to self-instruct: A brief report. *Education and Training in Mental Retardation, 23,* 51–58.

Rusch, F. R., & Menchetti, B. M. (1981). Increasing compliant work behaviors in a non-sheltered work setting. *Mental Retardation, 19,* 107–111.

Rusch, F. R., Morgan, T. K., Martin, J. E., Riva, M., & Agran, M. (1985). Competitive employment: Teaching mentally retarded employees self-instructional strategies. *Applied Research in Mental Retardation, 6,* 389–407.

Sabin, J. E., & Daniels, N. (2002). Strengthening the consumer voice in managed care: IV. The leadership academy program. *Psychiatric Services, 53*, 405–411.

Safren, S. A., Hollander, G., Hart, T. A., & Heimberg, R. G. (2001). Cognitive-behavioral therapy with lesbian, gay, and bisexual youth. *Cognitive and Behavioral Practice, 8*, 215–223.

Safren, S. A., & Rogers, T. (2001). Cognitive-behavioral therapy with gay, lesbian, and bisexual clients. *Psychotherapy in Practice, 57*, 629–643.

Saleebey, D. (1996). The strengths perspective in social work practice: Extensions and cautions. *Social Work, 41*, 296–305.

Saleebey, D. (2002). Power in the people. In D. Saleebey (Ed.), *The strengths perspective in social work practice* (3rd ed., pp. 1–22). Boston, MA: Allyn & Bacon.

Salend, S. J., Ellis, L. L., & Reynolds, C. J. (1989). Using self-instruction to teach vocational skills to individuals who are severely retarded. *Education and Training in Mental Retardation and Developmental Disabilities, 24*, 248–254.

Salmento, M., & Bambara, L. M. (2000). Teaching staff members to provide choice opportunities for adults with multiple disabilities. *Journal of Positive Behavior Interventions, 2*, 12–21.

Sauter, A. W., Jr., & Nevid, J. S. (1991). Work skills training with chronic schizophrenic sheltered workers. *Rehabilitation Psychology, 36*, 255–264.

Schinke, S. P. (1982). School-based model for preventing teenage pregnancy. *Social Work in Education, 4*, 34–42.

Schinke, S. P., Bythe, B. J., & Gilchrist, L. D. (1981). Cognitive-behavioral prevention of adolescent pregnancy. *Journal of Counseling Psychology, 28*, 451–454.

Schinke, S. P., Gilchrist, L. D., Smith, T. E., & Wong, S. E. (1978). Improving teenage mothers' ability to compete for jobs. *Social Work Research and Abstracts, 14*, 25–29.

Schleien, S. J., Kiernan, J., & Wehman, P. (1981). Evaluation of an age-appropriate leisure skills program for moderately retarded adults. *Education and Training of the Mentally Retarded, 16*, 13–19.

Schloss, P. J., Santoro, C., Wood, C. E., & Bedner, M. J. (1988). A comparison of peer-directed and teacher-directed employment interview training for mentally retarded adults. *Journal of Applied Behavior Analysis, 21*, 97–102.

Schloss, P. J., & Wood, C. E. (1990). Effect of self-monitoring on maintenance and generalization of conversational skills of persons with mental retardation. *Mental Retardation, 28*, 105–113.

Schwartz, I. S., & Baer, D. M. (1991). Social validity assessments: Is current practice state of the art? *Journal of Applied Behavior Analysis, 24*, 189–204.

Seekins, T., & Fawcett, S. B. (1987). Effects of a poverty-clients' agenda on resource allocations by community decision makers. *America Journal of Community Psychology, 15*, 305–320.

Seekins, T., Fawcett, S. B., & Mathews, R. M. (1987). Effects of self-help guides on three consumer advocacy skills: Using personal experiences to influence public policy. *Rehabilitation Psychology, 32*, 29–38.

Seekins, T., Mathews, R. M., & Fawcett, S. B. (1984). Enhancing leadership skills for community self-help organizations through behavioral instruction. *Journal of Community Psychology, 12*, 155–163.

Shevin, M., & Klein, N. K. (1984). The importance of choice-making skills for students with severe disabilities. *Journal of the Association for Persons with Severe Handicaps, 9*, 159–166.

Sievert, A. L., Cuvo, A. J., & Davis, P. K. (1988). Training self-advocacy skills to adults with mild handicaps. *Journal of Applied Behavior Analysis, 21*, 299–309.

Simmons, T. J., & Flexer, R. W. (1992). Community based job training for persons with mental retardation: An acquisition and performance replication. *Education and Training in Mental Retardation, 27*, 261–272.

Simon, B. L. (1994). *The empowerment tradition in social work: A history.* New York: Columbia University Press.

Sisson, L. A., Van Hasselt, V. B., Hersen, M., & Strain, P. S. (1985). Peer interventions: Increasing social behaviors in multihandicapped children. *Behavior Modification, 9*, 293–321.

Snyder, E. P. (2002). Teaching students with combined behavioral disorders and mental retardation to lead their own IEP meetings. *Behavioral Disorders, 27*, 340–357.

Solomon, B. B. (1976). *Black empowerment: Social work in oppressed communities.* New York: Columbia University Press.

Sowers, J., & Powers, L. (1995). Enhancing the participation and independence of students with severe physical and multiple disabilities in performing community activities. *Mental Retardation, 33*, 209–220.

Sowers, J., Verdi, M., Bourbeau, P., & Sheehan, M. (1985). Teaching job independence and flexibility to mentally retarded students through the use of a self-control package. *Journal of Applied Behavior Analysis, 18*, 81–85.

Spiegler, M. D., & Guevremont, D. C. (2003). *Contemporary behavior therapy* (4th ed.). Belmont, CA: Wadsworth & Thomson.

Staab, S., & Lodish, D. (1985). Reducing joblessness among disadvantaged youth. In L. D. Gilchrist & S. P. Schinke (Eds.), *Preventing social and health problems through life skills training* (pp. 63–72). Seattle: Center for Social Welfare Research, University of Washington.

Staples, L. H. (1990). Powerful ideas about empowerment. *Administration in Social Work, 14*, 29–42.

Stevenson, C. L., Krantz, P. J., & McClannahan, L. E. (2000). Social interaction skills for children with autism: A script-fading procedure for nonreaders. *Behavioral Interventions, 15*, 1–20.

Stidham, H. H., & Remley, T. P., Jr. (1992). Job Club methodology applied in a workfare setting. *Journal of Employment Counseling, 29*, 69–76.

St. Lawrence, J. S., Bradlyn, A. S., & Kelly, J. A. (1983). Interpersonal adjustment of a homosexual adult: Enhancement via social skills training. *Behavior Modification, 7*, 41–55.

St. Lawrence, J. S., Brasfield, T. L., Jefferson, K. W., Alleyne, E., O'Bannon R. E., III, & Shirley, A. (1995). Cognitive-behavioral intervention to reduce African American adolescents' risk for HIV infection. *Journal of Consulting and Clinical Psychology, 63*, 221–237.

St. Lawrence, J. S., Wilson, T. E., Eldridge, G. D., Brasfield, T. L., & O'Bannon, R. E., III. (2001). Community-based interventions to reduce low income, African American women's risk of sexually transmitted diseases: A randomized controlled trial of three theoretical models. *American Journal of Community Psychology, 29,* 937–964.

Stokes, T. F., & Osnes, P. G. (1989). An operant pursuit of generalization. *Behavior Therapy, 20,* 337–355.

Storey, K., Bates, P., & Hanson, H. B. (1984). Acquisition and generalization of coffee purchase skills by adults with severe disabilities. *Journal of the Association for Persons with Severe Handicaps, 9,* 178–185.

Storey, K., & Garff, J. T. (1999). The effect of coworker instruction on the integration of youth in transition in competitive employment. *Career Development for Exceptional Individuals, 22,* 69–84.

Stringfellow, J. W., & Muscari, K. D. (2003). A program of support for consumer participation in systems change: The West Virginia Leadership Academy. *Journal of Disability Policy Studies, 14,* 142–147.

Taras, M. E., Matson, J. L., & Leary, C. (1988). Training social interpersonal skills in two autistic children. *Journal of Behavior Therapy and Experimental Psychiatry, 19,* 275–280.

Test, D. W., Mason, C., Hughes, C., Konrad, M., Neale, M., & Wood, W. M. (2004). Student involvement in Individualized Education Program meetings. *Exceptional Children, 70,* 391–412.

Test, D. W., & Neale, M. (2004). Using the self-advocacy strategy to increase middle graders' IEP participation. *Journal of Behavioral Education, 13,* 135–145.

Thomas, E. J. (1967). *The socio-behavioral approach and applications to social work.* New York: Council on Social Work Education.

Thurston, L. (1990). Women surviving: An alternative approach to "helping" low-income urban women. *Women & Therapy, 8,* 109–127.

Thurston, L. *Survival skills for women: Facilitator manual & materials.* Manhattan, KS: Survival Skills Education and Development.

Thurston, L. P., Dasta, K., & Greenwood, C. R. (1984). A program of survival skills workshops for urban women. *Journal of Community Psychology, 12,* 192–196.

Thyer, B. A. (1991). Behavioral social work: It is not what you think. *Aretê, 16,* 1–9.

Thyer, B. A., Himle, J., & Santa, C. (1986). Applied behavior analysis in social and community action: A bibliography. *Behavior Analysis & Social Action, 5,* 14–16.

Tice, C. (1994). A community's response to supported employment: Implications for social work practice. *Social Work, 39,* 728–736.

Truax, C. B. (1966). Reinforcement and nonreinforcement in Rogerian psychotherapy. *Journal of Abnormal Psychology, 71,* 1–9.

Tsang, H. W. H. (2001). Applying social skills training in the context of vocational rehabilitation for people with schizophrenia. *Journal of Nervous and Mental Disease, 189,* 90–98.

Tsang, H. W. H. (2003). Augmenting vocational outcomes of supported employment with social skills training. *Journal of Rehabilitation, 69,* 25–30.

Tumlin, K. C., & Zimmermann, W. (2003). *Immigrants and TANF: A look at immigrant welfare recipients in three cities* (Occasional Paper No. 69). Washington, DC: The Urban Institute.

Twamley, E. W., Jeste, D. V., & Lehman, A. F. (2003). Vocational rehabilitation in schizophrenia and other psychotic disorders: A literature review and meta-analysis of randomized controlled trials. *Journal of Nervous and Mental Disease, 191,* 515–523.

Ulman, J. D. (1995). Marxist theory and behavior therapy. In W. O'Donohue & L. Krasner (Eds.), *Theories of behavior therapy: Exploring behavior change* (pp. 529–552). Washington, DC: American Psychological Association.

U.S. Census Bureau. (2001). *Overview of race and Hispanic origin: 2000* (Census 2000 Brief, C2KBR-01-1). Washington, DC: U.S. Government Printing Office.

U.S. Census Bureau. (2003). *Disability status: 2000* (Census 2000 Brief, C2KBR-17). Washington, DC: U.S. Government Printing Office.

U.S. Census Bureau. (2004). *We the people: Aging in the United States* (Current Population Reports, P23–211). Washington, DC: U.S. Government Printing Office.

U.S. Census Bureau. (2005). *65+ in the United States: 2005* (Current Population Reports, P23–209). Washington, DC: U.S. Government Printing Office.

U.S. Census Bureau. (2006). *Income, poverty, and health insurance coverage in the United States: 2005* (Current Population Reports, P60–231). Washington, DC: U.S. Government Printing Office.

U.S. Department of Health and Human Services. (2000). *Vol. 1. Healthy people 2010* (2nd ed.). Washington, DC: U.S. Government Printing Office.

U.S. Department of Labor. Bureau of Labor Statistics. (2006, May). *Employment situation summary* (USDL 06–777). Retrieved May 6, 2006, from http://www.bls.gov/news.release/empsit.nr0.htm

Valenti-Hein, D. C., Yarnold, P. R., & Mueser, K. T. (1994). Evaluation of the dating skills program for improving heterosocial interactions in people with mental retardation. *Behavior Modification, 18,* 32–46.

Van Acker, R., Boreson, L., Gable, R. A., & Potterton, T. (2005). Are we on the right course? Lessons learned about current FBA/BIP practices in schools. *Journal of Behavioral Education, 14,* 35–56.

VanBiervliet, A., Spangler, P. F., & Marshall, A. M. (1981). An ecobehavioral examination of a simple strategy for increasing mealtime language in residential facilities. *Journal of Applied Behavior Analysis, 14,* 295–305.

Van Den Bergh, N. (2002). Feminist social work practice: Where have we been . . . Where are we going? In N. Van Den Bergh (Ed.), *Feminist practice in the 21st century* (pp. xi–xxxix). Washington, DC: National Association of Social Workers.

Van den Pol, R. A., Iwata, B. A., Ivancic, M. T., Page, T. J., Neef, N. A., & Whitley, F. P. (1981). Teaching the handicapped to eat in public places: Acquisition, generalization and maintenance of restaurant skills. *Journal of Applied Behavior Analysis, 14,* 61–69.

Van Hasselt, V. B., Hersen, M., Kazdin, A. E., Simon, J., & Mastanuono, A. (1983). Training blind adolescents in social skills. *Journal of Visual Impairment and Blindness, 77,* 199–203.

Van Reusen, A. K., Bos, C. S., Schumaker, J. B., & Deshler, D. D. (1994). *The self-advocacy strategy.* Lawrence, KS: Edge Enterprises.

Wacker, D. P., Fromm-Steege, L., Berg, W. K., & Flynn, T. H. (1989). Supported employment as an intervention package: A preliminary analysis of functional variables. *Journal of Applied Behavior Analysis, 22,* 429–439.

Wall, M. E., & Gast, D. L. (1997a). Caregivers as teachers: Using constant time delay to teach adults how to use constant time delay. *Education and Training in Mental Retardation and Developmental Disabilities, 32,* 213–228.

Wall, M. E., & Gast, D. L. (1997b). Caregivers' use of constant time delay to teach leisure skills to adolescents or young adults with moderate or severe intellectual disabilities. *Education and Training in Mental Retardation and Developmental Disabilities, 32,* 340–356.

Wallace, C. J., Tauber, R., & Wilde, J. (1999). Teaching fundamental workplace skills to persons with serious mental illness. *Psychiatric Services, 50,* 1147–1153.

Wehman, P., Hill, J. W., & Koehler, F. (1979). Placement of developmentally disabled individuals into competitive employment: Three case studies. *Education and Training of the Mentally Retarded, 14,* 269–276.

Wehmeyer, M. L., & Palmer, S. B. (2003). Adult outcomes for students with cognitive disabilities three-years after high school: The impact of self-determination. *Education and Training in Developmental Disabilities, 38,* 131–144.

Weinhardt, L. S., Carey, M. P., Carey, K. B., & Verdecias, R. N. (1998). Increasing assertiveness skills to reduce HIV risk among women living with a severe and persistent mental illness. *Journal of Consulting and Clinical Psychology, 66,* 680–684.

Westbrook, L. E., Silver, E. J., & Stein, R. E. K. (1998). Implications for estimates of disability in children: A comparison of definitional components. *Pediatrics, 101,* 1025–1030.

Whang, P. L., Fawcett, S. B., & Mathews, R. M. (1984). Teaching job-related social skills to learning disabled adolescents. *Analysis and Intervention in Developmental Disabilities, 4,* 29–38.

Wheeler, J. J., Bates, P., Marshall, K. J., & Miller, S. R. (1988). Teaching appropriate social behaviors to a young man with moderate mental retardation in a supported competitive employment setting. *Education and Training in Mental Retardation, 23,* 105–116.

White, G. W., Paine-Andrews, A., Mathews, R. M., & Fawcett, S. B. (1995). Home access modifications: Effects on community visits by people with physical disabilities. *Journal of Applied Behavior Analysis, 28,* 457–463.

White, G. W., Thompson, R. J., & Nary, D. E. (1997). An empirical analysis of the effects of a self-administered advocacy letter training program. *Rehabilitation Counseling Bulletin, 41,* 74–87.

Wilson, A., Arnold, M., Rowland, S. T., & Burnham, S. (1997). Promoting recreation and leisure activities for individuals with disabilities: A collaborative effort. *Journal of Instructional Psychology, 24,* 76–79.

Wilson, P. G., Schepis, M. M., & Mason-Main, M. (1987). In vivo use of picture prompt training to increase independent work at a restaurant. *Journal of the Association for Persons with Severe Handicaps, 12,* 145–150.

Wodarski, J., & Horme, J. (1981). *Behavioral social work.* New York: Human Services Press.

Wolf, M. M. (1978). Social validity: The case for subjective measurement or how applied behavior analysis is finding its heart. *Journal of Applied Behavior Analysis, 11,* 203–214.

Wolfe, J. L. (1995). Rational emotive behavior therapy women's groups: A twenty year retrospective. *Journal of Rational-Emotive and Cognitive-Behavior Therapy, 13*, 153–170.

Wolford, P. L., Heward, W. L., & Alber, S. R. (2001). Teaching middle school students with learning disabilities to recruit peer assistance during cooperative learning group activities. *Learning Disabilities Research & Practice, 16*, 161–173.

Wolpe, J. (1977). Inadequate behavior analysis: The Achilles heel of outcome research in behavior therapy. *Journal of Behavior Therapy and Experimental Psychiatry, 8*, 1–3.

Wolpe, J. (1986). Individualization: The categorical imperative of behavior therapy practice. *Journal of Behavior Therapy and Experimental Psychiatry, 17*, 145–153.

Wong, S. E., & Woolsey, J. E. (1989). Re-establishing conversational skills in overtly psychotic, chronic schizophrenic patients: Discrete trials training on the psychiatric ward. *Behavior Modification, 13*, 415–430.

Wu, C., & Eamon, M. K. (in press). Public and private sources of assistance for low-income households. *Journal of Sociology and Social Welfare*.

Yu, D. C. T., Spevack, S., Hiebert, R., Martin, T. L., Goodman, R., Martin, T. G., et al. (2002). Happiness indices among persons with profound and severe disabilities during leisure and work activities: A comparison. *Education and Training in Mental Retardation and Developmental Disabilities, 37*, 421–426.

Zedlewski, S. R. (2002). Family economic resources in the post-reform era. *The Future of Children, 12*, 121–145.

Zirpoli, T. J., Hancox, D., Wieck, C., & Skarnulis, E. R. (1989). Partners in policymaking: Empowering people. *Journal of the Association for Persons with Severe Handicaps, 14*, 163–167.

Zirpoli, T. J., Wieck, C., Hancox, D., & Skarnulis, E. R. (1994). Partners in policymaking: The first five years. *Mental Retardation, 32*, 422–425.

Index

Accommodations
  educational, 255–259
  workplace, 253–255
Action Letter Portfolio training manual, 294–295
Adolescent mothers, social and emotional support interventions for, 120–121
Adults. *See* Vulnerable adults, interventions for
Advocacy activities, 292–297
Affection activities, 54–55
African American youths
  attaining individually defined goals and, 136–137
  job-seeking skills interventions for, 156–157
  sexual behavior interventions for, 266–267
  SST programs for goal attainment, 136–137
"A-iBs-C" model (Ellis), 16
Americans with Disabilities Act (ADA) (1990), 4
Assertiveness training, 21, 250
Assessment. *See* Cognitive-behavioral (CB) assessment
Autism, social interaction interventions for vulnerable children/youths with, 54–59
Aversive events, 14

Backup reinforcers, 24
Bandura, Albert, 15
Beck, A. T., 15
Beck, J. S., 15–16
Beck's cognitive therapy, 26
Behavioral interventions, 19–25
  changing antecedent conditions based on operant conditioning, 19–22
  changing antecedent conditions based on respondent conditioning, 22–23
  defined, 12
Behavioral theories
  operant conditioning, 13–14
  respondent conditioning, 14–15
Behavior rehearsal, 21
Behavior therapy, 11–12

CB. *See under* Cognitive-behavioral
Children. *See* Vulnerable children/youths, interventions for
Children/youths with behavioral/emotional disorders, social interaction interventions for, 59–61
Children/youths with hearing impairments, social interaction interventions for, 49–51
Children/youths with learning disabilities, social interaction interventions for, 51–53
Children/youths with mental retardation/developmental delays, interventions for
  recreational/leisure activities, 97–99
  social interaction, 53–54

Children/youths with multiple disabilities, interventions for, 61–66
  recreational/leisure activities and, 99–102
Children/youths with physical disabilities, interventions for, 47–49
  recreational/leisure activities and, 96–97
Cognitions, 18
Cognitive-behavioral (CB) assessment, 17–18
Cognitive-behavioral (CB) coping skills therapy, 15–16
Cognitive-behavioral (CB) interventions, 3, 4–5, 12, 25–27
  characteristics of, 12–13
  constraints on individual freedom through expert control and, 30–34
  criticisms of, 30–39
  for females, 6–7
  for individuals with disabilities, 4–5
  for individuals with low incomes, 7–8
  for older individuals, 7
  for racial/ethnic minorities, 5
  for sexual minorities, 5–6
  social justice perspective and, 34–37, 86, 326–328
  social relevance and, 37–39
  summary of effectiveness of, 319–322
  values and, 37
Cognitive-behavioral (CB) theories, 13–16
  behavioral theories, 13–15
  social learning and cognitive theory, 15–16
Cognitive rehearsal, 262
Cognitive restructuring, 26
Cognitive restructuring therapy, 15–16
Communication books, 65
Communication skills, acquiring, 45–46
Community residences, choosing, interventions
  client's freedom and control in, 243–244
  effectiveness of, 242–243
  generalization and, 247–248

individuals with multiple disabilities and, 240
  maintenance and, 247–248
  socially relevant goals and, 244–245
  socially relevant procedures of, 245–247
Community rights, 252
Competitive employment, 178–183
Conditioned stimulus (CS), 15
Conditioning
  operant, 13–14
  respondent, 14–15
Constant time delay (CTD) procedure, 98–99
Consumer rights, 252
Control, individual freedom and, 322–326
Cooperative learning group (CLG), 132

Daily/long-term decisions, interventions
  client's freedom and control in, 243–244
  for community residences, 240–242
  effectiveness of, 242–243
  generalization and, 247–248
  maintenance and, 247–248
  for recreational/leisure activity, 229–234
  for routine/daily activities, 234–240
  socially relevant goals and, 244–245
  socially relevant procedures and, 245–247
Decision making. *See also* Macro decision making; Self-determination
  client's freedom and control and, 223–224
  effectiveness of intervention for, 222–223
  enhancing control over personal, 212–221
  for establishing/attaining personal goals, 216–221
  generalization and, 226–227
  maintenance and, 226–227
  socially relevant goals and, 224–225
  socially relevant procedures and, 225–226

students with developmental/learning, health, and emotional/behavioral disabilities, 214–216
students with mental retardation and, 213–214
Desirable events, 14
Disabilities, 4–5
 learning, 4
 mental health, 4
 multiple, 4
 physical, 4
Disability rates, 4
Discrimination training, 252–253

Economic assistance
 assisting vulnerable populations in accessing, 199–202
 for females with low income, 200–202
 interventions
  for adults with severe mental illness, 199
  effectiveness of, 202–204
  for minority youths, 200
  public and private sources of, 197–199
  for youths with disabilities, 200
Educational accommodations, 255–259
Elderly, interventions for, 78–80
 for medical and emergency needs, 128–129
 performing routine or daily activities, 133
 recreational/leisure activities and, 108–109
 for social interaction, 78–80
Ellis, A., 16
Emergency needs. See Medical and emergency needs
Emotional support. See Social and emotional support, interventions for
Employment. See also Job-related social skills, interventions for enhancing; Job-seeking skills interventions; Productivity, work, CB interventions for increasing
 competitive, 178–183
 learning job-seeking skills and, 152–163
 older adults and, 151
 supported, 171–173
Empowerment
 cognitive-behavioral interventions and, 322–326
 defined, 28–29
 Job Club method and, 157
 levels of, 29–30
 selection of intervention goals and, 28–30
Events, 14
Exposure therapies, 22–23
 graduated, 23
Extinction, 14

Fading, 20
Fading (thining) reinforcers, 24
Females
 CB interventions for, 6–7
 right to refuse unwanted/unprotected sexual behavior and, 261–266
Flooding, 23
Freedom, individual, control and, 322–326
Freedom Self-Advocacy Curriculum, 274–275
Friendship circles, 59–60
Functional assessment, 17
Functional contingencies, taking advantage of current, 340–344
Functional mediators, using, 345–346

Gay men, interventions for, 80–82
 for high-risk sexual behavior, 267–270
 for social interaction, 80–82
Generalization
 community residence interventions and, 247–248
 daily/long-term decision interventions and, 247–248
 decision making interventions and, 226–227
 enhancing job-related social skills interventions and, 194–196

Generalization (*continued*)
  job-seeking skills interventions and, 168–170
  macro decision making interventions and, 316–317
  medical/emergency needs interventions and, 143–145
  recreational/leisure interventions and, 116–118, 247–248
  routine/daily activities interventions and, 247–248
  self-determination and, 226–227
  sexual behavior interventions and, 281–283
  social interaction interventions and, 90–93
Goals
  attaining individually defined, 133–138
  establishing/attaining personal, 216–221
  selection of intervention, 28–30
  socially relevant, establishing, 328–330
Graduated exposure therapies, 23

Hearing impairments, children with, social interaction interventions for, 49–51
Hess, Robert, 306
High-probability requests, 62–63
Homework assignments, 21
Human services rights, 252

Idaho Leadership Academy (ILA), 303–307
IEP. *See* Individual Education Programs (IEPs)
ILA. *See* Idaho Leadership Academy (ILA)
Individual Education Programs (IEPs), 209
Individuals with Disabilities Education Act (IDEA) (1997), 209
Individuals with low incomes, CB interventions for, 7–8

Interactive Hypermedia Program (IHP), 215
Interventions. *See also* Cognitive-behavioral (CB) interventions; specific intervention
  behavioral, 19–25
  cognitive-behavioral, 25–27
  socially valid, 333–339
Interviewing skills, 153–156
In Vivo Amplified Skills Training (IVAST), 92
I-PLAN, 214–215

Job Club method, 157–159, 161–162, 168–169, 338
Job-Finding Club, 159–160
Job-related social skills, interventions for enhancing, 184–190
  client's freedom and control and, 191–192
  effectiveness of, 190–191
  generalization and, 194–196
  maintenance and, 194–196
  socially relevant goals and, 192–193
  socially relevant procedures and, 193–194
  for workers with developmental/physical disabilities, 185–187
  for workers with severe mental illness, 188–190
Job-seeking skills interventions, 152–163
  for adults with severe mental illness, 159–160
  client's freedom and control in, 165–166
  for clients receiving public assistance, 160–162
  effectiveness of, 163–165
  generalization and, 168–170
  interviewing skills
    adults with severe mental illness and, 155
    adults/youths with mental retardation and, 153–154
    recent immigrants and, 155–156
  Job Club method, 157–159

maintenance and, 168–170
for older workers, 162–163
recruiting skills, 156–157
socially relevant goals and, 166–167
socially relevant procedures and, 167–168
for unemployed, 160–162
"Joining in," 48–49

Language Master Cards, 56, 89
Leadership training, 139. *See also* Macro decision making
Learning disabilities, 4
Legal rights
responding to violation of, 253
securing, 251–259
types of, 252
Leisure activities. *See* Recreational and leisure interventions
Leisure skills programs, for adults with mental retardation, 103–105
Lesbian, gay, and bisexual (LGB) individuals, CB interventions for, 5–6
Lesbian, gay, and bisexual (LGB) youths, 47
for social interaction interventions for, 66–67
Lesbians, social and emotional support interventions for, 124–125
Liberman, Robert, 73
Loose training, 345
Low-probability requests, 62–63

Macro decision making. *See also* Decision making
benefits of involving vulnerable groups in, 290–291
client's freedom and control and, 312–313
effectiveness of interventions, 311–312
generalization and, 316–317
government/foundation sponsored programs, 300–310
Idaho Leadership Academy (ILA), 303–307
maintenance and, 316–317

Oklahoma Aging Advocacy Leadership Academy (OAALA), 307–308
PPM program, 301–303
skills training for, 291–300
socially relevant goals and, 313–315
socially relevant procedures and, 315–316
vulnerable populations and, 288–290
West Virginia Leadership Academy (WVLA), 306–307
Maintaining antecedents, 17–18
Maintaining consequences, 18
Maintenance, of interventions
for community residences, 247–248
for daily/long-term decisions, 247–248
for decision making, 226–227
for enhancing job-related social skills, 194–195
job-seeking skills, 168–170
for medical/emergency needs, 143–145
for recreation/leisure, 116–118
for routine/daily activities, 247–248
for self-determination, 226–227
for sexual behaviors, 281–283
for social interactions, 90–93
for vulnerable adults, 90–93
Medical and emergency needs, interventions for
adults with chronic disease and, 125–126
adults with mental retardation and, 126–127
adults with severe mental illness and, 127–128
client's freedom and control and, 140–141
elderly and, 128–129
generalization and, 143–145
maintenance and, 143–145
performing routine or daily activities, 129–133
socially relevant procedures and, 142–143
social relevant goals and, 141–142

Medication Communication Skills Program (MCSP), 127–128
Medication Self-Management module, 127
Mental health disabilities, 4
Modeling, 21
Mothers, adolescent, social and emotional support interventions for, 120–121
Multiple disabilities, 4

National Breast Cancer Coalition (NBCC), 308–309
Natural supports, 66
Negative punishment, 14
Negative reinforcement, 13–14, 23

Observational learning, 15
Oklahoma Aging Advocacy Leadership Academy (OAALA), 307–308
Operant conditioning, 12, 13–14
  changing antecedent conditions based on, 19–22
Outcomes, socially relevant, 330–333

Peer network interventions, for autism, 57–59
Personal Effectiveness for Successful Living (PESL), 220–221
Personal Responsibility and Work Opportunity Reconciliation Act (PRWORA), 6, 151
Personal rights, 252. *See also* Legal rights
PESL. *See* Personal Effectiveness for Successful Living (PESL)
Physical disabilities, 4
Populations. *See* Vulnerable populations
Positive punishment, 14, 23
Positive reinforcement, 13, 23, 34
Positive reinforcers
  activities, 23
  social, 23
  tangible, 23
Poverty, 149–152
PPM program, 301–303
Prerequisites, 17

Princeton Child Development Institute, 56
Problem-solving therapy, 16
Problem-solving training (PST), 25–26, 46
Productivity, work, CB interventions for increasing, 173–184. *See also* Employment
  competitive employment, 178–183
  for workers with mental retardation, 175–178
  for workers with physical disabilities, 174–175
  for workers with severe mental illness, 183–184
Project LEAD, 308–310
Prompt-fade teaching strategy, 65–66
Prompt hierarchy, 19–20
Prompting, 19
Prompts, 17, 19
PRWORA. *See* Personal Responsibility and Work Opportunity Reconciliation Act (PRWORA)
PST. *See* Problem-solving therapy
Psychosocial rehabilitation work programs, 172
Public benefits. *See* Economic assistance
Punishment, 14
  negative, 14
  positive, 14

Racial/ethnic minorities, CB interventions for, 5
Rational emotive behavior therapy (REBT), 15–16, 26
Recreational and leisure interventions
  choices for, 229
  individuals with mental retardation and, 230–232
  individuals with multiple disabilities, 232–234
  client's freedom and control in, 111–112, 243–244
  effectiveness of, 110–111, 242–243
  for elderly, 108–109
  generalization of, 116–118, 247–248
  maintenance of, 116–118, 247–248

social justice and, 113
socially relevant goals and, 244–245
socially relevant goals of, 113–114
socially relevant procedures of, 114–116, 245–247
for vulnerable adults, 102–109
for vulnerable children/youths, 95–102
Recruiting skills, 156–157
Reinforcement, 13
  negative, 13–14, 23
  positive, 13, 23, 34
Reinforcers, 23–24, 34
  backup, 24
  positive, 23
Resources. *See* Economic assistance
Respondent conditioning, 12, 14–15
  changing antecedent conditions based on, 22–23
Results, socially relevant, 330–333
Rights. *See* Legal rights
Risk factors, of vulnerable populations, 8–9
Rogers, Carl, 34
Role playing, 21
Routine/daily activities, interventions choices for
  individuals with mental retardation and, 234–236
  client's freedom and control in, 243–244
  effectiveness of, 242–243
  generalization and, 247–248
  individuals with multiple disabilities and, 236–240
  maintenance and, 247–248
  socially relevant goals and, 244–245
  socially relevant procedures of, 245–247
Routine/daily activities, performing, interventions for
  adults with learning disabilities, 131–132
  adults with mental retardation, 131
  adults with multiple disabilities, 132–133

  adults with physical disabilities, 129–130
  adults with visual impairments, 130
"RSVP" procedure, 79

Schizophrenia, 72
Script-fading, 56–57
SDLMI. *See* Self-Determined Learning Model of Instruction (SDLMI)
Self-advocacy, 250
Self-Advocacy Strategy, 214–215, 251
Self-control assessment/intervention methods, 31
Self-determination, 209–210. *See also* Decision making
  client's freedom and control and, 223–224
  effectiveness of intervention for, 222–223
  generalization and, 226–227
  maintenance and, 226–227
  socially relevant goals and, 224–225
  socially relevant procedures and, 225–226
  of vulnerable populations, 210–212
Self-Determined Learning Model of Instruction (SDLMI), 217–220
Self-Directed IEP Program, 216, 251
Self-Help Behavioral Assessment Instrument, 122–123
Self-instructional training, 16, 26
  for work productivity, 179
Self-management strategies, 24, 86, 247
  for work productivity, 179–183
Self-recording, 31
Self-reinforce, 24
Self-tallk, 121
Setting events, 17
Sexual assertion training, 268
Sexual behavior interventions
  for African American youths, 266–267
  client's freedom and control in, 275–276
  effectiveness of, 272–275
  for females, 261–266
  generalization and, 281–283

Sexual behavior interventions (*continued*)
  for individuals with severe mental illness, 270–271
  maintenance and, 281–283
  right to refuse unwanted/unprotected, 259–271
  for sexual minorities, 267–270
  socially relevant goals and, 276–278
  socially relevant procedures and, 278–281
SHARE behaviors, 215
Sheltered workshop employment, 171–172, 175–178
Skills training, 20
  for macro decision making, 291–300
Social and emotional support, interventions for, 119–125
  for lesbians, 124–125
  for poor, minority pregnant or parenting adolescent mothers, 120–121
  for women with low income, 121–124
Social interaction interventions
  client's freedom and control in, 85–86
  effectiveness of, 82–85
  for the elderly, 78–80
  for gay men, 80–82
  generalization and, 90–93
  for LBG youths, 66–67
  maintenance and, 90–93
  socially relevant goals and, 86–88
  socially relevant procedures and, 88–90
  for vulnerable adults, 67–78
  for vulnerable children/youths, 46–66
Social justice perspective
  cognitive-behavioral interventions and, 34–37, 86, 326–328
  enhancing social/emotional support interventions and, 141
  enhancing social interaction interventions and, 86
  increasing choice making in daily/long-term decisions interventions, 244
  increasing involvement in macro decision making interventions and, 313

  increasing leisure/recreational activity interventions and, 113
  maintaining/advancing employment interventions and, 192
  obtaining employment interventions and, 165–166
  securing legal/personal rights interventions and, 276
  self-determination interventions and, 224
Social learning theory, 15
"Social life" program, 69–71
Social reinforcers, 23
Social relevance, cognitive-behavioral interventions and, 37–39
Social skills, acquiring, 45–46
Social skills training (SST), 20–21, 46, 49, 82–83
  meta-analysis of studies evaluating, 84–85
  for youth skills, 133–138
Social validity, 347–348
  of enhancing social/emotional support interventions, 141–145
  of enhancing social interaction interventions, 86–93
  of increasing choice making in daily/long-term decisions interventions, 224–248
  of increasing involvement in macro decision making interventions, 313–317
  of increasing leisure/recreational activity interventions, 113–118
  of maintaining/advancing employment interventions, 192–196
  of obtaining employment interventions, 166–170
  of securing legal/personal rights interventions, 276–283
  of self-determination interventions, 224–228
  summary of, 328–339
SST. *See* Social skills training (SST)
Stimulus control, 14, 17
Stress inoculation therapy, 16

Supported employment programs, 171–173
Survival Skills for Women (SSW) program, 201
Systematic desensitization, 22

Tangible reinforcers, 23
Target behavior, 12
Task analysis, 17
Teaching diversely, 344–345
Temporary Assistance to Needy Families (TANF), 151
Theories
  behavioral, 13–15
  cognitive, 15–16
  social learning, 15
Thining (fading) reinforcers, 24
Time-out procedures, 24
Token economies, 23–24
Tokens, 23
Touch Talker, 68, 89, 103
Transgender population, 5–6

Unconditioned response (UR), 15
Unconditioned stimulus (US), 15

Values, cognitive-behavioral models and, 37
Video modeling, 55
Visual impairments, 253–255
Vocational rehabilitation programs, 171–172
Vulnerable adults, interventions for
  analysis and critique of, 82–83
  with chronic disease, 125–126
  client's control and freedom in, 85–86
  effectiveness of, 83–85
  elderly, 78–80
    medical and emergency needs of, 128–129
    performing routine or daily activities, 133
    recreational/leisure activities and, 108–109
  gay men, 80–82
  with learning disabilities
    performing routine or daily activities, 131
  maintenance of, 90–93
  with mental retardation, 69–72
    medical and emergency needs of, 126–127
    performing routine or daily activities, 131
    recreational/leisure activities and, 103–106
  with multiple disabilities, 77–78
    performing routine or daily activities, 132–133
    recreational/leisure activities and, 107–108
  with physical disabilities, 68–69
    performing routine or daily activities, 129–130
    recreational/leisure activities and, 103
  recreational/leisure activities and, 102–109
  with severe mental illness, 72–77
    medical and emergency needs of, 127–128
    recreational/leisure activities and, 106–107
  for social interaction, 67–78
  socially relevant goals and, 86–88
  socially relevant interventions, 88–90
  with visual impairments, performing routine or daily activities, 130
Vulnerable children/youths, interventions for, 46–66
  with autism, 54–59
  with hearing impairments, 47–51
  with learning disabilities, 51–53
  with mental retardation/developmental delays, 53–54
  with physical disabilities, 47–49, 95–97
  for recreational/leisure activities, 96–102
  for social interaction, 46–66
Vulnerable populations
  benefits of involving, in macro decisions, 290–291

Vulnerable populations (*continued*)
  defined, 3–8
  economic resources of, 149–152
  macro decision making and, 288–290
  risk factors for, 8–9
  self-determination of, 210–212

Wallace, Charles, 73
West Virginia Leadership Academy (WVLA), 306–307

Women with low income, social and emotional support interventions for, 120–121
Workplace accommodations, 253–255
Workshops, sheltered, 175–178

Youths. *See* Vulnerable children/youths, interventions for
Youth skills, SST programs for, 133–138